MEDICATION ADMINISTRATION & I.V. THERAPY MANUAL

Process and Procedures

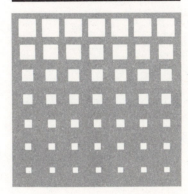

MEDICATION ADMINISTRATION & I.V. THERAPY MANUAL

Process and Procedures

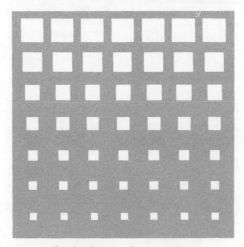

Springhouse Corporation
Springhouse, Pennsylvania

STAFF FOR THIS VOLUME

CLINICAL STAFF

Clinical Editors
Helen Hahler D'Angelo, RN, MSN;
Nina P. Welsh, RN

Drug Information Manager
Larry Neil Gever, RPh, PharmD

ADVISORY BOARD

Lillian S. Brunner, RN, MSN, ScD, FAAN, Nurse/Author, Brunner Associates, Inc., Berwyn, Pa.

Donald C. Cannon, MD, PhD, Resident in Internal Medicine, Univ. of Kansas, Wichita

Luther Christman, RN, PhD, Dean, Rush College of Nursing; Vice-President, Nursing Affairs, Rush–Presbyterian–St. Luke's Medical Center, Chicago

Kathleen A. Dracup, RN, DNSc, FAAN, Assoc. Prof., Univ. of California at Los Angeles

Stanley J. Dudrick, MD, FACS, Prof., Dept. of Surgery, and Director, Nutritional Support Services, Univ. of Texas Medical School at Houston; St. Luke's Episcopal Hospital, Houston

Halbert E. Fillinger, MD, Asst. Medical Examiner, Philadelphia County, Pa.

M. Josephine Flaherty, RN, PhD, Principal Nursing Officer, Dept. of National Health and Welfare, Ottawa

Joyce LeFever Kee, RN, MSN, Assoc. Prof., College of Nursing, Univ. of Delaware, Newark

Dennis E. Leavelle, MD, Assoc. Prof., Mayo Medical Laboratories, Mayo Clinic, Rochester, Minn.

Roger M. Morrell, MD, PhD, FACP, Prof., Neurology and Immunology/Microbiology, Wayne State University, Detroit; Chief, Neurology Service, Veterans Administration Medical Center, Allen Park, Mich.

Ara G. Paul, PhD, Dean, College of Pharmacy, Univ. of Michigan, Ann Arbor

Rose Pinneo, RN, MS, Assoc. Prof. of Nursing and Clinician II, Univ. of Rochester, N.Y.

Thomas E. Rubbert, BSL, LLB, JD, Attorney-at-Law, Pasadena, Calif.

Maryanne Schreiber, RN, BA, Product Manager, Hewlett-Packard Co., Waltham (Mass.) Division

Frances J. Storlie, RN, PhD, ANP, Director, Personal Health Services, Southwest Washington Health District, Vancouver

Claire L. Watson, RN, Clinical Documentation Associate, IVAC Corp., San Diego

PUBLICATION STAFF

Executive Director, Editorial
Stanley Loeb

Executive Director, Creative Services
Jean Robinson

Design
John Hubbard (art director), Stephanie Peters (associate art director), Elaine K. Ezrow, Darcy Feralio

Editing
Regina Daley Ford, acquisitions; Roberta Kangilaski

Copy Editing
David Moreau (manager), Edith McMahon (supervisor), Nick Anastasio, Keith de Pinho, Diane Labus, Doris Weinstock, Debra Young

Art Production
Robert Perry (manager), Mark Marcin, Loretta Caruso, Anna Brindisi, Donald Knauss, Robert Wieder, Christina McKinley, Christopher Buckley

Typography
David Kosten (manager), Diane Paluba (assistant manager), Nancy Wirs, Brenda Mayer, Joyce Rossi Biletz, Alicia Dempsey

Manufacturing
Deborah Meiris (manager), Lisa Weiss

Project Coordination
Aline S. Miller (supervisor), Maureen Carmichael

The drug selections and dosages in this textbook are based on research and current recommendations by medical and nursing authorities. These selections and dosages comply with currently accepted standards, although they cannot be considered conclusive. For each patient, any drug or dosage recommendation must be considered in conjunction with clinical data and the latest package-insert information. This is particularly essential with new drugs. The authors and the publisher disclaim responsibility for any untoward effects caused by these suggested selections and dosages or from the reader's misinterpretation of this information.

Authorization to photocopy items for internal or personal use, or the internal or personal use of specific clients, is granted by Springhouse Corporation for users registered with the Copyright Clearance Center (CCC) Transactional Reporting Service, provided that the base fee of $00.00 per copy, plus $.75 per page, is paid directly to CCC, 27 Congress St., Salem, Mass. 01970. For those organizations that have been granted a photocopy license by CCC, a separate system of payment has been arranged. The fee code for users of the Transactional Reporting Service is 0874340837/88 $00.00 + $.75.

© 1988 by Springhouse Corporation. All rights reserved. No part of this book may be used or reproduced in any manner whatsoever without written permission except for brief quotations embodied in critical articles and reviews. Printed in the United States of America. For information write Springhouse Corporation, 1111 Bethlehem Pike, Springhouse, Pa. 19477.

MAIT-031290

Library of Congress Cataloging-in-Publication Data
Medication administration & I.V. therapy manual.
Includes bibliographies and index. 1. Drugs—Administration—Handbooks, manuals, etc. 2. Intravenous therapy—Handbooks, manuals, etc. 3. Nursing—Handbooks, manuals, etc.

I. Springhouse Corporation. II. Title: Medication administration and I.V. therapy manual. [DNLM: 1. Drugs—administration & dosage—nurses' instruction. 2. Infusions, Parenteral—nurses' instruction. WB 340 M4885]
RM147.M43 1987 615'.6 87-7113
ISBN 0-87434-083-7

CONTENTS

Contributors and Consultants vii

Foreword ix

I Nurse's Role in Drug and I.V. Therapy

1 The Nursing Process in
  Medication Administration and I.V. Therapy 2

2 Legal Risks and Responsibilities in
  Administering Drug and I.V. Therapy 8

II Basics of Drug Administration

3 Principles of Pharmacology 26
4 Medication Orders and Distribution Systems 47
5 Calculations and Measurements 52
6 Preparation and Administration Guidelines 60

III Medication Administration Procedures

7 Administering Oral Medications 84
8 Parenteral Administration of Medication 92
9 Application of Medication to the Eye, Ear, Nose, and Throat 128
10 Topical Application of Medication 138
11 Inhalation Administration of Medication 159

v

IV Principles and Procedures in I.V. Therapy

12	Preparing for I.V. Therapy	168
13	Performing I.V. Therapy Procedures	195
14	Maintaining I.V. Therapy	210
15	Parenteral Nutrition	232
16	Blood and Blood Component Therapy	256

V Pediatric and Geriatric Considerations

17	Pediatric Drug and I.V. Therapy	286
18	Geriatric Drug and I.V. Therapy	308

Appendices

A	Guidelines for I.V. Drug Administration	318
B	Standard Infusion/Piggyback List	330
C	Answers to Review Questions	331
Index		343

CONTRIBUTORS AND CLINICAL CONSULTANTS

Contributors

Peggy Boyle, RN, CRNI
Unit Leader, I.V. Therapy
Doylestown (Pa.) Hospital

Carol A. Calianno, RN, ADN
Staff Nurse
Warminster (Pa.) General Hospital

Patricia L. Carroll, RN, RRT, BS
Independent Nurse Consultant
Fellow of the Litchfield (Conn.) Institute

Glynis Smith Chadwick, RN, BSN
Coordinator, Division of Clinical Nursing
    Education
Anne Arundel General Hospital
Annapolis, Md.

Belinda Pruitt Childs
Diabetic Research Nurse
University of Kansas School of Medicine
Wichita

Michael R. Cohen, RPh, BS
Director of Pharmacy
Quakertown (Pa.) Hospital

Joanne DaCunha, RN, BSN
Clinical Editor
Springhouse Publishing Company
Springhouse, Pa.

Helen Hahler D'Angelo, RN, MSN
Freelance Clinical Editor
Springhouse Publishing Company
Springhouse, Pa.

Sue Donahue, RN, BSN
Staff Nurse—ICU/CCU
Rolling Hill Hospital
Elkins Park, Pa.

DeAnn M. Englert, RN, MSN
Instructor, Specialty Teams
M.D. Anderson Hospital and Tumor Institute
Houston

Anne Marie Frey, CRNI, BSN
I.V. Nurse Clinician
St. Christopher's Hospital for Children
Philadelphia

Bruce M. Frey, PharmD
Clinical Pharmacist
Thomas Jefferson University Hospital, Pharmacy
    Department
Philadelphia

Susan M. Glover, RN, BSN
Williams & Wilkins Publishing Co.
Baltimore

Carol Ann Gramse, RN, CNA, PhD
Associate Professor of Nursing
Hunter-Bellevue School of Nursing
New York

Margaret J. Griffiths, RN, MSN
Assistant Professor
Department of Baccalaureate Nursing
Thomas Jefferson University
Philadelphia

Delores Heckenberger, RN
Community Health and Nursing Services of
    Greater Camden County
Collingswood, N.J.

Jane Ellen Helfant, RN
Vice-President—Marketing
Corpak Company—A Thermedics Inc. Company
Wheeling, Ill.

Alan W. Hopefel, PharmD
Assistant Professor of Clinical Pharmacy
St. Louis College of Pharmacy

Sheila Scannell Jenkins, RN, BSN
Instructor, Nursing of Children
Bridgeport (Conn.) Hospital School of Nursing

Sue M. Jones, RNC, FNC, MSN
Assistant Professor of Community Health
    Nursing
Vanderbilt University
Nashville, Tenn.

Joann Kaalaas, RN, MSN
Clinical Nurse Specialist—Oncology
Salt Lake City

Lora McGuire, RN, BSN, MS
Nursing Instructor
Joliet (Ill.) Junior College

Patrica Gonce Miller, RN, MS
Instructor
University of Maryland School of Nursing
Baltimore

Patrice N. Nasielski, RN
Staff Nurse
Los Robles Regional Medical Center
Thousand Oaks, Calif.

Helen Ritting Nawrocki, RN
Director, Education and Training
Delaware Valley Medical Center
Bristol, Pa.

Mary Ellen Pike, RN, CS, MSN
Lecturer
Allan and Donna Lansing School of Nursing,
  Education and Health Sciences
Bellarmine College
Louisville

Jean Rabinow, JD
Attorney
McMillan and Rabinow
Trumbull, Conn.

William Simonson, PharmD
Associate Professor
Oregon State University, College of Pharmacy
Corvallis

Harold H. Simpson III, JD
Attorney
Gill, Skokos, Simpson, Buford & Graham
Little Rock, Ark.

Rae Nadine Smith, RN, MS
Clinical Nursing Specialist
Sorenson Research Company
Salt Lake City

Judy L. Speciale, RN, AHN
Assistant Head Nurse—Oncology Unit
Providence Medical Center
Portland, Ore.

Joseph F. Steiner, PharmD
Associate Professor of Clinical Pharmacy/
  Director of Clinical Pharmacy Program
University of Wyoming
Casper

Robin Tourigian, RN, MSN
Nurse Clinician, Oncology Unit
Thomas Jefferson University Hospital
Philadelphia

Karen Dyer Vance, RN, BSN
Freelance Author
East Aurora, N.Y.

Susan Vigeant, RN, BSN
Public Health Nurse
Department of Corrections, Bucks County Prison
Warrington, Pa.

Nina P. Welsh, RN
Freelance Clinical Editor
Springhouse Publishing Company
Springhouse, Pa.

Alexandra Wright-Beebe, RN, MS
Nurse Consultant and Lecturer
Washington, D.C.

Consultants

Judith R. Brown, RN, JD
Attorney
Hershey, Pa.

Karen E. Burgess, RN, MSN
Neuro/Ortho/Rehab Clinical Specialist
Huntington Memorial Hospital
Pasadena, Calif.

Anne Marie Frey, CRNI, BSN
I.V. Nurse Clinician
St. Christopher's Hospital for Children
Philadelphia

Marion Newton, RN, BSN, MN
Assistant Professor, Undergraduate Programs
University of Nebraska Medical Center, College
  of Nursing
Omaha

FOREWORD

No matter what the clinical setting, the rapid changes in the complexity of care are apparent to every nurse. Medication administration is one of the most complicated activities. Constant attempts to refine specific drug actions, combined with the never-ending search for new drugs, make the correct administration of drugs and keen observation of outcomes main components of clinical care. These components help ensure the clinical protection of every patient. To accomplish this end safely and effectively, each nurse has an ethical and a personal responsibility for acquiring the in-depth knowledge necessary for precise clinical actions. Because this ongoing search for clinical knowledge is a way of life for each nurse, the need for a text such as this one is critical. As a strong tool for the active nurse who desires to stay current, it is clearly written, well organized, comprehensive, and up to date.

Medication Administration and I.V. Therapy Manual is a practical reference that covers both the scientific theory and principles of medication administration and I.V. therapy, stating each procedure clearly. Chapter 1, The Nursing Process in Medication Administration and I.V. Therapy, discusses an orderly method of assessment. Chapter 2, Legal Risks and Responsibilities in Administering Drug and I.V. Therapy, covers the legal aspects of performing these tasks, as well as the National Intravenous Therapy Association's standards for I.V. home therapy and hyperalimentation therapy. Chapter 5, Calculations and Measurements, is helpful to students learning about measurement systems and drug calculations and conversions.

Chapter 6, Preparation and Administration Guidelines, and Chapter 12, Preparing for I.V. Therapy, are useful to beginning nursing students, their instructors, and nurses returning to practice. These chapters cover nursing tasks and responsibilities performed in the medication room or before entering the patient's room to give a medication or begin I.V. therapy. They include the selection and use of equipment, use of sterile techniques, preparation of admixtures, types of I.V. solutions, setting up a fluid system, calculating flow rates, preparing for venipuncture, and documenting medication and I.V. therapy. These chapters are unique because they contain the basics, which frequently are excluded from or not compiled and organized by subject in textbooks.

Several later chapters comprehensively describe approximately 50 basic, complex, or new medication administration or I.V. therapy procedures. They cover equipment used, steps performed, and nursing considerations relative to the performance or outcome of each procedure, including home care procedures. Parenteral nutrition and blood and blood component therapy are addressed in one chapter, as well as pediatric and geriatric considerations in drug and I.V. therapy in another.

The review questions at the end of each chapter will help students assess learning. Answers to the review questions are provided in the Appendix.

Students and instructors will find *Medication Administration and I.V. Therapy Manual* useful in all patient care settings. Nurses in active practice can use it as a reliable, accurate reference or a learning tool.

LUTHER CHRISTMAN, RN, PhD
Dean Emeritus, College of Nursing
Rush University
Chicago

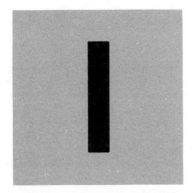

Nurse's Role in Drug and I.V. Therapy

1 The Nursing Process in Medication
  Administration and I.V. Therapy 2

2 Legal Risks and Responsibilities in
  Administering Drug and I.V. Therapy 8

The Nursing Process in Medication Administration and I.V. Therapy

Today, nurses work in a variety of roles and settings. They constantly make decisions concerning medication administration and I.V. therapy. To ensure the safety of the patient and to meet medical and legal concerns, it is essential that this important part of nursing practice be carried out in a deliberate and organized manner. The nursing process directs purposeful and planned actions for patient care. This chapter explains the use of the nursing process in medication administration and I.V. therapy.

Although this manual's emphasis is on the methods of giving medications and performing I.V. therapy, it supports the use of the nursing process. The foundation of thorough assessment, appropriate nursing diagnosis, purposeful planning, accurate implementation, and constant evaluation provided by the nursing process is vital to the safe and effective administration of medication and I.V. therapy.

Assessment

Before you administer medication or I.V. therapy, take note of factors in the patient's health history that can affect drug or I.V. therapy. Using data from the health history, you can then identify actual or potential problems. It is not always necessary or possible to obtain all of the relevant information in a standard health history. However, the questions in the health history section that follows can be useful because they focus on identifying problems associated with drug and I.V. therapy. You can obtain the answers from the patient, a family member, other health care professionals involved with the patient, or the medical record.

Assessment is also an ongoing part of the nursing process. You and other health care professionals will continue to add to the patient's data base during and even after the administration of medication or I.V. therapy. You must continually assess the patient's response.

Health history
Past history
What major illnesses has the patient had? Has he been hospitalized or had surgery? Does he have any medical or surgical conditions that would contraindicate the use of a particular drug or alter the dosage or the method of administration?

Family history
Does any member of the patient's family have a current or hereditary illness? What were the causes of death of deceased family members? This information is important in deciding if the benefits of using a drug outweigh the possible adverse reactions. For example, a patient with a strong family history of cancer may not want to take an estrogen supplement after a hysterectomy, and a woman considering birth control methods needs to be aware of the connection between a family history of cardiovascular problems and the adverse reactions of birth control pills.

Drug use
What medications have been prescribed for the patient? What dose? How often? What is he actually taking?

What over-the-counter (OTC) medications, if any, does the patient take? What dose? How often? Ask about the use of OTC medications since their use may reduce or enhance the response to other medications. (See "Drug-drug interactions," p. 37, in Chapter 3.) OTC medications also can be abused, as in the abuse of OTC laxatives by women with anorexia nervosa.

Does the patient use alcohol, caffeine, or nicotine? How much? How often? These drugs can also alter the response to some medications. Explore the use of illegal drugs, when suspected, to prevent possible drug interactions and withdrawal complications.

Allergies
Is the patient allergic to any drugs? Foods? Environmental substances? Are there any drugs he cannot take? If so, what effects do the drugs have? Is anyone in his family allergic to the prescribed medication? Note allergies in red ink in the cardex and on the front of the patient's chart.

Diet
Is the patient on a special diet? What does he eat on a typical day? What did he eat yesterday? Are there any foods he cannot tolerate? Information about his diet can be helpful in reducing unpleasant side effects and in improving compliance. (See "Drug-food interactions," p. 37, in Chapter 3.)

Family support system
Does the patient live alone? If he lives with someone, is that person able and willing to assist with the medication or I.V. therapy? If the patient lives alone, does someone regularly check on him?

This information is important in evaluating a patient's ability to comply with the prescribed medication schedule at home in a safe, effective manner. It is also important in deciding when he can be discharged from the hospital. Many patients can be discharged early if there is someone at home to help them with medication or I.V. therapy. For example, the cancer patient needing total parenteral nutrition (TPN) has the option of using it at home if someone can and will assist him. An early discharge is desirable to the patient and cost-effective for the hospital.

Finances
Can the patient pay for prescribed drugs and supplies? The patient who has no money for medications cannot be compliant. He will need nursing intervention to seek financial assistance.

Motivation toward wellness
Is the patient interested in getting well and doing what it takes to get well? For example, will a patient taking an antihypertensive medication continue to do so even though he "feels fine" without it?

Level of intelligence and education
Does the patient have the intelligence to follow directions? Directions may be complex, and the ability to follow them is necessary for safe administration of medication or I.V. therapy at home. For example, a patient who lacks the intelligence to follow directions would not be able to use a glucometer to measure his blood glucose level and then safely change his insulin dose as indicated by the results.

Can the patient read? If not, he will need to be taught about his medications in a very creative fashion, and he will need nursing intervention for follow-up assessment and instruction at home.

Religious and cultural beliefs
Does the patient hold beliefs that may influence his attitude about medications or I.V. therapy? For example, a Christian Scientist may refuse prescription drugs based on his belief that one is healed only through prayer, and a parent who is a Jehovah's Witness may refuse a blood transfusion for a sick child because of religious beliefs.

Life-style
How does the patient's life-style affect his ability to safely and effectively take medication or receive I.V. therapy at home? What factors other than his family support system affect his ability to do so?

Is the patient's vision adequate? If not, how will this affect self-administration of medication? For example, a diabetic patient with deteriorating vision will need assistance in measuring and injecting insulin.

Does the patient have any impairment in mobility or dexterity that would affect his ability to give himself medications at home? For example, a person with decreased dexterity may not be able to manipulate a tube of nitroglycerin paste and correctly measure the prescribed amount; a 24-hour transdermal patch could be used instead.

Are there any environmental impediments, such as lack of refrigeration for TPN solutions or drugs that need to be refrigerated?

How does the medication or I.V. therapy schedule fit into the patient's work schedule or activities of daily living? Do alterations need to be made? For instance, a patient who works on a night shift will not be able to take medications at 9 a.m., 1 p.m., and 6 p.m., and the schedule will have to be altered.

Physical assessment

The patient's age, height, weight, and underlying diseases can affect drug action and therefore must be considered when determining drug choice and dosage. (See "Factors that affect drug action," p. 36, in Chapter 3.) These factors are important in determining a therapeutic dosage range and in preventing adverse reactions and drug toxicity.

Nursing diagnosis

Gordon defines nursing diagnosis as "...actual or potential health problems which nurses, by virtue of their education and experience, are capable and licensed to treat." (See Selected References.) A nursing diagnosis often necessitates the administration of medication and I.V. therapy as a nursing intervention. For example, one intervention for the nursing diagnosis "Impaired gas exchange related to altered oxygen supply" would be to administer medications, as ordered, and to monitor and record the effectiveness of and adverse reactions to the medication.

There are times, however, when medication administration may result in a nursing diagnosis. For example, birth control pills are prescribed for a patient with a history of hypermenorrhea. From a brief health history, the nurse finds that the patient has a family history of cardiovascular disorders, has an intense desire to get well, is an intelligent person, and is a strict Roman Catholic. The patient is visibly upset and expresses a conflict between the desire not to violate religious beliefs and the need and desire to get well. Possible nursing diagnoses for this patient might include the following:

A problem diagnosis:
 Anxiety related to conflict between religious beliefs and prescribed medication

A potential-problem diagnosis:
 Potential for drug-induced phlebitis or hypertension related to adverse reactions to medication and family history of cardiovascular disease

The problem diagnosis is based on a patient problem that occurs as a result of the prescribed drug therapy. It demonstrates the nurse's ability to assess all factors related to administering medications in this patient.

The potential-problem diagnosis is based on assessment data that details a family history of cardiovascular problems. The nurse's knowledge about the medication's potential adverse reactions of phlebitis and hypertension confirms the relevance of this nursing diagnosis.

Planning

Once a nursing diagnosis has been made, goals and nursing interventions are developed to alleviate the problem. The diagnosis "Anxiety related to conflict between religious beliefs and prescribed medication" is an actual problem.

Suggested goals for this diagnosis:
• The patient will discuss conflict concerning religious beliefs and medication.
• The patient will exhibit no signs of anxiety, such as crying, when leaving the clinic.

Possible nursing interventions to meet these goals:
• Listen to patient's feelings about the conflict.
• Discuss with patient primary purpose of the prescribed medication.
• Remind patient that other attempts at treatment were unsuccessful.
• Refer patient to priest or chaplain.

- Telephone later in week to see if patient has resolved or at least begun to resolve conflict.

The second nursing diagnosis states a potential problem that requires observation. The goals and nursing interventions are directed toward preventing that problem. They relate to the patient's risk for developing the cardiovascular disorders found in the family history: varicose veins, hypertension, and stroke.

Suggested goals for this diagnosis:
- The patient will maintain diastolic blood pressure less than 90 mm Hg.
- The patient will remain free of pain, tenderness, redness, or heat in calves.
- The patient will remain free of edema.
- The patient will have no complaints of headache.

Possible nursing interventions to meet these goals:
- Instruct patient to have blood pressure checked twice weekly while on medication and to report any diastolic reading greater than 90 mm Hg.
- Instruct patient on how to examine calves for tenderness, redness, or heat, and tell her to report any such symptoms.
- Instruct patient to report any edema or headache.

The planning phase concludes with the documentation of the proposed nursing interventions. This documentation should be a written care plan in the cardex or outpatient record.

Implementation

During the implementation phase of the nursing process, the proposed nursing interventions take place and the prescribed medication and I.V. therapy are administered.

Patient/family teaching

A common nursing intervention related to administration of medication and I.V. therapy is providing the patient/family with the information for safe, effective administration at home. The administration of eye drops, the technique for flushing a heparin lock, the use of inhalants, observation of an I.V. site, the variety of ways to administer nitroglycerin, and insulin injection techniques are a few examples of the topics taught.

A teaching plan designed for the patient's needs should be devised, carried out, and documented. In developing the plan, consider what the patient/family needs to know for safe, effective home administration. The patient taking digoxin at home every day must be taught how to take a radial pulse, for example. The patient also should be instructed not to take the medication and to notify the physician if the pulse rate is below a specified level. In addition, if the patient shows interest in knowing more about the specific action of digoxin, that information should be taught. However, if the patient is not interested, there is no need to include it because it is not essential to ensure safe administration of the drug.

A patient/family teaching plan related to the administration of medication and I.V. therapy should include at least:
- the name and dose of the medication
- the medication's predicted effect
- directions on when and how to take the medication
- possible acceptable side effects
- unacceptable side effects
- indications of when health care personnel should be notified and who should be notified.

Patient/family understanding of the material should be evaluated throughout your teaching and again at completion. That may be done with such methods as questioning, patient/family explanation, or return demonstration. Evaluation helps you determine the effectiveness of the teaching plan and identifies areas where revision or reinforcement is necessary.

When your teaching is completed, it must be documented on the patient record. Documentation might include a completed, signed checklist of all the necessary points. If you do not use a checklist, then include documentation in the nurses' notes, as shown below. State what was taught, and evaluate the patient's learning.

Sample nurses' note:
Explained how nitroglycerin works, why patient is on the medication, importance of taking every day, and how to apply transdermal patch. Patient verbalized

adequate understanding of all the above information. Demonstrated how to properly apply and remove transdermal patch.
M. Smith, R.N.

Evaluation

Evaluation is especially critical in the administration of medication and I.V. therapy. It measures the success of the treatment regimen and also helps the nurse identify strengths and weaknesses in the plan of care. Because there is no room for error, the safest and most appropriate plan must be sought.

The plan
Evaluate the plan of care by examining if the patient goals were met. If they were, then it is likely that you identified an accurate nursing diagnosis, set realistic goals, and ordered effective nursing interventions.

The intervention
Most nursing diagnoses and care plans include giving an ordered medication or I.V. therapy as an intervention. When evaluation of a plan shows that the goals were not met, the effectiveness of each nursing intervention must be evaluated. That means that the patient's response to medication or I.V. therapy must be evaluated.

Evaluating patient response
In evaluating a patient's response to medication or I.V. therapy, ask the following questions:
- Did the desired or therapeutic effect occur? For example, did the pain medication relieve the pain? If the desired effect did not occur, why not? You should be aware of the factors that affect drug action when evaluating a patient's response. (See Chapter 3, Principles of Pharmacology.)
- Did factors other than the drug perhaps result in the desired effect? For example, a patient with frequent migraine headaches is taking methysergide maleate (Sansert) daily. She also changes her diet by avoiding chocolate, cheese, and peanut butter. It would not be clear in this case whether the drug or the diet change resulted in the desired effect.
- Did an undesired or adverse reaction occur? For example, the effect of diazepam in an elderly patient may be to excite rather than calm him.
- Is the adverse reaction potentially life-threatening, as in a blood transfusion reaction or an allergic response to a drug? Does the medication need to be discontinued? Do the charge nurse and physician need to be notified about the response?
- Is there a lack of response? For example, a patient with a urinary tract infection is not responding if his temperature remains high and his urine has sediment and a foul smell after he has received I.V. antibiotic therapy for a week.

Collecting data
Completing the evaluation of patient response to medication or I.V. therapy requires collecting subjective and objective data. You can do this in several ways.

Direct patient observation is a basic, yet beneficial, evaluation method. How does the patient regard the medication or I.V. therapy? Does his subjective view correlate with your objective view? For example, some antihypertensive medications cause impotence. You may note a decrease in blood pressure, which is the desired effect. However, a patient may reject the medication because of its unacceptable side effect.

The family often identifies changes that go unnoticed by health care professionals and the patient. Their insight can be invaluable and should be solicited when necessary. For example, a patient who has been on a high dose of an aminoglycoside such as tobramycin may experience diminished hearing. The family would be the best resource to help you evaluate the patient's hearing loss.

Clinical measurements also provide objective data with which to evaluate a patient's response. Blood pressure, temperature, pulse, and laboratory test results all help in determining the efficacy of medication or I.V. therapy.

Evaluation of the patient's response should not be based on any single factor. A combination of data from direct patient observation, discussions with the patient or family, and clinical measurements is necessary to complete the evaluation.

Review Questions

1. The most essential component of the assessment phase of the nursing process is:
   A. Identifying the patient's medications
   B. Reading the patient's record
   C. Talking with the patient's family
   D. Eliciting a health history from the patient

2. The act of administering medications or I.V. therapy is usually done in which phase of the nursing process?
   A. Assessment
   B. Nursing diagnosis
   C. Implementation
   D. Evaluation

3. Documentation of proposed nursing interventions is best done by:
   A. Telling the patient
   B. Writing a nursing care plan
   C. Making an anectodal note in the patient record
   D. Writing it on the medication cardex

4. Which of the following includes inappropriate information for a basic teaching plan on medication administration?
   A. When and how to take the medication, name of medication, predicted effect, and chemical structure
   B. Name of medication, dose, acceptable side effects, and unacceptable side effects
   C. Dose, purpose, when health care personnel should be notified, and unacceptable side effects
   D. All of the above

5. Which of the following is (are) acceptable way(s) to assess the patient's knowledge of material taught by the nurse?
   1. Return demonstration
   2. Having the patient explain the material
   3. Asking the patient if he understands the material
   4. Asking the patient specific questions about the material
   A. 1 only
   B. 1 and 2
   C. 1, 2, and 3
   D. 1, 2, and 4

6. To evaluate the patient's response to medication or I.V. therapy, which of the following resources is (are) recommended?
   A. Discussion with the family
   B. Direct patient observation
   C. Clinical measurements
   D. All of the above

Selected References

Alfaro, R. *Application of Nursing Process: A Step-by-Step Guide to Care Planning.* Philadelphia: J.B. Lippincott Co., 1986.

Carpenito, L.J. *Nursing Diagnosis: Application to Clinical Practice.* Philadelphia: J.B. Lippincott Co., 1983.

Edmunds, M.W., ed. *Nursing Drug Reference: A Practitioner's Guide.* East Norwalk, Conn.: Appleton & Lange, 1985.

Gordon, M. *Manual of Nursing Diagnosis, 1984-1985.* New York: McGraw-Hill Book Co., 1984.

Hahn, A.B., et al. *Pharmacology in Nursing,* 16th ed. St. Louis: C.V. Mosby Co., 1985.

Iyer, P.W., et al. *Nursing Process and Nursing Diagnosis.* Philadelphia: W.B. Saunders Co., 1986.

Legal Risks and Responsibilities in Administering Drug and I.V. Therapy

Administering drugs and performing I.V. therapy continue to be two of the most important and most frequently performed nursing duties. They also involve much legal risk. This chapter addresses the most important legal issues that affect you in dealing with medication administration, I.V. therapy, incident reporting, and risk management.

The nurse's role in medication administration

For many years, U.S. and Canadian registered nurses (RNs) were permitted to give drugs only orally or rectally. If a patient needed to receive a drug by injection, the prescribing physician injected it. Gradually, however, the nurse's role expanded. Today, RNs give subcutaneous and intramuscular injections, induce anesthesia, and give drugs intravenously. In some states, RNs may even prescribe drugs, within certain limitations.

In a few states and Canadian provinces, nurse practice acts do not permit licensed practical nurses (LPNs) or licensed vocational nurses (LVNs) to administer drugs to patients at all, even under supervision. Most nurse practice acts, however, now permit them to give drugs under the supervision of an RN, a physician, or a dentist, assuming that the LPN or LVN has the appropriate educational background or on-the-job training. No clear-cut definitions of appropriate background or training exist, but most courts probably would be satisfied if an LPN or LVN could prove that her supervising nurse or physician had watched her administer drugs and had judged her competent.

In general, the law has kept pace with the nurse's expanding role in administering drugs. Nurses must meet high practice standards and adhere to the long-standing five-rights formula:
- The right drug
- To the right patient
- At the right time
- In the right dosage
- By the right route.

It is wise to add two rights to this list:
- The patient's right to know about the medication he is receiving
- The patient's right to refuse the medication or I.V. therapy.

Drug control laws

Legally, a *drug* is any substance listed in an official state, Canadian provincial, or national formulary. It may also be any substance other than food "intended to affect the structure or any function of the body... (or) for use in the diagnosis, cure, mitigation, treatment, or prevention of disease" (N.Y. Education Law).

A *prescription drug* is any drug restricted from regular commercial purchase and sale. It has been restricted because the state, provincial, or national government has determined that it is, or might be, unsafe unless used under a qualified medical practitioner's supervision.

In the United States, two federal laws mainly govern the use of drugs: the Comprehensive Drug Abuse Prevention and Control Act (incorporating the Controlled Substances Act), which regulates drugs thought to be most subject to abuse; and the Food, Drug, and Cosmetic Act, which restricts interstate shipment of drugs not approved for human use and outlines the process by which drugs are tested and approved.

On the state and (in Canada) provincial level, the main laws affecting the distribution of drugs are pharmacy practice acts. These give pharmacists (and sometimes physicians, in Canada) the sole legal authority to prepare, compound, preserve, and dispense drugs. *Dispensing* refers to taking a drug from the pharmacy supply and giving or selling it to another person. This contrasts with *administering,* which is the act of giving the drug to the patient.

Nurse practice acts are laws that most directly affect how nurses administer drugs. In general, most state and provincial practice acts first define the tasks that belong uniquely to the profession being regulated and then state that anyone who performs such tasks without being a licensed or registered member of the profession is breaking the law.

In many states, if a nurse prescribes a drug, she is practicing medicine without a license. If she goes into the pharmacy or drug supply cabinet, measures out doses of a drug, and puts the powder into capsules, she is practicing pharmacy without a license. For either action, she can be prosecuted or lose her license (or both), even if no one is harmed by what she does. In most states and provinces, practicing a licensed profession without a license is, at the very least, a misdemeanor.

In *Stefanik v. Nursing Education Committee* (1944), a Rhode Island nurse lost her nursing license in part because she had been practicing medicine illegally. She had changed a physician's drug order for a patient because she did not agree with what had been prescribed. No one claimed she had harmed the patient. However, changing a prescription is the same as writing a new prescription. Rhode Island's nurse practice act did not—and still does not—consider that to be part of nursing practice.

The Food, Drug, and Cosmetic Act and federal and state drug abuse laws are less important to nursing practice than the professional practice acts. That is because most nurses do not test drugs, prescribe them, compound them, or dispense them.

TAKING DRUG ORDERS AND CARRYING THEM OUT: HOW TO PROTECT YOURSELF

When a physician writes a drug order for his patient and signs it—or when another health care professional writes an order and the physician countersigns it—the courts usually will not question the legality of the order. But if a physician gives you a verbal drug order—either in person or by telephone—protect yourself legally, as follows:

- Write down the order *exactly* as he gives it.
- Repeat the order back to him so that you are sure you heard him correctly.

Once you have given the drug to the patient, make sure you document all necessary information.

- Record *in ink* the type of drug, the dose, the time you administered it, and any other information your facility's policy requires.
- Sign or initial your notes.

If your facility keeps drug orders in a special file, make sure that you transfer the physician's drug order, which you wrote on the patient's chart, to that file.

If a physician gives you a verbal drug order during an emergency, your first duty is to carry it out at once. When the emergency is over, document what you did.

Here is what can happen if you do not document drug orders:

- You could face disciplinary measures for failing to document.
- You could damage your facility's defense or your defense in any malpractice lawsuit.
- Other nurses, not knowing what drugs have been given, may administer other drugs that could have harmful interactions.

However, you should know what the drug abuse laws do. They categorize drugs by how dangerous they are (forbidding the use of some, limiting the use of others), and they provide for rehabilitating drug abuse victims.

Liability for dispensing drugs

In rare instances, adequate patient care may require you to give a drug that is not available on the floor. Normally, you would call your facility's pharmacist and ask that the drug be sent. But what would you do if you were working on the night or weekend shift and no pharmacist were available? In this situation, you cannot escape liability if you dispense the drug yourself and a lawsuit results.

Some facilities have written policies that permit the charge nurse, under special circumstances, to go into the pharmacy and dispense an emergency dose of a drug. But whether the facility has a written policy or not, a nurse who dispenses drugs is doing so unlawfully unless her state or provincial pharmacy practice act specifically authorizes it. If she makes an error in dispensing the drug and the patient later sues, the fact that she was practicing as an unlicensed pharmacist can be used as evidence against her.

You can, of course, choose to disregard the laws that govern nursing practice and dispense a drug if you think a patient's well-being requires it. But clearly you do so at your own risk. Even if you do not harm the patient, you can still be prosecuted and can still lose your license. In extraordinary circumstances—when ethics and the law conflict and you have to weigh concern for a patient's life or health against concern for your license—you must make up your own mind about what action you are going to take.

Common bases of drug-related lawsuits

Unfortunately, lawsuits involving nurses' medication errors are common.

Derrick v. Portland Eye, Ear, Nose, & Throat Hospital (1922) involved an Oregon nurse who gave a young boy a pupil-contracting drug when the physician had ordered a pupil-dilating drug. As a result of the error, the boy lost his sight in one eye, and the nurse and the hospital were found negligent.

Giving the wrong drug for diagnostic purposes can also prompt a lawsuit. A 1967 case in Tennessee, *Gault v. Poor Sisters of St. Francis Seraph of Perpetual Adoration*, involved a nurse who was supposed to give a gastric lavage using salt water. Instead, she gave the patient dilute sodium hydroxide, causing severe internal injuries. The hospital lost the initial verdict and an appeal.

Giving the wrong dosage can be the cause of a lawsuit. A Louisiana case, *Norton v. Argonaut Insurance Company* (1962), involved a nurse who inadvertently gave a 3-month-old infant a digitalis overdose that resulted in the infant's death. In the malpractice trial that followed, the nurse, the hospital, and the attending physician were found liable.

Similarly, *Dessauer v. Memorial General Hospital*, a 1981 New Mexico case, involved an emergency department physician who ordered 50 mg of lidocaine for a patient. A nurse who normally worked in the hospital's obstetrics ward gave the patient 800 mg. The patient died, the family sued, and the hospital was found liable.

A mistake in the administration route was the basis of *Moore v. Guthrie Hospital*, a 1968 West Virginia case. A nurse gave a patient two drugs intravenously rather than intramuscularly. The patient suffered a seizure, sued, and won.

The court decisions in these cases were based on, and in turn helped to define, the standard of nursing care to be applied in administering drugs to patients. In some of these court cases, it is clear that if the nurse had known more about the proper dose, administration route, or procedure for giving the drug, she might not have made a mistake. But even when a nurse can demonstrate her competence, another point remains clear: The courts will not permit carelessness that harms a patient.

Responsibility in drug experimentation

Your legal duties in administering experimental drugs to patients, or in administering established drugs in new ways or at

AVOIDING COMMON MEDICATION ERRORS

You have probably heard the statistic that one out of every six medications given in a hospital is associated with an error.

A number of studies have tried to calculate how many patients are actually harmed by such errors. These studies demonstrate that injuries from medication errors are far from rare.

In four independent studies published between 1972 and 1978, researchers reported that 9% to 30% of all malpractice claims arose from drug-related injuries. The average amount paid to settle such a claim in 1976 was $25,480.

A 1981 study of 815 consecutive hospital admissions showed that drugs were the major cause of iatrogenic illness and injury in hospitalized patients. Nearly 20% of the patients developed a serious disability from a drug-related complication.

Another study, published in 1979, analyzed the type of drug-related incidents reported in a Michigan hospital. That study showed seven kinds of errors with these occurrences:

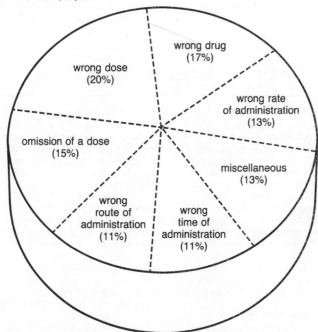

Three safeguards against giving the wrong drug:
• Avoid distractions during preparation and administration.
• Separate look-alike medications, and separate medications from toxic chemicals.
• Discard out-of-date drugs.
Three safeguards against giving a medication by the wrong route:
• Use only accepted injection sites.
• Aspirate before giving an I.M. injection.
• Use the right length needle.
Two suggestions regarding the importance of labels and package inserts:
• Know the peculiarities and particular dangers of a drug before giving it.
• Read and follow warnings on drug labels.

Reprinted with permission from Fink, Joseph L., III, "Preventing Lawsuits—Medication Errors to Avoid," *NursingLife*, 26-29, March/April 1983.

experimental dosage levels, are the same as your legal duties in administering drugs customarily. In addition, you must make sure no drug is given to a patient who has not consented to take part in the experimentation. (Consent must be in writing if the research is federally funded.)

Obtain answers to any questions you or the patient may have about experimental drugs or dosages in the experimental protocol, not in the usual books, product labels, or package inserts.

Responsibility for knowing about drugs

Once you have your nursing license, you are expected—by law—to know about any drugs you administer. You are expected to know a drug's safe dosage limits, toxicity, side effects, potential adverse reactions, and indications and contraindications for use. If you are an LPN or LVN, you assume the same legal responsibility as an RN once you have taken a pharmaceutical course or have received some other authorization to administer drugs.

LaMade v. Wilson (1975) involved a nurse who applied Ophthaine [proparacaine] to the eye of an ophthalmology unit patient. The anesthetic stopped his eye from hurting, but it also stopped it from healing. The hospital and the attending nurses were sued.

When the case was appealed, the court presumed that a reasonably experienced nurse on an ophthalmology unit would know a great deal about the drugs she was

WHEN YOUR PATIENT IS ABUSING DRUGS

If you suspect your patient is abusing drugs, you have a duty to do something about it. If such a patient harms himself or anyone else, and a lawsuit results, the court may hold you liable for his actions. However, your legal responsibilities vary, depending on how much you know about the patient's drug or alcohol abuse.

For instance, suppose you know for certain that a patient is abusing drugs—if you're an emergency department nurse, you may find drugs in a patient's clothes or handbag while looking for identification. Your facility's policy may obligate you to confiscate the drugs and take steps to see that the patient does not acquire more.

What if a patient's erratic or threatening behavior makes you *suspect* he is abusing drugs, but you have no evidence? Your facility's policy may require that you conduct a drug search. The legal question here is whether your search is justified. As a rule of thumb, if you strongly believe the patient poses a threat to himself or others, and you can document your reasons for searching his possessions, you are probably safe legally.

Before you conduct a search, review your facility's guidelines on the matter.

Then follow those guidelines carefully. Most guidelines will first direct you to contact your supervisor and explain why you have legitimate cause for a search. If she gives you her approval, next ask a security guard to help you. Besides protecting you, he will serve as a witness if you do find drugs. When you are ready, confront the patient, tell him you intend to conduct a search, and tell him why.

Depending on your facility's guidelines, you can search a patient's belongings as well as his room. If you find illegal drugs during your search, confiscate them. Remember, possession of illegal drugs is a felony. Depending on your facility's guidelines, you may be obligated to report the patient to the police.

If you find alcoholic beverages, take them from the patient and explain that you will return them when he leaves the facility.

After you have completed your search, tell the patient's physician about it and record your findings in your nurses' notes and in an incident report. Your written records will be an important part of your defense (and the facility's defense) if the patient decides to sue.

ordered to give, including contraindications. The burden was on the nurse and on the hospital to prove that the appropriate standard of care was lower. The appellate court decided that the lower court should have heard evidence to determine whether the nurse knew, or should have known, that Ophthaine might be contraindicated after trauma or after surgery. This decision implied that if she knew, or should have known, and did not at least question the order, she and the hospital would be liable.

Increasingly, judges and juries also expect nurses to know what the appropriate observation intervals are for a patient receiving any type of medication—even if the physician does not know or does not write an order stating how often to check on the newly medicated patient. A case that was decided on this basis is *Brown v. State*, a 1977 New York case. After a patient was given 200 mg of Thorazine [chlorpromazine], the nurses on duty left him largely unobserved for several hours. When someone finally checked on the patient, he was dead. The hospital and the nurses lost the resulting lawsuit.

Questioning drug orders

Follow your facility's policy when questioning a drug order. Usually, the policy suggests pursuing the following steps until you obtain a satisfactory answer:
• Look up the answer in a standard drug reference.
• Ask the charge nurse.
• Ask the facility's pharmacist.
• Ask the prescribing physician.
• Ask the prescribing physician's supervisor (service chief).

Refusing to administer a drug

You have the legal right not to administer drugs you think will harm patients. You may exercise this right in a variety of situations:
• When you think the dosage prescribed is incorrect
• When you think the drug is contraindicated because of possible dangerous interactions with other drugs or with substances such as alcohol
• When you think the patient's physical condition contraindicates using the drug.

In limited circumstances, you may also legally refuse to administer a drug on grounds of conscience. Some states and provinces have enacted right-of-conscience laws that excuse medical personnel from the requirement to participate in any abortion or sterilization procedure. Under such laws, you may, for example, refuse to give any drug you believe is intended to induce abortion.

When you refuse to carry out a drug order, you must be sure to do the following:
• Notify the immediate supervisor so she can make alternative arrangements (assigning a new nurse, clarifying the order).
• Notify the prescribing physician if the supervisor has not done this already.
• If the drug was not given (sometimes a supervisor, physician, or substitute nurse will give the drug), document that the drug was not given and explain why.

Protecting yourself from liability

If you make an error in giving a drug, or if a patient reacts negatively to a properly administered drug, you must protect yourself by documenting the incident thoroughly. (See *Taking Drug Orders and Carrying Them Out: How to Protect Yourself*, p. 9.) Some of the documentation belongs in the patient's chart, including information on the patient's reaction and any medical or nursing interventions taken to minimize harm to the patient. Other documentation should be confined to the incident report. Here, you should identify what happened, the names and functions of all persons involved, and the actions taken to protect the patient after the error was discovered.

An incident report does not become part of the patient's medical record, nor does it take the place of proper documentation in the patient's chart. The medical record should not even mention that an incident report has been filed, but should include only clinical observations relating to the incident. (Value judgments should be avoided.) Entering these observations in the patient's record, however, does not take the place of completing an incident report.

Incident reports

Many times, despite the best training and intentions, incidents occur in a health care facility. These are events that are inconsistent with the facility's standards of care or its routine operations. In most facilities, any patient injury or complaint, medication error, or injury to an employee or visitor requires an incident report.

The report serves two main purposes:

• To inform administrators about the incident so they can consider changes that will help prevent similar incidents (risk management)
• To alert administrators and the facility's insurance company to potential liability claims and the need for further investigation (claims management).

Even when the incident is not investigated, the report helps to identify witnesses if a lawsuit is filed months or even years later.

ADMINISTERING CONTROLLED DRUGS: PRECAUTIONS TO TAKE

Government agencies regulate certain drugs that have a high potential for abuse. In the United States, the Food and Drug Administration divides these controlled substances into five groups, Schedules I to V. In Canada, the Health Protection Branch groups all controlled drugs into one group, Schedule G.

Schedule I drugs have the highest potential for abuse and are not accepted for any medical use. You may administer Schedule II to V drugs, or Schedule G drugs in Canada.

Remember that all these drugs are potentially habit-forming and addictive. Before administering them, take these precautions:
• Check your facility's policy for special procedures.
• Sign out, on the narcotics form, any drugs you remove from the narcotics cabinet.
• Follow the proper disposal procedures if any part of the drug remains after use.
• Never leave any drugs lying on the counter.
• Relock the narcotics cabinet after you have removed the drugs you need.

SCHEDULE	EXAMPLES
In the United States:	
I	heroin, lysergic acid diethylamide (LSD), marijuana derivatives, mescaline, peyote, and psilocybin
II	amobarbital, amphetamine, cocaine, codeine, hydromorphone, meperidine, methadone, methamphetamine, methaqualone, methylphenidate, morphine, opium, oxycodone, oxymorphone, pentobarbital, phenmetrazine, and secobarbital
III	barbituric acid derivatives (except those listed in another schedule), benzphetamine, glutethimide, mazindol, methyprylon, paregoric, and phendimetrazine
IV	barbital, benzodiazepine derivatives, chloral hydrate, diethylpropion, ethchlorvynol, ethinamate, fenfluramine, meprobamate, methohexital, paraldehyde, phenobarbital, and phentermine
V	diphenoxylate compound and expectorants with codeine
In Canada:	
G	all salts and derivatives of the following: amphetamine, barbituric acid, benzphetamine, butorphanol, chlorphentermine, diethylpropion, methamphetamine, methaqualone, methylphenidate, pentazocine, phendimetrazine, phenmetrazine, and phentermine

LEGAL IMPLICATIONS OF I.V. THERAPY

The legal basis for nursing practice in I.V. therapy is determined by:
1. State nurse practice acts. Each state has a nurse practice act that defines which duties a nurse may or may not perform relative to I.V. therapy. These acts serve as guidelines for practice and place limits on practice.
2. Joint policy statements. These statements are position papers developed by the state nurses' association in collaboration with at least two other organizations, such as the state medical society and the state hospital association. Common to joint policy statements are the requirements that you will be held liable in relation to your knowledge, skill, and judgment, and that you may refuse to perform an I.V. therapy procedure if in your judgment you feel you are not qualified or competent. Joint policy statements also serve as guidelines for practice and place limits on practice.
3. Institutional policy. Every health care facility has developed I.V. therapy policies that determine which duties you may or may not perform in that work setting. These policies may *not* expand what the state nurse practice acts and joint policy statements permit, but they may further limit your duties. The policy of your facility is the final determinant of what you may or may not do.

The above statutes and policies provide legal protection as long as you act *correctly* and *within* the limitations they set up.

An incident report is useful only if it is filed promptly, thoroughly, and appropriately. Whether you are an RN, an LPN, or an LVN, and whether you are in a staff or management position, your legal duty is to report any incident of which you have firsthand knowledge. Failure to report an incident not only can lead to being fired, but also can expose you to personal liability for malpractice, especially if failing to report the incident causes injury to a patient.

Only a person with firsthand knowledge of an incident should report it, and only the person making the report should sign it. Each person with firsthand knowledge should fill out and sign a separate report. You should never sign a report describing circumstances or events that you have not witnessed personally.

Why you must report
If an incident results from an error you make, you have the duty to file an incident report immediately. Making a mistake is serious and may invite corrective action, but attempting to cover it up is worse—and so are the potential consequences. Most facilities will reprimand a nurse severely for not filing an incident report if irreversible injury is done to the patient.

The likelihood that an incident report will be used against a nurse is slight. A facility's administration wants nurses to report incidents and to keep proper records, but is usually aware that they may not do this consistently if they are always reprimanded even for small errors. However, if an incident results from a nurse's act of gross negligence or irresponsibility or is one of a series of incidents resulting from her actions, then the facility may take action against her. That possibility increases if the patient sustains irreversible injury.

If a fellow employee's error causes a reportable incident, your safest course is to report factually and objectively what you observed. The truth is not libel. By properly fulfilling your duty to the patient and the facility, you also minimize potential liability if the employee files a lawsuit against you. Most states have laws granting qualified privilege to those who have a duty to discuss or evaluate their co-workers, employees, or fellow citizens. That means that no liability for libel exists unless the person giving the information knows it is false or has acted with a reckless disregard for the truth.

What to include and omit
A patient-related incident report should include only the following:
- The identities of the patient and any witnesses

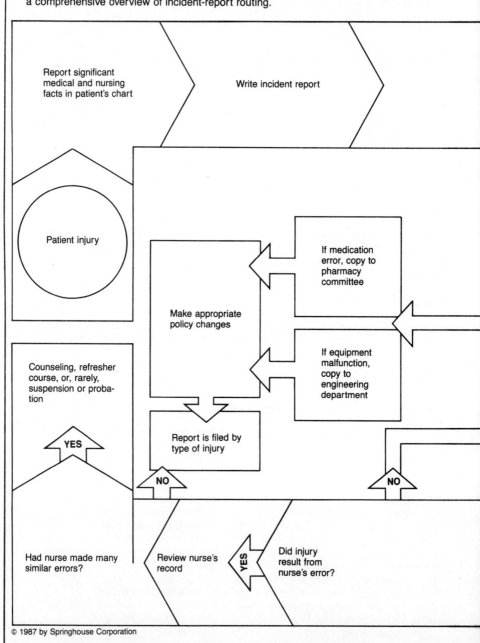

Legal Risks and Responsibilities 17

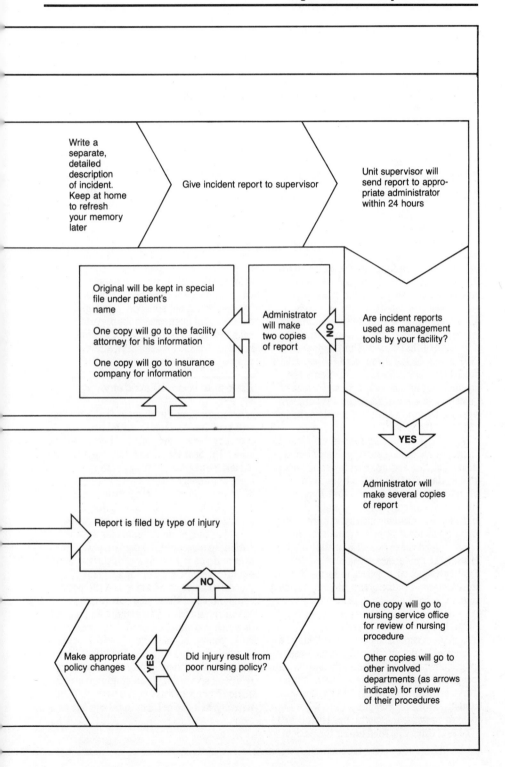

- Information about what happened and how it affected the patient (supply enough information so that administrators can decide if the matter needs further investigation)
- Any other relevant facts.

Information such as the following should never be included:
- Statements about events not seen by the reporter (such as something another employee said happened)
- Opinions (such as the reporter's opinion of the patient's prognosis)
- Conclusions or assumptions (such as what caused the incident)
- Suggestions of who caused the incident
- Suggestions to prevent such an incident from happening again.

Including such information in an incident report could seriously hinder the defense in any lawsuit arising from the incident.

The incident report serves only to notify the administration that an incident has occurred. In effect it says, "Administration: Please note that this incident happened, and please decide if you want to investigate it further." Such items as detailed statements from witnesses and descriptions of remedial action are normally part of an investigative follow-up and should not be included in the report.

A facility's reporting system may lead to improper incident reporting. For example, some facilities require nursing supervisors to correlate reports from witnesses and then to file a single report. And some incident report forms invite inappropriate conclusions and assumptions by asking, "How can this incident be prevented in the future?" Avoid these potential pitfalls by following the guidelines given above. If a facility's reporting system or forms contain such potential pitfalls, the administration should be notified about them.

What happens to the report

An incident report, once it is filed, may be reviewed by the nursing supervisor, the physician called to examine the patient, appropriate department heads and administrators, the health care facility's attorney, and its insurance company. (See *What Happens to an Incident Report?*, pp. 16 and 17.) The report may be filed under the patient's name or the type of injury, depending on the facility's policy and the insurance company's regulations. Reports are rarely placed in a reporting nurse's employment file.

A currently controversial issue is whether a patient's attorney may discover (request and receive a copy of) an incident report and introduce it as evidence in a malpractice lawsuit. The law on this issue varies from state to state. To avoid discovery, the health care facility may send copies of the incident report to its attorney, or its attorney may write a letter stating that the report is being made for his use and benefit only.

Concern about discovery should be minimal if an incident report contains only properly reportable material. The information reported is readily available to the patient's attorney through many other sources. Only when an incident report contains secondhand information, opinions, conclusions, accusations, or suggestions for preventing such incidents does discovery become an important issue for attorneys and the courts.

Risk-management strategy

What minimizes the chances that a patient will sue after an incident? And how can you protect yourself and your facility in case he does? The best way is to follow the three Rs of risk-management strategy: rapport, record, and report.

Maintain rapport with the patient. Answer questions honestly, but do not offer any explanation if you were not personally involved in the incident. Instead, refer the patient to someone who can supply answers. If you try to answer questions without direct knowledge of the incident, inconsistencies could arise and the patient could interpret these as a cover-up.

You should not try to explain an incident in which you were involved if doing so might make you visibly nervous. Continue to try to maintain rapport with the patient, but ask your supervisor, your facility's patient-relations specialist, or an administrator for advice on how to answer the patient. Alternatively, ask one of them to talk to the patient.

In talking with the patient, do not blame anyone for the incident if you feel someone else was at fault. Tell the charge nurse or supervisor, not the patient.

If an incident necessarily changes the way a patient is cared for, tell the patient about it, and clearly explain the reasons for the change.

Record the incident in the medical records. Truthfulness is the best protection against lawsuits. If you try to cover up or play down an incident, you could end up in far more serious trouble than if you had reported it objectively. Never write in the medical record that an incident report has been completed. An incident report is not clinical information, but an administrative tool.

Report every incident. Some nurses think incident reports are more trouble than they are worth and, furthermore, that they are a dangerous admission of guilt. That is false.

Incident reports are important for the following reasons:
- They jog our memories. Much time may pass between the dates of an incident and any legal actions arising from it. Memories cannot be trusted, but incident reports can be.
- They help administrators act quickly. A policy or procedure that contributed to or caused an incident can be changed. An administrator can also talk with families and offer assistance, explanation, or other appropriate support. Sometimes, helpful communication with an injured patient and his family can be the balm that soothes their anger and prevents a lawsuit.
- They provide the information needed to decide if restitution should be made. When a patient is harmed instead of helped, administrators sometimes decide the facility has a moral obligation to compensate the patient.

N.I.T.A. STANDARDS FOR I.V. NURSING CARE

The National Intravenous Therapy Association (NITA) has developed the following standards for practice in I.V. therapy, which are used as models in policy development.

Description of practice
The registered professional I.V. nurse utilizes the nursing process (assessment, care planning, implementation and evaluation) as the framework for providing I.V. nursing care. The nursing process begins with assessment by collection of subjective and objective data to arrive at an I.V. nursing diagnosis. The second step in the nursing process is to formulate a plan of nursing care. Implementation of the plan is the nursing management of the patient's needs and problems. The evaluation of the process and outcome of the nursing care plan is used to adjust or change nursing care as required by the patient's condition. The registered professional I.V. nurse shall coordinate the delivery and monitor, with an established quality control program, all aspects of I.V. therapy. I.V. nursing practice requires integration of basic nursing knowledge and skills with advanced knowledge of psycho-social, physiological and therapeutic components specific to I.V. care.

The I.V. nurse shall establish I.V. policies and procedures and evaluate I.V. equipment for utilization which best serves the needs of the patient and health care facility. Participation on hospital committees relating to I.V. therapy, establishment of I.V. orientation and educational curriculums, continuing education, I.V. nursing responsibilities and performance evaluations shall encompass the registered professional I.V. nurse's practice. Collaboration with other health care professionals provides a comprehensive approach to the intravenous nursing management of the patient. The registered professional I.V. nurse shall use a holistic approach to the patient, insure safe I.V. practice and clinical competency and shall be professionally accountable for I.V. care.

A. Management
The registered professional I.V. nurse is the specialist in the management of I.V. nursing. The registered professional I.V.

(continued)

N.I.T.A STANDARDS FOR I.V. NURSING CARE *(continued)*

nurse shall establish parameters of I.V. care and services and be accountable for I.V. nursing management decisions. Other management decisions that establish criteria for care and services delivered to patients receiving I.V. therapy need I.V. nursing input to achieve optimal outcome.

B. Supervision
The registered professional I.V. nurse shall be aware of basic management skills, be capable of supervising others and be held accountable for all work performed under his/her supervision.

C. Consultation
The registered professional I.V. nurse is an essential consultant to the health care profession, the family, the community and related industry. The consultant and dominant themes of this consultation are patient advocacy and delivery of optimal I.V. nursing care.

D. Technology
Sophisticated technology related to I.V. nursing is continually advancing. The registered professional I.V. nurse shall continuously evaluate and control regimes and products for clinical application used in this nursing specialty.

E. Research
Research is an inherent component of I.V. nursing to continually investigate, validate and develop this nursing practice. Through research and its dissemination, the art and science of the I.V. nursing specialty will be advanced.

F. Quality assurance
All registered professional I.V. nurses are responsible for quality assurance as it relates to this specialty. This is achieved by identifying the structures associated with quality, utilizing the I.V. therapy nursing process of assessment, planning, implementation, evaluation and monitoring the desired outcome. Deviation from optimal care in I.V. nursing practice requires corrective action. Observation of patient's condition and reevaluation of the nursing care plan shall be done on a continual basis. The patient receiving I.V. nursing shall be guaranteed the highest level of care.

G. Legal
Development of national standards for the specialty of I.V. therapy will:
1. Protect the patient from unnecessary trauma by receiving specialty I.V. care.
2. Assist the medical profession by reducing risk of malpractice claims against the doctor, nurse or hospital.
3. Assist the manufacturers by reducing the risk of product liability claims against their companies.
4. Establish a framework for monitoring of acceptable standards for care and products used in I.V. therapy by federal and state agencies.

The registered professional I.V. nurse and the health care facility shall be responsible for I.V. care rendered by licensed personnel, i.e. LPN/LVN involved in this specialty.

The registered professional I.V. nurse and the health care facility shall be responsible for I.V. care rendered by unlicensed personnel in this specialty.

With the establishment of standards, the patient will have a frame of reference so as to be able to distinguish between malpractice or product failure and a poor medical result.

The development of standards may help to resolve ethical conflict between the I.V. nurse's duty to the patient and the nurse's position as an employee in the hospital.

H. Communication
The registered professional I.V. nurse shall have verbal and written communication skills in translating ideas and facts to a variety of persons within and beyond the limits of the specialty.

I. Continuing education
Continuing education and staff development is essential to sustain and advance I.V. nursing. Active participation in continuing education is vital for the continual growth of this specialty and the profes-

(continued)

N.I.T.A STANDARDS FOR I.V. NURSING CARE (continued)

sion. Sharing this knowledge with other collaborative disciplines improves care. Continuing education in this specialty is the responsibility of all registered professional I.V. nurses.

J. Patient education
In keeping with the holistic approach to patient care, it is the registered professional I.V. nurse's responsibility to educate the patients and significant others who are involved in delivery of this therapy on the aspects of I.V. therapy. Education and the patient's comprehension is documented, communicated to the appropriate person(s) and stored in a retrievable and accessible system.

Education and teaching of I.V. therapy encompasses the health care facility and the community.

Effectiveness of teaching methods will be periodically evaluated and continually assessed by the registered professional I.V. nurse.

K. Clinical
The registered professional I.V. nurse shall be proficient in all clinical aspects of I.V. therapy with validated competency in clinical judgement and practice.

L. Procedures
Performing procedures include, but are not limited to, the following:
1. Interpreting the physician's order for I.V. therapy.
2. Performing venipuncture and arterial puncture and insertion of *all* types of needles and catheters commercially available but excluding the insertion of subclavian and cut-down catheters, in accordance with established hospital policy.
3. Initiation, monitoring and termination of all I.V. solutions and subsequent additives.
4. Preparing I.V. solutions with the addition of medications in the absence of an admixture service.
5. The administration of I.V. medications as ordered by the physician and in accordance with established hospital policy.
6. Administration of medications via A-V shunts and arterial lines as ordered by the physician and in accordance with established hospital policy.
7. Initiation and monitoring of investigational drugs in accordance with established hospital policy.
8. Administration of I.V. push medications in accordance with established hospital policy.
9. The recognition of medication and solution incompatibilities.
10. Maintenance and replacement of sites, tubing and dressing changes in accordance with established hospital policy.
11. To establish flow rates for all I.V. solutions, medications, blood and blood components as ordered by the physician and in accordance with established hospital policy.
12. The administration of all blood and blood components as ordered by the physician and in accordance with established hospital policy.
13. Performing phlebotomies.
14. Evaluation of I.V. equipment.
15. Thorough knowledge and proficient technical ability in the use of I.V. equipment.
16. Care and maintenance of I.V. equipment.
17. Observation of equipment prior to use.
18. Nursing management of total parenteral nutrition.
19. Nursing management of out-patient and home I.V. care.
20. Maintenance of established infection control and aseptic practices.
21. Assist in cardiac arrests in accordance with established hospital policy.
22. Observation and assessment of all adverse reactions related to I.V. therapy and initiation of appropriate nursing intervention.
23. To maintain documentation associated with the preparation, administration and termination of all forms of I.V. therapy.

Reprinted with permission from *NITA Standards of Practice*, Cambridge, Mass.: National Intravenous Therapy Association, March 1981.

N.I.T.A. STANDARDS FOR HOME I.V. THERAPY

Home I.V. therapy standards are written for nurses delivering intravenous care outside of the hospital. The nurse's practice shall comply with state laws and all standards set forth by NITA which are applicable to the delivery of home I.V. therapy. The primary goals of home I.V. therapy are to achieve the highest level of self care and quality of life for the patient by providing patient teaching and follow-up nursing care.

1. A physician's order shall be written regarding patient referral(s) for home I.V. therapy.
2. A medical order shall be written and signed by a physician to initiate and direct home I.V. therapy.
3. The written medical order(s) shall be reviewed and updated by the physician routinely.
4. Only physicians shall initiate a verbal medical order(s). Verbal medical order(s) shall be documented immediately by the registered nurse and brought to the physician's attention to be countersigned by the physician as soon as possible.
5. To insure that prescribed care is administered safely, the registered nurse shall have the knowledge and skills to interpret and implement the written medical order.
6. A consent form should be established and signed by the patient and/or legal guardian.
7. The patient shall be assessed for his/her ability to safely administer the prescribed home I.V. therapy.
8. If after the nursing assessment the patient is unable to achieve a determined level of self care, a significant other(s) shall be incorporated into the home I.V. therapy care plan and the physician shall be notified.
9. The significant other(s) shall be assessed for his/her ability to safely administer the prescribed home therapy treatment(s).
10. As the primary educator, the registered nurse shall address indication(s), benefits, methods and risks of therapy.
11. The teaching process for the patient and/or significant other(s) shall include written instructions, verbal explanations, demonstrations, evaluation and documentation of competency, proficiency in performing therapy-related procedures, self-monitoring, scope of physical activities, necessary intervention(s), safe discard of disposable equipment and specific actions to be taken in a possible emergency situation.
12. Therapy-specific teaching instructions will be utilized during the educational process and shall be given to and remain with the patient and/or significant other(s).
13. All supplies and equipment necessary for therapy shall be available in the home before therapy is initiated.
14. Supply and equipment needs shall be continuously evaluated and met.
15. By the date of discharge, a registered nurse shall perform a home assessment and assist the patient and/or significant other(s) to determine an appropriate area for clean, safe storage of supplies/equipment, select a suitable area for procedures to be performed, and determine a safe discard of disposable equipment.
16. An ongoing assessment of patient and/or significant other(s) compliance in performing therapy-related procedures shall be done at periodic intervals depending on patient condition and therapy.
17. All communication(s) with and/or site visit(s) to the patient shall be documented.
18. A summary of patient care shall be communicated to the physician at regular intervals.
19. Any pertinent observation that requires medical intervention shall be reported to the physician immediately.
20. The patient and/or significant other(s) shall be provided 24-hour access to appropriate health care professional(s).
21. It is recommended that the patient carry and/or wear appropriate identification indicative of therapy.
22. Psycho-social concerns of home I.V. therapy should be evaluated.

Reprinted with permission from *Home I.V. Therapy Nursing Standards of Practice*, Cambridge, Mass.: National Intravenous Therapy Association, March/April 1984.

N.I.T.A. STANDARDS FOR HYPERALIMENTATION THERAPY

NITA has established the following nursing standards of practice as a model for those practicing PNIV (parenteral nutrition intravascular) nursing.

I. Education
A. For NITA recognition to practice PNIV nursing, the registered professional nurse must complete the educational requirements as set forth by the Association. Education is fundamental to preparation for nursing practice in the art and science of parenteral nutrition.

Continuing education and staff development is essential to sustain and advance PNIV nursing. Sharing this knowledge with other collaborative disciplines improves care.

B. In keeping with the holistic approach to patient care, it is the registered professional nurse's responsibility to educate the patient and significant others who are involved in delivery of this PNIV specialty. Education and the patient's comprehension is documented, communicated to the appropriate person(s), and stored in a retrievable and accessible system.

C. Effectiveness of teaching methods will be continually assessed and periodically evaluated by the registered professional PNIV nurse.

II. Practice
Collaboration with other health care professionals provides a comprehensive approach to the PNIV nursing management of the patient. The registered professional nurse uses a holistic approach to the patient. The nursing process is the primary tool for delivery of PNIV nursing.

III. Management
The PNIV nurse is the specialist in the management of PNIV nursing. Other management decisions that establish criteria for care and services delivered to patients receiving parenteral nutrition need PNIV nursing input to achieve optimal outcome.

IV. Consultation
The PNIV nurse is an essential consultant to the health care profession, the community, and related industry. The constant and dominant themes of this consultation are patient advocacy and delivery of optimal PNIV care.

V. Technology
Sophisticated technology related to PNIV nursing is continually advancing. The PNIV nurse should continuously evaluate regimens and products used in this nursing specialty.

VI. Research
Research is an inherent component of PNIV nursing. Through research and its dissemination, the art and science of this nursing specialty will be advanced.

VII. Quality Assurance
All PNIV nurses are responsible for quality assurance as it relates to this specialty. The components of PNIV nursing associated with quality assurance and with monitoring the desired outcome must be identified. The patient receiving PNIV nursing must be guaranteed the highest level of care.

Reprinted with permission from *NITA Standards of Practice*, Cambridge, Mass.: National Intravenous Therapy Association, March 1981.

Review Questions

1. What are the five rights of medication administration?

2. What are the two rights of medication administration that should be added?

3. Define prescription drug.

4. What are the two federal laws that govern the use of drugs in the United States?

5. Explain the difference between dispensing and administering a drug.

6. What four steps should be followed when taking an oral drug order from a physician?

7. What are the three Rs of risk management?

8. What source should be checked for information on an experimental drug you are administering?

9. List the five resources to use when questioning a drug order.

10. What determines the legal basis for nursing practice in I.V. therapy?

Selected References

Fink, J.L. "Preventing Lawsuits: Medication Errors to Avoid," *NursingLife* 3(2):26-29, March/April 1983.

"Home Intravenous Care," *National Intravenous Therapy Association* 7(1):10-11, January/February 1984.

National Intravenous Therapy Association, Inc. "NITA's I.V. Standards/CDC's I.V. Guidelines,"*National Intravenous Therapy Association* 5:8-11, January/February 1982.

Nurse's Legal Handbook. Springhouse, Pa.: Springhouse Corp., 1985.

Plumer, A. *Principles and Practices of Intravenous Therapy,* 3rd ed. Boston: Little, Brown & Co., 1982.

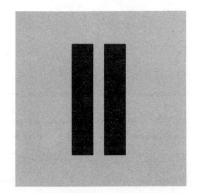

Basics of Drug Administration

3 Principles of Pharmacology 26

4 Medication Orders and Distribution Systems 47

5 Calculations and Measurements 52

6 Preparation and Administration Guidelines 60

Principles of Pharmacology

A basic understanding of pharmacology is required of all nurses, since medication administration is a nursing responsibility in almost all health care settings. This chapter discusses drug nomenclature, principles of drug action, factors that affect drug action, and adverse reactions to drug therapy. This information is the foundation for safe medication administration and for education of patients about their medications.

Drug names

Generally, drugs are identified by their generic or trade names. A *generic name* is the original name given to a drug by the company that developed it. A *trade name* or brand name is the name under which the company markets the drug.

Different drug companies have different trade names for the same generic drug. The generic name begins with a lower-case letter; the trade name begins with a capital letter. Sometimes generic drugs may be substituted for more expensive trade-name counterparts. (See *Generic Drugs: A Safe Substitute?*)

A drug also has a *chemical name,* which is the chemical description of its ingredients. This is not used clinically. (See *Examples of Drug Names,* p. 28.)

Drug classifications

Drugs are classified according to their therapeutic action (for example, antihypertensive) or the body system on which they act (for example, cardiovascular). The drugs in each class are prescribed for similar health problems, but a drug may belong to one or more classes. For instance, propranolol can be classified as an antiarrhythmic, an antianginal, an antihypertensive, or a beta-adrenergic blocking drug.

Drug forms and routes of administration

Drugs are prepared in a variety of forms, and the form determines the route of administration. Many drugs are available in more than one form. For example, many antibiotics are available in tablet, capsule, suspension, or solution. (See *Major Drug Forms and Routes of Administration,* p. 29, and *Comparing Drug Routes,* pp. 30 to 32.)

Pharmacokinetics

Understanding the principles of pharmacokinetics (the characteristic actions and movement of drugs in the body during absorption, distribution, metabolism, and excretion) helps you know the proper drug and dosage form required to produce a desired drug effect. The following summaries explain these pharmacokinetic processes.

Absorption
Since absorption may take place over several hours, the processes of absorption, distribution, metabolism, and excretion can occur simultaneously. A drug that is absorbed and circulating in the bloodstream is *bioavailable,* or ready to produce its effect. Several factors determine the rate and degree of absorption: various patient characteristics and the drug's physiochemical effects, dosage form, route of administra-

GENERIC DRUGS: A SAFE SUBSTITUTE?

Generic versus trade names. A generic drug name is the chemical description of the drug; a trade name (or brand name) is the name chosen by a drug company for marketing purposes. For example, *phenytoin sodium* is a generic name; *Dilantin* is a trade name.

Although generic drugs are usually less expensive than their trade-name counterparts, using them can cause problems—especially if they are used interchangeably with a trade-name counterpart during a course of therapy. Why? Surprisingly, generic and trade-name drugs are *not* always bioequivalent, even though they contain the same amount of the same drug. The reason could be differences in nondrug ingredients, such as diluents or disintegrants. Or the drugs may be subject to different manufacturing processes. These and other factors can cause drugs to become bioavailable at different rates.

Although some experts disagree, most generic drugs are roughly bioequivalent with their trade-name counterparts, and substitutions can be made safely. But some drugs should not be substituted after a course of therapy begins. This is especially important for drugs with a narrow therapeutic range, such as digoxin and levothyroxine.

Your role. By all means, encourage the patient to ask his physician or pharmacist about generic drug use, especially for long-term therapy. And, if possible, suggest to the physician that he *begin* therapy by ordering a generic drug, to avoid the problems that a later substitution may cause. By prescribing a generic drug, the physician may save the patient a substantial amount of money.

If the physician prescribes a generic drug, give the patient this advice:
• Instruct him to check with the pharmacist (or physician) if the pharmacist refills the prescription with a drug that is a different color than the one your patient is accustomed to. The pharmacist may have substituted one formulation of the generic drug for another. If so, he and the physician must make sure that the new generic drug will affect the patient in the same way as the one he took previously.
• Tell him to inform the physician if the generic drug does not seem to be as effective as the trade-name drug—or if he notices any effects that the previous drug did not cause.

---

tion, and interactions with other substances in the gastrointestinal (GI) tract.

Drugs in solution, such as syrups, elixirs, and injectables, are usually absorbed more rapidly than other dosage forms. That explains why some drugs, such as digoxin, reach higher blood levels when administered as solutions than they do as tablets.

A drug in tablet or capsule form must first disintegrate. Small particles of the disintegrated drug can then dissolve in gastric juices and be absorbed into the bloodstream.

Drugs administered intramuscularly are absorbed through the muscle before entering the bloodstream. This relatively fast process can be prolonged by administering a drug in an oil solution or as a suspension—forms that decrease its solubility. For example, after intramuscular (I.M.) injection, penicillin G potassium is absorbed almost immediately, but penicillin G procaine takes several hours to be absorbed because its oily base makes it relatively lipid-insoluble.

Drugs administered intravenously enter the circulation directly and are immediately bioavailable. Drugs administered by any other route must first pass through membranes by such methods as active (carrier) transport and passive diffusion before they can enter the bloodstream.

Active transport plays a minor role in drug absorption. The drug combines with a "carrier" on one side of the membrane and is taken through to the other side, where it dissociates from the carrier and is deposited in the bloodstream.

Passive diffusion is the more common method of drug absorption. The rate of

EXAMPLES OF DRUG NAMES

Generic	Trade	Chemical
aspirin	Bufferin, Ecotrin, St. Joseph Aspirin for Children	acetylsalicylic acid
furosemide	Lasix, Uritol, Novosemide	4-chloro-N-furfuryl-5-sulfamoylanthranilic acid
digoxin	Lanoxin, Lanoxicaps	$C_{41}H_{64}O_{14}$

transfer during passive diffusion depends on the *concentration gradient* and the *lipid solubility* of the drug.

The concentration gradient necessary for passive diffusion is set up when a drug's concentration—for instance, in the GI tract—is greater than its concentration in the bloodstream. The drug will continue to pass through the GI membrane into the bloodstream until the concentrations are equal. The higher concentration of drug in the GI tract maintains the concentration gradient until the drug is completely absorbed.

A drug's lipid solubility has an important effect on passive diffusion and absorption: the higher the solubility, the more rapid the rate of diffusion and the greater the absorption. Lipid solubility depends on several factors, including the degree of ionization of the drug in solution. Nonionized (uncharged) drugs are more lipid-soluble and are therefore more readily absorbed than ionized (charged) drugs, which are lipid-insoluble.

Since most drugs are either weak acids or weak bases, their degree of ionization depends on their location in the GI tract. Weak acids such as aspirin have a higher ratio of nonionized to ionized molecules in the acidic environment of the stomach, and thus are more readily absorbed from this area. Weak bases such as quinidine, however, have a higher proportion of nonionized molecules in the more alkaline medium of the small intestine. Because of this, such drugs are more readily absorbed there than in the stomach. Absorption of acids and bases occurs in both locations, however, since some nonionized molecules are present in both the stomach and the intestine. Also, since the small intestine has a larger surface area than the stomach, a good blood supply, and a pH of 6.0 to 8.0, more absorption occurs there.

Gastric emptying time also affects absorption of medications from the GI tract. For instance, food or antacids in the stomach may prolong gastric emptying time and delay a drug's movement to the small intestine. However, if GI motility is increased, as in diarrhea, a drug may travel through the GI tract so rapidly that it is not completely absorbed. This condition would particularly undermine absorption of sustained-release preparations that are intended to be absorbed over 8 to 12 hours. (See *Factors Affecting Oral Drug Absorption*, p. 33, for a summary of patient condition and drug composition factors that influence the way an oral drug is absorbed.)

Distribution

Once absorption starts, a drug moves from the bloodstream into other body fluids and tissues; this is distribution. Initially, the drug reaches tissues in highly vascularized organs, such as the heart, liver, kidneys, and brain. It takes longer to reach less vascularized areas, such as muscle, fat, and skin.

A drug's ability to cross the lipid layer of cell membranes influences distribution to various sites in the body. Since some drugs cannot cross it, their distribution is limited.

Other drugs, such as ethyl alcohol, can pass through virtually all cell membranes.

Plasma protein binding

Plasma protein binding can greatly influence distribution and therefore the effectiveness and duration of drug action. Many drugs are insoluble in plasma and are bound as weak complexes to plasma proteins, especially albumin. Binding can occur at sites of absorption, at extravascular sites, or, most commonly, in the blood. Some drugs are highly bound to plasma protein, many are moderately bound, and others may not be bound at all.

All drugs bound to plasma proteins have a ratio of free, or unbound, drug to bound drug. For example, warfarin is 97% bound to plasma proteins. Only free drug is pharmacologically active, or able to produce an effect at the drug receptor site; only free drug can be metabolized or excreted. Bound drug acts as a reservoir; it is released as free drug is eliminated. The binding process regulates the amount of free drug in circulation and prevents a drug from reaching its site of action fully concentrated.

Volume of distribution

The volume of distribution—the total area to which a drug is distributed—depends on characteristics of the patient and the drug. For example, in an edematous patient, a given dose must be distributed to a larger volume than in a nonedematous patient; therefore, the dose may have to be increased. Conversely, in an extremely dehydrated patient, the drug is distributed to a much smaller volume, and the dose must be decreased.

Obese patients may present another problem. Some drugs, such as digoxin, gentamicin, and tobramycin, are not well distributed to fatty tissue; therefore, dosage based on actual body weight may lead to overdose and serious toxicity. In some cases, dosage must be based on lean body weight, which may be estimated from actuarial tables that give average weight ranges for body height.

Metabolism

Most drugs are metabolized (biotransformed) by the liver before they are excreted by the kidneys. Hepatic metabolism usually

MAJOR DRUG FORMS AND ROUTES OF ADMINISTRATION

Route	Form
Oral (solid)	Tablet Capsule Powder
(liquid)	Suspension Emulsion Syrup Elixir Solution
Parenteral	Solution
Rectal	Suppository Solution
Vaginal	Suppository Solution Tablet Foam Gel
Topical (skin)	Cream Ointment Lotion Liniment Paste Powder Aerosol

produces a metabolite of the drug that is less lipid-soluble and more water-soluble and thus can be readily excreted by the kidneys. A metabolite may be pharmacologically active or inactive. An active metabolite may produce effects similar to those of the drug itself or other, possibly toxic, effects.

Some drugs are pharmacologically inactive and must be metabolized to be effective. Examples are cyclophosphamide, a cytotoxic drug, and chloral hydrate, a hypnotic. These inactive drugs must undergo a second biotransformation before they can be excreted.

The liver is the main site of drug metabolism, but other tissues, such as the lungs, kidneys, blood, and intestines, may also metabolize drugs. Orally administered drugs traverse the liver before reaching the

COMPARING DRUG ROUTES

A drug's administration route influences absorption and distribution, which, in turn, affect drug action and patient response. Consider the following points.

Topical
Advantages
- Drugs are easily administered.
- They provide fast relief for itching and topical pain.
- They are not likely to cause severe allergic reactions, as in systemic administration.
- They cause fewer adverse reactions than drugs administered by systemic routes.
- Some drugs (for example, nitroglycerin and scopolamine) may be applied topically (in a form called transdermal skin patches) for prolonged systemic effects.

Disadvantages
- Dosage accuracy may be difficult to achieve.
- Drugs may stain clothing or bedding.
- Drugs applied for systemic effect may cause unexpected adverse reactions if administered carelessly. For example, scopolamine applied as an antiemetic may cause more pupil dilation than usual if the drug is accidentally transferred to the eyes from the fingertips.
- Drugs applied for topical effect may be absorbed systemically, causing problems.

Oral
Advantages
- Self-medication is easy.
- Drug retrieval or dilution is possible by lavage or vomiting in cases of overdose.

Disadvantages
- Drugs cannot be given in most emergencies because of relatively slow absorption.
- They may be metabolized during first pass through the liver.
- They may irritate the GI tract, discolor the teeth, or taste unpleasant.
- They may be accidentally aspirated if patient has difficulty swallowing or is combative.
- Unpredictable absorption may limit drug reliability.
- Self-medication is impossible if patient cannot manage his own therapy.

Sublingual or Buccal
Advantages
- Drugs take effect quickly, since they are absorbed directly into the bloodstream.
- They can be taken if patient cannot swallow, if he is intubated, or if he cannot take anything by mouth for any other reason.
- There is no first-pass effect in the liver.
- There is no GI tract irritation.

Disadvantages
- Only drugs that are highly lipid-soluble may be given.
- Drugs with unpleasant taste are not suitable.
- Oral mucosa may be irritated.

Rectal
Advantages
- Administration is safe if patient is vomiting, unconscious, or unable to swallow for any other reason.
- It is an effective route to treat vomiting.
- Drugs do not irritate the patient's upper GI tract, as some oral medications do.
- They are not destroyed by digestive enzymes in the stomach and small intestine.

Disadvantages
- Administration may be uncomfortable and embarrassing for the patient.
- It is usually contraindicated when the patient has a disorder affecting the lower GI tract; for example, rectal bleeding or diarrhea.
- Drug absorption may be irregular or incomplete, depending on patient's ability to retain medication and presence of feces in his rectum.
- Because absorption may be incomplete, rectal doses of some medications may be larger than oral doses.
- Drugs cannot be given in most emergencies because absorption is unreliable.
- Rectal mucosa may be irritated.
- Patient's vagus nerve may be stimulated by stretching of anal sphincters. This may be dangerous for cardiac patients.

Respiratory
Advantages
- Drugs are absorbed and distributed

(continued)

COMPARING DRUG ROUTES (continued)

rapidly because of the lungs' large surface area and rich capillary network.
• Smaller doses of potent drugs can be given to minimize their adverse reactions.
• The route is easily accessible, providing a convenient alternative when other routes are unavailable. In emergencies, some injectable drugs (such as epinephrine) can be given directly into the lungs.
• Drugs that are both lipid-soluble and available as gases can be administered.

Disadvantages
• Dosage accuracy may be difficult to achieve.
• Some drugs may cause nausea and vomiting.
• Tracheal or bronchial mucosa may be irritated, resulting in coughing or bronchospasm.
• Hand-held nebulizer dependency may result (for example, in an asthmatic patient).
• Full drug dose may be difficult to administer by hand-held nebulizer; for example, if patient is an uncooperative child.
• Hand-held nebulizers are a potential infection source.
• Relatively few drugs can be given by this route.

PARENTERAL
All parenteral routes are potentially useful for treating a patient who cannot receive medication orally, for example, because he is unconscious. And all of them avoid the risk of decreased drug absorption from vomiting or gastric activity. Listed here are some specific advantages and disadvantages for each parenteral route.

Intravenous
Advantages
• Bioavailability is immediate, making this route the first choice for emergency drug administration and for immediate or long-term pain relief.
• Absorption into the bloodstream is complete and reliable.
• Some medications, such as dopamine (Intropin), cannot be given by any other route.
• Large drug doses can be delivered at a continuous rate.

• Muscle tissue damage from potentially irritating drugs can be avoided.
• There is no first-pass effect in the liver.

Disadvantages
• Life-threatening adverse reactions may result if drugs are administered too rapidly, if I.V. flow rate is not carefully monitored, or if incompatible drugs are mixed. (Mixing incompatible drugs may also cause precipitation, lessening the drug's effectiveness.)
• There is increased risk of complications, such as extravasation, vein irritation, systemic infection, or air embolism.

Intramuscular
Advantages
• Aqueous suspensions, solutions in oil, or medications that are not available in oral form can be administered.
• I.M. medication administration ensures long-term absorption of suspensions or solutions in oil.
• Parenteral medications can be administered in relatively large doses (up to 5 ml).
• Need for an I.V. site is eliminated.
• Drug effect is relatively rapid.

Disadvantages
• Medication may precipitate in the muscle, reducing absorption.
• Medication may not be properly absorbed if the patient is hypotensive or has poor blood supply to the muscle for any other reason.
• It may be accidentally injected into the bloodstream, possibly causing overdose or an adverse reaction.
• Injection may damage blood vessels, causing bleeding.
• It may damage nerves, causing unnecessary pain or paralysis.
• It may damage bone.
• It may cause pain and local tissue irritation.
• By damaging muscle tissue, it may interfere with cardiac isoenzyme reading ordered to help diagnose myocardial infarction.

Subcutaneous
Advantages
• Self-administration of insulin is easy for diabetic patients.

(continued)

COMPARING DRUG ROUTES *(continued)*

- A drug such as insulin can be absorbed slowly, prolonging the effects.
- Drug is absorbed rapidly without the need for an I.V. site.

Disadvantages
- Injection may damage skin tissue.
- It may not be used when patient has occlusive vascular disease with poor perfusion, since decreased peripheral circulation delays absorption.
- It may not be used when patient's skin tissue is grossly adipose, edematous, burned, hardened, swollen at all the common injection sites, damaged by previous injections, or diseased.

---

systemic circulation. If they are significantly metabolized in this process, only a fractional amount of unmetabolized drug ever reaches the circulation. This first-pass effect explains why oral doses of many drugs are much higher than parenteral doses. Oral doses of propranolol, for example, range from 10 to 80 mg; I.V. doses range from 1 to 3 mg.

The rate at which a drug is metabolized varies with the patient. In some patients, the rate is so rapid that blood and tissue levels prove therapeutically inadequate. In others, metabolism is so slow that ordinary doses can produce toxic results.

Some drugs alter the metabolism of other drugs. For example, a drug such as phenobarbital can stimulate hepatic enzymes that speed the metabolism of other drugs, thereby changing their effects.

Hepatic diseases may affect liver function, resulting in increased, decreased, or unchanged drug metabolism. Patients with hepatic diseases, therefore, must be closely monitored for drug effect and toxicity.

Excretion

Slight elimination of drugs takes place in perspiration, saliva, tears, feces, and breast milk. Certain volatile anesthetics, such as halothane, are eliminated primarily by exhalation. But most drugs are excreted by the kidneys, usually as metabolites.

Some drugs (digoxin, gentamicin) are largely unmetabolized before they are excreted by the kidneys. For safe use, renal function must be adequate or these drugs will accumulate and produce toxic effects.

Renal excretion of drugs follows the usual pattern of excretion: passive glomerular filtration, active tubular secretion, and tubular reabsorption. In a patient with renal impairment, the route of drug excretion should be reviewed and dosage modifications made as necessary. Also, if a patient's renal function changes, all current medications in his regimen must be reevaluated.

Some drugs can alter the effect and excretion of other drugs. For example, probenecid can block renal excretion of penicillin, causing it to accumulate and enhancing its effects. Antacids speed excretion of salicylates (aspirin) and thus diminish their effects.

A drug's excretion is also affected by its blood concentration, half-life, and accumulation in the body.

Blood concentration

The ongoing processes of absorption, distribution, metabolism, and excretion continuously affect blood concentration of a drug. Absorption of an oral drug is greater than excretion until its peak blood level is reached. After this, more drug is excreted than is absorbed, and the blood concentration of the drug falls. A drug administered by I.V. push is immediately bioavailable at peak level; it is rapidly distributed and excreted.

Half-life

Half-life is the time required for the blood concentration of a drug to decrease by 50%. For every half-life, the concentration of a drug is halved. After five half-lives a drug is 95% eliminated. (See *The Importance of Half-Life,* p. 34.)

Half-life is used to establish optimal dosage regimens, such as loading dose, mainte-

FACTORS AFFECTING ORAL DRUG ABSORPTION

FACTOR	EFFECT
Patient Conditions	
Rate of gastric emptying	Increased gastric emptying speeds the absorption rate of all but poorly or erratically absorbed drugs.
GI motility	In most cases, increased motility speeds the drug absorption rate. However, with very rapid motility, the total amount of drug absorbed may decrease.
pH of GI tract	A changing pH has variable effects, depending on the drug. Certain drugs require a specific pH for optimal absorption.
Presence of food in GI tract	Food slows absorption rate and may prevent drug absorption in some cases.
Presence of antacids in GI tract	Antacids alter absorption by changing pH. They decrease absorption of most acidic drugs and increase absorption of basic drugs. They also react with some drugs, forming complexes that are not well absorbed.
Fluid intake	Fluid intake with medication prevents drugs from lodging in the esophagus, promotes dissolution, and enhances drug passage to the small intestine. As a result, absorption increases.
Blood flow	Decreased blood flow to the GI tract decreases absorption.
Drug Composition	
Drug form	Liquid forms are absorbed more quickly than solid forms, because drug dissolution has already occurred.
Amount and type of inert ingredients	Disintegrants speed absorption; buffers may slow absorption.
Enteric coating	A coating prevents drug dissolution in the stomach and delays absorption.

nance dose, and interval between doses. A drug with a short half-life, such as penicillin G, must be given several times daily to maintain its therapeutic effect. A drug such as digoxin, which has a long half-life, can be given once daily.

Accumulation
Many drugs reach a therapeutic blood level after the same dose is repeated several times. When an immediate response is required, a large loading dose is given, followed by smaller maintenance doses. The

THE IMPORTANCE OF HALF-LIFE

What it is
Half-life is the time required for the blood level of a drug to fall to half its peak amount. This diagram shows the time required (2½ hours) for the blood level of gentamicin to fall to 3 mcg/ml, one-half its peak level of 6 mcg/ml. Intravenous injections, of course, produce peak blood levels immediately.

How it is determined
Blood samples are taken from the patient at specific time intervals to determine the amount of drug in the blood. Standard data on drug half-life have helped establish the drug dosages required to achieve and maintain desired blood levels.

Thus, standard dosage intervals, such as every 4 hours, every 6 hours, and so on, give an indication of half-life. For some drugs, it is 30 minutes or less; for others, 8 hours or more.

What to watch for
Watch for body changes that may increase standard half-life, such as decreased ability to metabolize or excrete drugs. Patients with hepatic or renal disease, for example, may retain the drug in the blood or tissues for a longer time than normal. The half-life of the drug is extended in these cases; the dosage or frequency can be adjusted to prevent accumulation and toxicity.

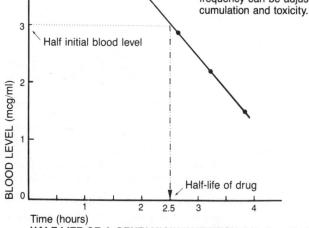

HALF-LIFE OF A GENTAMICIN INJECTION (I.V., 1 mg/kg)

drug will accumulate if each successive dose is given before the previous dose has been completely excreted.

Accumulation continues until the dose given is equal to the amount being excreted. At that time a steady state exists; the blood level will remain in this range as long as consecutive doses are given and no physiologic or pharmacokinetic processes change. (See *Achieving Steady-State Blood Concentrations.*)

The process of accumulation explains why the full effects of a drug may not be demonstrated for a few days to several weeks after therapy has started. It also explains how toxicity occurs. When a drug is excreted more slowly than it is absorbed, its level in blood and organs increases. Unless the dosage is adjusted, cumulative toxicity results.

Pharmacodynamics

Certain drugs have an affinity for certain cells; their biologic effect is produced selectively and specifically. When a drug combines with a receptor at a specific site, a series of biochemical and physiologic changes begins. Pharmacodynamics is the process by which a drug combines with cell receptors and exerts its effect.

Most receptors are proteins, including the receptors for regulatory chemicals, such as hormones and neurotransmitters; the enzymes of metabolic or regulatory pathways; and the intracellular proteins of infecting bacteria. Drugs can mimic endogenous chemicals and enzymes or block their effects at receptor sites. The receptor for penicillin, for example, is the enzyme transpeptidase. Penicillin renders this enzyme incapable of making bacterial cell walls strong and rigid. The cell walls then break down, and the bacteria die.

Affinity refers to a drug's ability to combine with a receptor; efficacy refers to its ability to activate the receptor. Drugs that have both characteristics are agonists. The degree of response to an agonist depends on the drug's affinity for the receptor site and its concentration there.

Drugs called antagonists may also combine with a receptor. These produce no pharmacologic response, but they inhibit actions of agonists for the receptor. An antagonist can be either competitive or noncompetitive. It is competitive if a sufficiently high dose of an agonist can overcome its effects. For example, histamine (agonist) can overcome antihistamine (antagonist). The process in this case is reversible. An antagonist is noncompetitive if an agonist cannot overcome it regardless of dose. For example, organophosphates noncompetitively block cholinergic receptors. The process in this case is irreversible since the antagonist inactivates the receptor.

ACHIEVING STEADY-STATE BLOOD CONCENTRATIONS

How quickly your patient receives the full effects of the drug you are giving him depends on many factors, including the drug's *accumulation.* The concentration of the drug in your patient's bloodstream must increase until the dose he is receiving equals the exact amount of drug he is eliminating; this level is *steady state.*

When a loading dose is given, the drug attains a steady state more quickly. In this graph, the broken line shows the effects of a loading dose, followed by smaller maintenance doses. The black solid line shows the effects of equal maintenance doses given at regular intervals (at the half-life), with no loading dose.

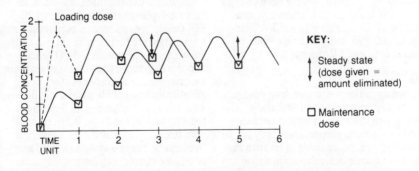

Graph adapted from Steven E. Mayer, et al., "Introduction: The Dynamics of Drug Absorption, Distribution, and Elimination," in *Goodman and Gilman's The Pharmacological Basis of Therapeutics,* 6th ed., edited by Alfred Goodman Gilman and Louis S. Goodman. Copyright © 1980 by Macmillan Publishing Co., Inc. Used with permission of the publisher.

Whether a drug is an agonist or an antagonist, its affinity for the receptor depends on its specific molecular structure. Relatively small changes in the drug molecule may leave its affinity relatively unchanged yet result in major differences in pharmacologic effect. This relationship between molecular configuration and pharmacologic effect is called the structure-activity relationship.

Investigations of the structure-activity relationships of drugs and of endogenous substances such as hormones have led to the discovery of new drugs that are safer, more effective, or more advantageous to use. For example, cefazolin and cefonicid are both cephalosporin antibiotics. The chemical structure of cefonicid is such that it is administered once every 24 hours. Cefazolin has to be given every 8 hours. Both drugs have the same therapeutic effect, but it is more time-efficient and cost-effective to administer cefonicid.

Factors that affect drug action

Age
Age is an important factor affecting a drug's action, particularly age extremes. Neonates excrete some drugs slowly because they have underdeveloped metabolic enzyme systems and reduced renal function. They need highly individualized dosing and careful monitoring. Elderly patients may have decreased muscle mass and diminished hepatic and renal function. Consequently, lower doses at longer intervals may be necessary to avoid toxicity. (See Chapter 17, Pediatric Drug and I.V. Therapy, and Chapter 18, Geriatric Drug and I.V. Therapy, for pediatric and geriatric considerations in drug and I.V. therapy.)

Sex
Sex has an indirect effect on drug dosage. The average woman has a lower body weight than the average man. A woman also has a greater proportion of body fat, so drugs that are more soluble in fat than in water are more quickly distributed in a woman than in a man. Finally, hormonal differences between men and women can alter the metabolism of some drugs.

Body weight
Drug dosage is usually based on a person's body weight. The greater the body weight, the greater the drug's dilution in the body, and the larger the dose needed to achieve a therapeutic effect. Conversely, the lower the body weight, the greater the drug's concentration in body tissues, and the more powerful its effects. However, the dosage of some drugs must be based on lean body weight to avoid overdose or toxicity. (See "Volume of distribution" in this chapter.)

Body weight is a critical factor in determining drug dosage in infants, children, and elderly or debilitated patients who have less than average body weight. Drug toxicity is more likely to occur in these patient populations. (See Chapter 17, Pediatric Drug and I.V. Therapy, and Chapter 18, Geriatric Drug and I.V. Therapy, for further information on body weight in pediatric and geriatric patients.)

Nutritional status
Adequate nutrition supports formation of enzymes and proteins necessary for drug distribution and metabolism. Poor nutritional status may impair drug action, since most drugs bind with proteins for distribution to cell receptors, where they exert their effect.

Pathologic and genetic conditions
An underlying disease can also markedly affect drug action. For example, acidosis may cause insulin resistance, and hyperthyroidism may speed the metabolism of some drugs. Genetic diseases—such as glucose-6-phosphate dehydrogenase (G-6-PD) deficiency and hepatic porphyria—may turn drugs into toxins, with serious consequences. A patient with G-6-PD deficiency may develop hemolytic anemia when given sulfonamides or a number of other drugs. A genetically susceptible patient can develop an acute attack of porphyria if given a barbiturate or a sulfonamide. When treated with isoniazid, a patient with a highly active hepatic enzyme system (a rapid acetylator, for example) can develop hepatitis from the rapid intrahepatic buildup of a toxic metabolite.

Route of administration
Routes of administration are not therapeutically interchangeable. For example, phenytoin (Dilantin) is readily absorbed orally, but slowly and erratically absorbed intramuscularly. Conversely, carbenicillin is usually given parenterally because oral administration yields inadequate blood levels to treat systemic infections. Carbenicillin is given orally only to treat urinary tract infections, since it concentrates in the urine.

Dosage form
Some tablets and capsules are too large for very ill patients to swallow readily. You may request an oral solution or elixir of the same drug, but remember that the liquid is usually more easily and completely absorbed and produces higher blood levels than the tablet. When a potentially toxic drug such as digoxin is given in solution, increased absorption can cause toxicity. Also, enteric-coated tablets and sustained-release preparations may affect the degree of absorption of a drug and necessitate a dosage change to produce the desired effect.

Drug-drug interactions
A drug-drug interaction takes place when one drug administered in combination with or shortly after another drug alters the effect of one or both drugs. Usually, the effect of one drug is increased or decreased. In rare instances, interaction yields an effect that cannot be attributed to either drug alone.

Drug interaction may result from a combination of two drugs' actions or effects or from one drug's alterations of another's absorption, distribution, metabolism, or excretion. For instance, one drug may displace another from plasma protein-binding sites, freeing it for further action, or it may inhibit or stimulate the metabolism or excretion of the other.

Drug interaction is sometimes used to prevent or minimize certain side effects. Hydrochlorothiazide and spironolactone, both diuretics, are administered in combination because the former is potassium-depleting and the latter, potassium-sparing.

Drug interaction can also be beneficial; it is the basis of *combination therapy.* One drug may be given to potentiate, or increase, the effects of another (potentiation). For example, probenecid blocks the excretion of penicillin and is sometimes given with it to maintain adequate blood levels for a longer period. Also, two drugs with similar actions may be given together precisely because of additive effect. For example, aspirin and codeine, both analgesics, may be given in combination because they provide greater pain relief than either does alone.

Antagonism is a reduced or absent pharmacologic response to a drug due to the presence of a second drug. A hypertensive patient well controlled with guanethidine (Ismelin) may see his blood pressure rise to its former high level if he takes the antidepressant amitriptyline (Elavil) at the same time. Drug combinations that produce antagonism should be avoided if possible.

Another kind of inhibiting effect occurs when tetracycline is administered with drugs or foods that contain calcium or magnesium (for example, antacids or milk). Calcium and magnesium ions combine with tetracycline in the GI tract and cause inadequate absorption of the drug.

Drug-food interactions
Food in the stomach may speed up, retard, or sometimes prevent drug absorption. And some foods may affect different drugs in different ways.

Drugs given orally go through several processes before entering the systemic circulation. Tablets, for example, must disintegrate and dissolve before they can be absorbed through the intestinal mucosa. Tablet breakdown is affected by the stomach's pH, and when food changes the pH, the rate and degree of breakdown—and of drug absorption—may also change.

Food stimulates various body secretions, including gastric acid and bile. For this reason, acid-labile drugs should be taken on an empty stomach, when gastric acid secretions are minimal. Fat-soluble drugs, however, should be administered with meals because bile helps dissolve them.

Food delays gastric emptying, so a drug given with meals may remain in the stomach longer and delay therapeutic effect. If a rapid effect is important, administer the drug when the patient's stomach is empty. Sometimes a food buffer may be useful. It can, for example, reduce the gastrointestinal distress, nausea, and mucosal damage caused by ulcerogenic drugs such as aspirin and indomethacin (Indocin).

Before you administer medications, check possible food and alcohol interactions. You may help patients reduce unpleasant drug side effects, such as nausea, vomiting, dyspepsia, and diarrhea. You may even improve patient compliance and reduce the length (and cost) of a patient's stay.

Psychological considerations

A patient's attitude toward taking a drug can influence its therapeutic effect. If he expects that a drug will be helpful, therapeutic effect may be enhanced. On the other hand, if he feels that the drug will not help, therapeutic effect may diminish, and adverse reactions may occur.

Your attitude about the effectiveness of a drug and the manner in which you administer it may shape the patient's attitude. Therefore, your attitude may indirectly affect the results of drug therapy.

Patient compliance

A common cause of failure or adverse reactions in drug therapy is poor patient compliance with the prescribed drug regimen. The patient may fail to take the prescribed doses, take inappropriate doses, forget to take doses at the correct times, prematurely discontinue his medication, or take medications prescribed for previous disorders. Such noncompliance is usually unintentional and may be prevented or corrected by patient education.

Drug effects

Therapeutic effect

Therapeutic effect is the effect that is desired from a drug. It may be local, affecting only the body tissue at the administration site, or systemic, affecting the whole body. A drug may also have combined local and systemic effects.

Adverse reactions

Any drug effect other than the intended therapeutic effect can be called an adverse reaction. It may be expected and benign, or unexpected and potentially harmful. Mild but predictable adverse reactions are sometimes called side effects. Drowsiness caused by antihistamines is an example. During hay fever season, a patient may have to contend with this drowsiness to get relief from hay fever symptoms. The dose may be adjusted up or down to balance therapeutic effect with side effect.

A more severe adverse reaction also may be tolerated for a necessary therapeutic effect, or it may be hazardous and unacceptable and require discontinuation of the drug. Some adverse reactions subside with continued use. For example, the drowsiness associated with methyldopa (Aldomet) and the orthostatic hypotension associated with prazosin (Minipress) usually subside after several days. But many adverse reactions are dose-related and lessen or disappear only if dosage is reduced.

Most adverse reactions are undesirable, but an occasional one can be put to clinical use. An outstanding example is the drowsiness associated with diphenhydramine (Benadryl), which makes it clinically useful as a mild hypnotic.

Drug hypersensitivity, a term sometimes used interchangeably with drug allergy, is the result of an antigen-antibody immune reaction that occurs when a drug is given to a susceptible patient. One of the most dangerous of all drug hypersensitivity reactions is penicillin anaphylaxis. In its severest form, it can be rapidly fatal. (See *Responding to Anaphylactic Shock;* and *Drugs Used to Reverse Anaphylaxis,* pp. 40 and 41, for more information.)

Rarely, idiosyncratic adverse reactions occur. These are highly unpredictable and individual. Probably the best-known idiosyncratic drug reaction is the aplastic anemia caused by the antibiotic chloramphenicol (Chloromycetin). This reaction appears in only 1 out of 40,000 patients; it is often fatal. More common idiosyncratic reactions are extreme sensitivity to very low doses of a drug or insensitivity to higher-than-normal doses.

RESPONDING TO ANAPHYLACTIC SHOCK

Recognizing signs and symptoms
Most anaphylactic reactions become evident within seconds or minutes after exposure to the antigen. A drug injection may cause symptoms 5 to 60 minutes later, but most of these reactions begin within 30 minutes. Occasionally, a reaction sets in hours later. The faster the reaction, the more severe it tends to be—and the more crucial the need for prompt identification of signs and symptoms and immediate intervention.

Typically, the reaction is preceded by one or more of the following prodromal signs and symptoms—vague complaints of uneasiness or impending doom, severe anxiety, headache, dizziness, paresthesia, disorientation, and even loss of consciousness. The most common initial signs and symptoms of the reaction itself are cutaneous, typically progressing from pruritus to diffuse erythema to generalized urticaria and angioedema (especially of the eyelids, lips, or tongue). The patient is likely to complain of feeling very warm.

Early respiratory changes include the feeling of having a lump in the throat, followed by hoarseness, coughing or sneezing, dyspnea, and stridor. The uvula, vocal cords, and posterior pharynx may appear swollen. On auscultation, you might detect diffuse wheezes and prolonged expirations.

Nursing interventions
• Top priority—assess the patient's respiratory status immediately. If he has stopped breathing, start pulmonary resuscitation; if he is not breathing *and* has no pulse, start cardiopulmonary resuscitation. Administer oxygen as needed and prepare for endotracheal intubation. If laryngeal edema has closed off the patient's airway, the physician will perform an emergency tracheostomy. Keep the patient in a sitting position unless contraindicated (by severe hypotension, for example).
• Call for help and notify the physician.
• Try to determine the cause of the reaction, but do not waste time. (You do not have to know the cause to assess the patient.) Look for obvious causes. If the patient was just given an injection, wrap a tourniquet (or blood pressure cuff) above the affected site to obstruct venous return. If the patient is receiving an infusion of I.V. medication, stop it immediately, since that would be a likely cause of the reaction. The same goes for a dye infusion and blood transfusion.
• Insert or maintain a patent I.V. line. You can expect the physician to order epinephrine, the drug of choice for acute anaphylaxis. Epinephrine can promptly reverse life-threatening conditions such as bronchoconstriction and hypotension.

A warning—epinephrine can be dangerous. Watch for tachycardia and other possible adverse effects, such as hypertension, dyspnea, and electrocardiogram changes. Other drugs may also have to be given, especially to patients who respond sluggishly to epinephrine. (See *Drugs Used to Reverse Anaphylaxis*, pp. 40 and 41.)
• Expect to administer normal saline or lactated Ringer's solution to restore fluid volume, increase blood pressure and cardiac output, and reverse lactic acidosis. Assess the patient for signs of fluid overload, such as crackles, dyspnea, coughing with frothy sputum, and jugular venous distention.

Monitor fluid intake and output hourly. If hypotension persists, be ready to start a continuous epinephrine infusion or to administer plasma or a vasopressor to raise blood pressure. Measure urine output; it should be at least 30 ml/hr.
• Check vital signs frequently (every 15 to 30 minutes) for the first 1 to 4 hours. Look for a change in respiratory or cardiovascular status. The patient will still be at risk for bronchospasms, upper respiratory obstruction, tachycardia, and hypotension. Following severe reactions, patients should be monitored closely for 24 hours. They are most likely to have another reaction within 12 to 24 hours.
• Reassure the patient and provide continual emotional support. Few experiences are as frightening as an anaphylactic reaction.

DRUGS USED TO REVERSE ANAPHYLAXIS

Drug	Classification	Indication	Dosage
diphenhydramine (Benadryl)	Antihistamine	*Mild anaphylaxis*	*P.O.:* 25 to 100 mg t.i.d. *I.M./I.V.:* 25 to 50 mg q.i.d.
epinephrine (Adrenalin)	Adrenergic	*Severe anaphylaxis (drug of choice)*	*Initial infusion:* 0.2 to 0.5 mg of epinephrine (0.2 to 0.5 ml of 1:1,000 strength diluted in 10 ml normal saline) given I.V. slowly over 5 to 10 minutes, followed by continuous infusion *Continuous infusion:* 1 to 4 mcg/min (Mix 1 ml of 1:1,000 epinephrine in 250 ml of dextrose 5% in water [D_5W] to get concentration of 4 mcg/ml.)
hydrocortisone (Solu-Cortef)	Corticosteroid	*Severe anaphylaxis*	*I.V.:* 100 to 200 mg q4h to q6h
aminophylline (Aminophyllin)	Methyl xanthine bronchodilator	*Severe anaphylaxis*	*I.V.:* 5 to 6 mg/kg loading dose, followed by 0.4 to 0.9 mg/kg/min infusion
cimetidine (Tagamet)	Antihistamine	*Severe anaphylaxis (experimental use in refractory cases)*	*I.V.:* 600 mg diluted in D_5W and administered over 20 minutes

Action	Nursing Considerations
• Competes with histamine for H₁ receptor sites • Prevents laryngeal edema • Controls localized itching	• Administer I.V. doses slowly to avoid hypotension. • Monitor patient for hypotension. • Drug causes drowsiness and slows reflexes, so caution patient about driving. • Give fluids as needed. Drug causes dry mouth.
Alpha-adrenergic effects: • Increases blood pressure • Reverses peripheral vasodilation and systemic hypotension • Decreases angioedema and urticaria • Improves coronary blood flow by raising diastolic pressure • Causes peripheral vasoconstriction *Beta-adrenergic effects:* • Causes bronchodilation • Causes positive inotropic and chronotropic cardiac activity • Decreases synthesis and release of chemical mediator	• Select large vein for infusion. • Use infusion controller to regulate drip. • Check blood pressure and heart rate. • Monitor patient for dysrhythmias. • Check solution strength, dosage, and label before administering. • Watch for signs of extravasation at infusion site. • Monitor intake and output. • Assess color and temperature of extremities.
• Prevents neutrophil and platelet aggregation • Inhibits synthesis of mediators • Decreases capillary permeability	• Monitor fluid and electrolyte balance, intake and output, and blood pressure closely. • Maintain patient on ulcer regimen and antacid prophylactically.
• Causes bronchodilation • Stimulates respiratory drive • Dilates constricted pulmonary arteries • Causes diuresis • Strengthens cardiac contractions • Increases vital capacity • Causes coronary vasodilation	• Monitor blood pressure, pulse, and respirations. • Monitor intake and output, hydration status, and aminophylline and electrolyte levels. • Monitor patient for dysrhythmias. • Use I.V. controller to reduce risk of overdose. • Maintain serum levels at 10 to 20 mcg/ml.
• Competes with histamine for H₂ receptor sites • Prevents laryngeal edema	• Tagamet is incompatible with aminophylline. • Dose may be reduced for patients with impaired renal or hepatic function.

To deal with adverse reactions correctly, you need to be alert to even minor changes in the patient's clinical status. These may be early warnings of toxicity. Listen to the patient's complaints about his reactions to a drug, and consider each complaint objectively.

You may be able to reduce adverse reactions in several ways. Obviously, dosage reduction often helps. Often so does rescheduling the same doses. For example, pseudoephedrine (Sudafed) may produce stimulation; that may not be a problem for the patient if the drug is given early in the day. Similarly, the drowsiness that occurs with antihistamines or tranquilizers can be totally harmless if they are given at bedtime.

Most important, the patient needs to be told what adverse reactions to expect so he will not become worried or even stop taking a drug on his own. Of course, the patient should report any unusual or unexpected adverse reactions to his physician.

Recognizing drug allergies or serious idiosyncratic reactions can be lifesaving. Ask each patient about drugs he is taking or has taken in the past and what, if any, unusual effects he experienced from taking them. If a patient claims to be allergic to a drug, ask him to tell you exactly what happens when he takes it. He may be calling a harmless side effect, such as upset stomach, an allergic reaction, or he may have a true tendency to anaphylaxis. In addition, ask about food allergies because they can be helpful in identifying a potential drug allergy. For example, an allergy to seafood is really an allergy to the iodine in the seafood; therefore, drugs that contain iodine would cause a hypersensitivity response.

Information about allergies must be recorded on the chart and in the medication and nursing cardex. Assess the patient's response to drug therapy throughout his hospital stay, and report any clinical changes. If you suspect an adverse reaction, withhold the drug until you can check with the pharmacist and the physician.

Toxic reactions

Toxic reactions to drugs can be acute, resulting from an excessive dose taken accidentally or deliberately, or they can be chronic, resulting from the cumulative effect of the drug buildup in the body. These reactions may be extensions of the desired pharmacologic effect. For example, barbiturates produce hypnotic and sedative effects by acting as nonspecific central nervous system (CNS) depressants. Toxic reactions to barbiturates are revealed by excessive CNS depression, decreased deep tendon reflexes, and possibly coma.

Toxicity may also occur when a drug's blood level rises because of impaired metabolism or excretion. For example, theophylline may reach a toxic level in blood when hepatic dysfunction impairs metabolism of the drug. Similarly, digoxin toxicity can follow impaired renal function. Digoxin is largely unmetabolized, and it accumulates when renal excretion of the drug slows.

Of course, toxic blood levels also result from excessive dosage. Tinnitus (ringing in the ears) caused by aspirin, for example, may be a sign that a safe level has been exceeded.

Most drug toxicity is predictable and dose-related; fortunately, it is also readily reversible with dosage adjustment. Monitor patients carefully for physiologic changes that may alter drug effect. Watch especially for impaired hepatic or renal function. Tell the patient the signs of toxicity, and explain what to do if a toxic reaction occurs. Emphasize the importance of taking a drug exactly as prescribed. Warn the patient that serious problems may arise if he changes the dose or schedule.

Tolerance

When a person must take larger and larger doses of a drug to achieve the therapeutic effect, drug tolerance has developed. Its cause is unknown. Tolerance commonly develops with the use of morphine, a narcotic analgesic, over a period of time. As a result, some patients with chronic pain will receive several times the recommended doses.

Physical dependence

Physical dependence is an altered physiologic state produced by the long-term use of narcotics or other drugs such as diazepam. Repeated use of the drug is needed to prevent withdrawal symptoms. In *addiction*, or psychological dependence, the addicted patient uses a drug compulsively to experience its psychic effects and perhaps to avoid withdrawal symptoms. He may or may not be physically dependent, but drug-seeking behavior occurs without physical need. The development of drug addiction is rare in patients with no history of addiction. Therefore, you should not fear causing addiction in chronic pain patients who are receiving narcotics.

Drugs and pregnancy

Ever since the thalidomide tragedy of the late 1950s—when thousands of infants were born malformed after their mothers used this mild sedative-hypnotic during pregnancy—use of drugs during pregnancy has been a source of medical concern and controversy.

To identify drugs that may be teratogenic (capable of producing physical defects in the fetus), preclinical drug studies always include tests on pregnant laboratory animals. These tests reveal gross teratogenicity but do not clearly establish safety. Different species react to drugs in different ways, and animal studies do not rule out possible teratogenic effects in humans. For example, the preliminary animal studies on thalidomide gave no warning of teratogenic effects, and it was subsequently released for general use in Europe.

To prevent such tragedies, a drug now must have its pregnancy category listed in the package insert. (See *FDA-Assigned Pregnancy Categories.*) Pregnancy categories classify drugs according to the results of human and animal studies. With the exception of vitamins and minerals, no drug is approved warning-free for use in pregnancy.

At one time, the placenta was thought to protect the fetus from drug effects, but today the idea of a placental barrier is considered a myth. Almost all drugs cross the placental membrane to some extent. Orally administered drugs that can cross the GI membrane probably can cross the placental membrane. Drugs with exceptionally large molecular structure, such as heparin, will not cross the placenta to a great extent, but use of these medications in pregnancy still requires caution.

Just because drugs cross the placenta, however, does not necessarily mean that the fetus will be harmed. Actually, only one factor seems to be clearly related to exag-

---

F.D.A.–ASSIGNED PREGNANCY CATEGORIES

A: Adequate and well-controlled studies have failed to demonstrate a risk to the fetus in the first trimester of pregnancy (and there is no evidence of risk in later trimesters).

B: Animal reproduction studies have failed to demonstrate a risk to the fetus and there are no adequate and well-controlled studies in pregnant women.

C: Animal reproduction studies have shown an adverse effect on the fetus and there are no adequate and well-controlled studies in humans, but potential benefits may warrant use of the drug in pregnant women despite potential risks.

D: There is positive evidence of human fetal risk based on adverse reaction data from investigational or marketing experience or studies in humans, but potential benefits may warrant use of the drug in pregnant women despite potential risks.

X: Studies in animals or humans have demonstrated fetal abnormalities and/or there is positive evidence of human fetal risk based on adverse reaction data from investigational or marketing experience and the risks involved in use of the drug in pregnant women clearly outweigh potential benefits.

Copied from the *USP-DI*, Volume I, *Drug Information for the Health Care Provider*, 6th ed. Copyright 1985, The United States Pharmacopeial Convention, Inc. Permission granted.

> **GUIDELINES FOR ADMINISTERING DRUGS TO A PREGNANT PATIENT**
>
> - Before administering any drug to a woman of childbearing age, ask the date of her last menstrual period and whether she could possibly be pregnant.
> - Avoid administering all drugs except those essential to maintain the pregnancy or the mother's health. Be particularly cautious during the first and third trimesters when the fetus is most vulnerable.
> - To minimize any harmful effect on the fetus, administer *the safest possible drug in the lowest possible dose.*
> - Apply topical drugs cautiously. Many topically applied drugs can be absorbed in amounts large enough to harm the fetus.
>
> As a precaution, remind the pregnant patient to check with her physician before taking any drug.
> *Remember:* Alcohol and caffeine are drugs, too. Caution her to use them judiciously.

gerated risk in drug therapy during pregnancy: the stage of fetal development. During the first and third trimesters, the fetus is especially vulnerable to damage from the mother's use of drugs. All drugs should be given with extreme caution during these times.

The most sensitive period for drug-induced fetal malformation is the first trimester, when fetal organs are differentiating (organogenesis). All drugs should be withheld during this time unless the mother's health is in jeopardy without them. Theoretically, even aspirin could harm the fetus during this sensitive time.

Drugs should be used with caution during the last 3 months of pregnancy, and only when absolutely necessary at term. At birth, the newborn must rely on his own metabolism to excrete any drug remaining in his body. Since his detoxifying systems are not fully developed, any residual drug may take a long time to be metabolized—and thus may induce prolonged toxic reactions.

Nevertheless, in many circumstances, pregnant women must continue to take certain drugs. For example, a woman with epilepsy who is well controlled with an anticonvulsant should continue to take it even during pregnancy. And a pregnant woman with a bacterial infection should receive antibiotics. In such cases, the potential risk to the fetus is outweighed by the mother's need for the drug. (See *Guidelines for Administering Drugs to a Pregnant Patient.*)

Drugs and lactation

Most drugs a nursing mother takes appear in breast milk. Drug levels in breast milk tend to be high when blood levels are high—generally, shortly after taking each dose. Therefore, advise the mother to breast-feed before taking her medication, not after. (See *The Breast-Fed Infant: Special Considerations.*)

Breast-feeding should be temporarily interrupted and replaced with bottle-feeding when the mother must take the following:
- Tetracyclines
- Chloramphenicol
- Sulfonamides (during first 2 weeks postpartum)
- Oral anticoagulants
- Iodine-containing drugs
- Antineoplastics
- Propylthiouracil.

Review Questions

1. Define "pharmacokinetics."

2. State three factors that affect oral drug absorption.

3. Distribution is the movement of the drug:
   A. From the stomach into the bloodstream
   B. From the bloodstream into body fluids and tissues
   C. From the bloodstream into the cell
   D. From the bloodstream into the kidneys

THE BREAST-FED INFANT: SPECIAL CONSIDERATIONS

In some circumstances, the physician may order one of the following drugs for a patient—even though these drugs may cause adverse reactions in the breast-fed infant. To ensure the infant's safety, closely monitor his condition. Watch for the following signs and symptoms.

Drug	Possible Adverse Reactions
Ampicillin	Rash, diarrhea, drug sensitivity, candidiasis
Analgesics	Lethargy, poor feeding, drowsiness
Anticonvulsants	Drowsiness
Cathartics	Gastrointestinal hypermotility
Isoniazid (INH)	Peripheral neuritis
Oral antidiabetic agents	Hypoglycemia
Penicillin G	Drug sensitivity, candidiasis
Propranolol (Inderal)	Bradycardia
Psychotropics	Lethargy, poor feeding, drowsiness
Salicylates	Internal bleeding

4. What is the main site of drug metabolism?
   A. The blood
   B. The kidneys
   C. The liver
   D. The lungs

5. Kidney disease would affect which pharmacokinetic process?
   A. Absorption
   B. Distribution
   C. Metabolism
   D. Excretion

6. What does the term "half-life" mean, and what is its significance?

7. Define "pharmacodynamics."

8. State three factors (other than age, sex, and body weight) that affect drug action.

9. Define potentiation and antagonism as the terms relate to drug therapy.

10. An adverse reaction is:
    A. The desired effect from a drug
    B. An unwanted effect from a drug
    C. The cumulative effect from a drug
    D. The tolerance effect from a drug

11. Anaphylactic shock is an example of:
    A. A therapeutic effect
    B. An adverse effect
    C. A toxic effect
    D. A tolerance effect

12. During which trimester(s) is the fetus especially vulnerable to damage from the mother's use of drugs?

Selected References

Drug Interactions. Nursing Now Series. Springhouse, Pa.: Springhouse Corp., 1984.

Drugs, 2nd ed. Nurse's Reference Library. Springhouse, Pa.: Springhouse Corp., 1984.

Gilman, A.G., et al., eds. *Goodman and Gilman's The Pharmacological Basis of Therapeutics,* 6th ed. New York: Macmillan Publishing Co., 1980.

Hahn, A.B., et al. *Pharmacology in Nursing,* 16th ed. St. Louis: C.V. Mosby Co., 1985.

Randall, B. "Reacting to Anaphylaxis," *Nursing86* 16(3):34-39, March 1986.

Rodman, M.J., and Karch, A. *Pharmacology and Drug Therapy in Nursing,* 3rd ed. Philadelphia: J.B. Lippincott Co., 1985.

United States Pharmacopeia Dispensing Information, 6th ed. Rockville, Md.: United States Pharmacopeial Convention, Inc., 1986.

Weiner, M., and Pepper, G.A. *Clinical Pharmacology and Therapeutics in Nursing,* 2nd ed. New York: McGraw-Hill Book Co., 1985.

Medication Orders and Distribution Systems

To prevent drug errors, you must understand the different types of medication orders and know how to transcribe them from the physician's order sheet to the medication cardex. This chapter discusses medication orders and their transcription, as well as the types of systems pharmacies use to distribute medication to patient care units.

Medication orders

A medication order is written by a physician on a special form on the patient's medical record. It includes the date the order was written, name and dose of medication, route of administration, frequency of administration, and the physician's signature. Abbreviations are commonly used, but they should be interpreted carefully since people attach different meanings to them. Seek clarification whenever you are unsure of an abbreviation or its use in a particular order. (See *Abbreviations Commonly Used in Medication Orders*, p. 48.)

Consult the physician *before* giving a medication if you have questions about any part of the order or cannot read the handwriting. Do not guess at what the order might be. Doing so could lead to a harmful drug error for which you will be held responsible.

Types of orders
Standard order without a termination date
A standard order is also called a routine order. It means that the medication is to be given until the physician writes an order to discontinue it or until institutional policy dictates that the order must be rewritten. Such a policy requires medication use to be reevaluated periodically and prevents continued administration of medication no longer needed by a patient.
Example:
digoxin 0.25 mg P.O. daily.

Standard order with a termination date
With this type of order, the medication is to be given for a determined number of times or days.
Example:
amoxicillin 250 mg P.O. q.i.d. × 10 days.

Single order
With this type of order, the medication is to be given only once, at a specific time or at the earliest possible time.
Example:
Dulcolax suppository before breakfast this a.m.

Stat order
Stat orders are to be used in emergencies, and the medication is to be given immediately and only once.
Example:
Vistaril 100 mg I.M. stat.

PRN order
PRN, or as needed, orders indicate that the medication may be given when nursing judgment determines it is needed and when enough time has passed since the last dose. PRN orders are discontinued according to the physician's written order or institutional policy, as with standard orders.
Example:
nitroglycerin 1/200 grams S.L. PRN chest pain.

ABBREVIATIONS COMMONLY USED IN MEDICATION ORDERS

Abbreviation	Meaning	Abbreviation	Meaning
a.c.	before meals	P.O. or p.o.	by mouth
ad lib.	as often as desired	P.R.N. or p.r.n.	as needed
b.i.d.	twice daily (while awake)	pt	pint
g, gm, or Gm	gram(s)	q	every
gr	grain(s)	q.d.	every day
gtt	drop(s)	q.h.	every hour
h or hr	hour(s)	q.i.d.	four times daily (while awake)
h.s.	at bedtime	q2h, q3h, etc.	every 2 hours, every 3 hours, etc.
I.M.	intramuscular		
I.V.	intravenous	q.o.d.	every other day
kg	kilogram	q.s.	quantity sufficient
Ⓛ	left	Ⓡ	right
L or l	liter	s̄	without
mcg or μg	microgram(s)	S.C., S.Q., or subq	subcutaneous
mEq	milliequivalent(s)	S.L. or s.l.	sublingual
mg	milligram(s)	s.o.s.	if needed
ml	milliliter(s)	s̄s̄	one-half
mm	millimeter(s)	stat	immediately
NPO	nothing by mouth	T, Tbl, or tbsp	tablespoon(s)
od	every day		
O.D.	right eye	tsp or t	teaspoon(s)
O.S.	left eye	t.i.d.	three times daily (while awake)
O.U.	both eyes		
oz	ounce(s)	U	unit(s)
p̄	after	VO	verbal order
p.c.	after meals	w/ or c̄	with

Medication Orders and Distribution Systems

Protocol
Protocol, or standing orders, is a list of orders set up to be followed automatically in certain clinical situations. You must decide whether or not the protocol should be used by applying specified criteria. Protocols are often used in critical care settings where nurses have been trained to respond to potential emergencies. They are sometimes used when a patient is admitted to a specialty unit. And they are used by community health nurses when it is not possible for a patient to be seen by a physician.

Verbal orders
Verbal orders are given orally, either in person or by telephone. In most health care settings, nurses may take verbal orders only in an emergency since a verbal order carries a greater risk for drug error than does a written order. (See *Taking Drug Orders and Carrying Them Out: How to Protect Yourself*, p. 9, for guidelines on taking a verbal order.) The verbal order should be written on the patient's chart and should be countersigned by the physician as soon as possible.

Transcribing medication orders
Medication orders must be copied clearly and accurately from the physician's order sheet to the medication cardex. Institutional policy determines who is permitted to transcribe medication orders. Usually a specially trained secretary does this job, but it often becomes the responsibility of an RN. The procedure varies, but these guidelines can be followed:
- Clarify unclear or incomplete orders with the physician before transcribing the order.
- Check that you have the right patient's medication cardex before you begin transcribing.
- Use ink to transcribe orders onto the medication cardex since the cardex is a legal document.
- Transcribe the order exactly as it appears on the physician's order sheet.
- Write out any abbreviation you think could be misinterpreted.
- Enter on the cardex the date the medication was ordered and the times it is to be given.
- Draw a diagonal line through the time block on the cardex to indicate when a drug is not to be given or has been discontinued.
- Keep the medication cardex neat and clean to minimize drug error and preserve it as a legal document.
- Check off each medication order after it has been transcribed.
- Recheck the accuracy of each transcription and check for omissions.
- Sign or initial each transcription on the physician's order sheet.

Drug distribution systems

The drug distribution methods used in most health care facilities today are almost always derived from one of these four basic systems:
- Floor stock system
- Individual prescription order system
- Combination floor stock and individual prescription order system
- Unit dose system.

Floor stock system
In this system, nearly all necessary medications are kept in stock at the nurses' station. Only special drugs, such as chemotherapeutic agents, certain antibiotics, and diagnostic agents, are ordered from the pharmacy as needed.

Individual prescription order system
In this system, medications for each patient are dispensed by the pharmacist based on individual prescription orders. Normally a 5-day supply of medications is dispensed at one time.

Combination floor stock and individual prescription order system
This combination system is probably the most common one used in health care facilities today. Most medications are dispensed as in the individual prescription order system, but the most frequently used medications are kept in floor stock.

Unit dose system
Many hospitals in the United States and Canada have initiated a unit dose system of drug distribution in the last 10 years. This system has been shown to be safer and more cost-effective and time-efficient than traditional systems. The following characteristics are common to unit dose systems:
- The pharmacist receives a copy of all physicians' orders.

COMPARING DRUG DISTRIBUTION SYSTEMS

System	Advantages	Disadvantages
Floor stock system	• Less delay because almost all drugs are readily available when ordered. Fewer orders need to be sent to the pharmacy.	• More work for the nurse, who must select the proper drug from a large floor stock • Chance of "pouring" errors because drugs are not stored in separate containers for individual patients • Chance of medication errors because the pharmacist and nurse do not double-check each other whenever a drug is reordered and dispensed. Also, drugs may be used inadvertently after their expiration dates. • Increased costs of larger drug inventory throughout the facility
Individual prescription order system	• Better pharmacy control of drug distribution than in the floor stock system • Less chance of medication errors. Medication containers are identified by patient name, and both the nurse and the pharmacist double-check each other whenever a drug is reordered and dispensed.	• Potential delays in initiating therapy while waiting for ordered drugs • Waste of prescription medications due to changes or discontinuations after a drug is dispensed • Possibility of hoarding discontinued drugs on the nursing unit and using them for other patients • Potential for administering deteriorated doses • Chance of "pouring" errors because doses are not stored individually • More nursing time spent in inventorying, ordering, and reordering prescribed drugs • Increased cost of inventory throughout the facility
Combination floor stock and individual prescription order system	• Less delay in obtaining the most commonly ordered drugs because they are in stock on the unit	• Same as those for the floor stock and individual prescription order systems
Unit dose system	• Less chance of medication and record-keeping errors because of numerous checks built into the system • Lower overall costs of drug distribution and inventory within the facility • Lower costs for the patient. Unopened, discontinued doses may be returned to the pharmacy stocks and credited to the patient's bill. • More effective utilization of nurses and pharmacists	• Danger of errors caused by overconfidence if the nurse neglects to double-check the pharmacy • More expensive packaging • Increased pharmacy staff

- The pharmacist maintains a medication profile for each patient. Before dispensing medications, he enters new orders on the profile, checking that each medication is appropriate.
- The pharmacist dispenses medication in properly labeled unit dose packages that contain the ordered amount of drug in a dosage form ready for administration to a particular patient by the prescribed route at a prescribed time.
- Medications are dispensed into patient-separated drug storage bins, usually in a drug cart.
- No more than a 24-hour supply of each medication is dispensed at one time.
- Floor stock of drugs is minimized. Emergency medications, mouthwash, antiseptics, and frequently used PRN medications are usually stocked.
- Nurses maintain a medication administration record. Before administering medication, they compare what is written on the medication administration record with what the pharmacist has dispensed. Any discrepancies (for example, extra doses, missing doses, or wrong drugs or doses) must be resolved with the pharmacist. In that way, dispensing, administration, and record-keeping errors by pharmacists and nurses are minimized.

Review Questions

True or False

1. There is little risk of drug error if a medication order is given verbally.

2. Consult the physician if you question any part of a medication order *before* you give the medication.

3. A single order is the type of order usually given in emergencies.

4. Nursing judgment is necessary when giving PRN medications.

5. Verbal orders taken by a nurse must be countersigned by a physician as soon as possible.

6. Always repeat a verbal order back to the physician to be sure you heard it correctly.

7. The medication cardex is a legal document.

8. The meaning of any abbreviation that could be misinterpreted in a medication order should be written out.

9. The unit dose system is safer and more cost-effective and time-efficient than any other distribution system.

Brief response

10. Which of the following is (are) incomplete order(s)? Why?
   A. Digoxin 0.25 mg daily
   B. Keflin 500 mg I.V. w/500 ml D_5W q6h
   C. Demerol 75 mg I.M. q4h PRN pain
   D. Motrin 300 mg P.O.

11. Besides the patient's name and room number and the date the medication order was written, what other information is necessary to complete the order?

12. What is the difference in the time of administration when a medication is to be given q.i.d. versus q6h? Both provide four doses within 24 hours.

Selected References

Abrams, A.C., et al. *Clinical Drug Therapy—Rationales for Nursing Practice.* Philadelphia: J.B. Lippincott Co., 1983.

Bayt, P.T. *Administering Medications.* Indianapolis: Bobbs-Merrill Co., 1982.

Drugs, 2nd ed. Nurse's Reference Library. Springhouse, Pa.: Springhouse Corp., 1984.

Lewis, L.W., *Fundamental Skills in Patient Care*, 3rd ed. Philadelphia: J.B Lippincott Co., 1984.

Weiner, M., and Pepper, G.A. *Clinical Pharmacology and Therapeutics in Nursing*, 2nd ed. New York: McGraw-Hill Book Co., 1985.

Worley, E. *Pharmacology and Medications*, 4th ed. Philadelphia: F.A. Davis Co., 1982.

Calculations and Measurements

The unit dose system, in which the pharmacist dispenses the prescribed amount of medication in individually labeled unit dose packages, eliminates some of the mathematics involved in administering medications. However, even if this system is used in your facility, you will sometimes have to make calculations and conversions yourself. Also, to double-check for accuracy, you will have to know how to calculate a dispensed dose. This chapter discusses the three most often used systems of measurement—the metric, apothecaries', and household systems—and how to make calculations and conversions within the same system and from one system to another.

Measurement systems

The *metric system*—also called the decimal system—is most commonly used because of its accuracy. It includes measures of weight, volume, and length. Any changes of units of measure can be made by multiplying or dividing by 10. (See *Table of Equivalents,* p. 54, for metric weights and volume scales.)

The *apothecaries' system,* an old English method, includes measures of weight and volume and is being replaced by the metric system. However, it is still used by some health care professionals.

The terms *fluidram* and *fluidounce* are usually shortened to *dram* and *ounce,* with the understanding that drugs in liquid form are measured by volume and those in solid form by weight. When symbols are used, quantity is expressed in small Roman numerals placed after the symbol, for example, ii. If a fraction of a measure is ordered, a symbol is not used; instead, the amount is written out with the fraction first, for example, ⅕ ounce. An exception to this is one half, which has its own symbol (s̄s̄). Thus an order for one-half ounce can be written as ℥ s̄s̄ or ½ ounce. (See *Numerical Symbols Commonly Used with the Apothecaries' System.*)

Household measure, the least accurate system, includes measures of weight, volume, and length. It is used only when it is impractical to calculate and measure doses by other systems. This may be the most convenient system for taking medications at home, for example. The household measure system is based on cooking utensils, such as the teaspoon and tablespoon. However, since a household teaspoon may hold from 3 to 8 ml, the American Standards Institute has established these standards:

60 drops (gtt) = 1 teaspoonful
3 teaspoonfuls = 1 tablespoonful
2 tablespoonfuls = 1 fluidounce
8 fluidounces = 1 glassful

Conversions

Setting up a proportion may be the least complex method for converting measures either within the same system or from one system to another. A proportion is made up of two ratios, each indicating the relationship one quantity has to the other. It can be written as whole units or as a fraction:

Calculations and Measurements 53

> **NUMERICAL SYMBOLS COMMONLY USED WITH THE APOTHECARIES' SYSTEM**
>
> | | | | | |
> |---|---|---|---|---|
> | $\overline{ss}$ | = ½ | vi | = | 6 |
> | i | = 1 | vii | = | 7 |
> | ii | = 2 | viii | = | 8 |
> | iii | = 3 | ix | = | 9 |
> | iv | = 4 | x | = | 10 |
> | v | = 5 | xv | = | 15 |
>
> When apothecary symbols are used, the quantity is expressed in lower-case Roman numerals, which are placed after the symbol: gr ii, ℨii, ℨiii. However, when fractions are indicated, or when pt, qt, and gal are written, Arabic numerals are always used: gr ¼, qt 9. The only exception to this rule is the quantity ½, which is expressed as the symbol $\overline{ss}$ (Latin *semi* or *semisis*, meaning half).

$$A : B :: C : D$$
$$2 : 3 :: 4 : 6$$
$$\frac{A}{B} = \frac{C}{D}$$
$$\frac{2}{3} = \frac{4}{6}$$

The first and fourth terms (A and D) are called the extremes, and the second and third terms (B and C) are called the means. The product of the means equals the product of the extremes.

$$A : B :: C : D \qquad \frac{A}{B} = \frac{C}{D}$$
$$2 : 3 :: 4 : 6 \qquad \frac{2}{3} = \frac{4}{6}$$
$$2 \times 6 = 3 \times 4 \qquad 2 \times 6 = 3 \times 4$$
$$12 = 12 \qquad 12 = 12$$

The proportion method can be helpful when one of your terms is unknown (x).
- Keep the unknown quantity on the left, the known on the right.
- Solve the proportion by equating the product of the means to the product of the extremes.
- For the value of x, simply divide the numerical value of the product containing the x into the product on the right of the equation.

Example:
2 : x :: 4 : 6 or

      Unknown   Known

$$\frac{2}{x} = \frac{4}{6}$$
$$4x = 2 \times 6$$
$$4x = 12$$
$$x = 3$$

- You can prove your answer when the problem is solved by substituting it in place of the x:

$$\frac{2}{3} = \frac{4}{6}$$
$$3 \times 4 = 2 \times 6$$
$$12 = 12$$

- When using proportion to solve medication problems, be sure the ratios are expressed in the same units of measure.

In the following practice problems, the proportions are set up as fractions.

Conversion within the same system
Example:
How many milligrams are in 4 grams?

Set up a proportion according to the information given.

$$\frac{g}{mg} = \frac{g}{mg}$$

Step 1: Check *Table of Equivalents* on p. 54 to determine the relationship between grams and milligrams.

$$1\ g = 1{,}000\ mg$$

Step 2:

      Unknown   Known

$$\frac{4\ g}{x\ mg} = \frac{1\ g}{1{,}000\ mg}$$
$$x = 4{,}000\ mg$$

TABLE OF EQUIVALENTS

WEIGHTS

APOTHECARIES'	METRIC	APOTHECARIES'	METRIC
1 ounce =	31.1 g	1/150 grain =	0.4 mg
15 grains =	1 g	1/200 grain =	0.3 mg
1 grain =	60 mg	1/250 grain =	0.25 mg
1/60 grain =	1 mg	1/300 grain =	0.2 mg
1/80 grain =	0.8 mg	1/400 grain =	0.15 mg
1/100 grain =	0.6 mg	1/500 grain =	0.12 mg
1/120 grain =	0.5 mg	1/600 grain =	0.1 mg

LIQUID MEASURE

HOUSEHOLD	APOTHECARIES'	APPROXIMATE METRIC
1 teaspoonful =	1 fluidram	= 5 ml
1 tablespoonful =	4 fluidrams	= 15 ml
2 tablespoonfuls =	1 fluidounce	= 30 ml
1 measuring cupful =	8 fluidounces	= 240 ml
1 pint =	16 fluidounces	= 500 ml
1 quart =	32 fluidounces	= 1,000 ml

TEMPERATURE

Centigrade to Fahrenheit
$(C.° \times 9/5) + 32 = F.°$

Fahrenheit to Centigrade
$(F.° - 32) \times 5/9 = C.°$

METRIC WEIGHT EQUIVALENTS

1 kg	=	1,000 g
1 g	=	1,000 mg
1 mg	=	0.001 g
1 mcg or µg	=	0.001 mg
1,000 mcg or µg	=	1 mg

CONVERSIONS

1 oz	=	28 g
1 lb	=	454 g
2.2 lb	=	1 kg
1 lb	=	0.454 kg

METRIC VOLUME EQUIVALENTS

1 liter	=	1,000 ml
1 deciliter	=	100 ml

Step 3: Prove your answer by substituting 4,000 for x.

$$\frac{4}{4,000} = \frac{1}{1,000}$$

$$4,000 = 4,000$$

Conversion from one system to another
Example:
How many grains are in 4 grams?

Set up a proportion.

$$\frac{\text{metric}}{\text{apothecaries'}} = \frac{\text{metric}}{\text{apothecaries'}}$$

Step 1: Check *Table of Equivalents* to determine the relationship between grains and grams.

$$15 \text{ gr} = 1 \text{ g}$$

Step 2:

$$\begin{array}{cc} \text{Unknown} & \text{Known} \\ \dfrac{4 \text{ g}}{x \text{ gr}} = & \dfrac{1 \text{ g}}{15 \text{ gr}} \end{array}$$

$$x = 60 \text{ gr}$$

Step 3: Prove your answer by substituting 60 for x.

Calculations and Measurements   55

$$\frac{4}{60} = \frac{1}{15}$$

$$60 = 60$$

Since reference tables are not always available, you should memorize at least the following approximate equivalents:

$$1 \text{ g} = \text{gr xv (15 grains)}$$
$$1 \text{ gr (gr i)} = 0.06 \text{ g or } 60 \text{ mg}$$

In the apothecaries' system, tablets and capsules are usually available in ½, 1, 1½, 5, or 7½ grains. Therefore, the preferable equivalent is one that provides an answer in terms of an available form.

Example:
How many grains are in 0.3 grams?

If you use the equivalent 1 g = gr xv, then 0.3 g = gr iv$\overline{\text{ss}}$, a dosage form that is not available.

Unknown		Known
$\frac{g}{gr}$	=	$\frac{g}{gr}$
$\frac{0.3 \text{ g}}{x \text{ gr}}$	=	$\frac{1 \text{ g}}{15 \text{ gr}}$
x	=	4.5 gr or gr iv$\overline{\text{ss}}$

However, if you use the equivalent gr i = 0.06 g, then 0.3 g = gr
$$x = 5 \text{ grains or gr v}$$

Drug calculations

Tablets or capsules
You can determine the number of tablets required for a specific amount of medication in two steps:

Within the same system
Example:
How many ampicillin capsules containing 250 mg each do you need to give 1 gram?

Step 1: Convert the amount desired and the size of the tablet on hand into a common unit.

$$1 \text{ g} = 1,000 \text{ mg}$$

Step 2: Set up a proportion.

$$\frac{\text{mg}}{\text{capsules}} = \frac{\text{mg}}{\text{capsules}}$$

Unknown		Known
$\frac{1,000 \text{ mg}}{x \text{ capsules}}$	=	$\frac{250 \text{ mg}}{1 \text{ capsule}}$
250 x	=	1,000
x	=	4 capsules

From one system to another
Example:
The physician ordered gr i$\overline{\text{ss}}$ of a medication. The tablets available are 0.2 grams each. How many tablets should you give?

Step 1: Convert size of the tablet on hand and amount desired into a common unit.

$$1 \text{ g} = 15 \text{ gr}$$

$$\frac{g}{gr} = \frac{g}{gr}$$

$$\frac{0.2 \text{ g}}{x \text{ gr}} = \frac{1 \text{ g}}{15 \text{ gr}}$$

$$x = 0.2 \times 15$$

$$x = 3 \text{ gr in each tablet}$$

Step 2: Set up a proportion according to the information given.

$$\frac{\text{gr}}{\text{tablets}} = \frac{\text{gr}}{\text{tablets}}$$

Unknown		Known
$\frac{1.5 \text{ gr}}{x \text{ tablets}}$	=	$\frac{3 \text{ gr}}{1 \text{ tablet}}$
3 x	=	1.5
x	=	0.5 or ½ tablet

Drugs in oral solution
Medications in dry form, such as crystals and powders, must first be weighed and then mixed into a solution. You are responsible for giving the volume of solution that contains (by weight) the amount of drug ordered for the patient. Oral solutions are prepared in many different concentrations. Therefore, double-check the prescribed con-

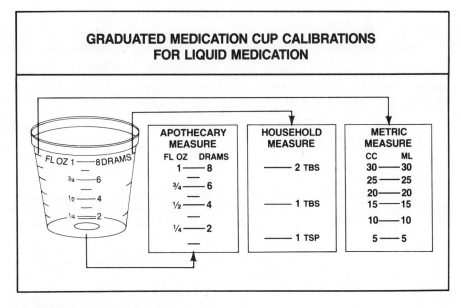

centration and then read the label carefully to determine the amount of drug according to volume. This information will always be indicated on the drug label.

One-ounce containers, such as the medicine cup, are generally used for administering oral medications. Most of these are calibrated in the three commonly used systems of measurement—metric, apothecaries', and household. (See *Graduated Medication Cup Calibrations for Liquid Medication.*) For measuring smaller units, minim glasses, medicine droppers, or syringes without needles may be used.

Calculating oral solutions

The method for calculating oral solutions is the same as for any other medication problem.

Example 1:
The physician ordered phenobarbital elixir gr xv. On hand is a bottle labeled 1 g/dram. How much medication should you give?

Step 1: Convert amount desired and solution on hand into a common unit.

$$1 \text{ g} = \text{gr xv}$$

Step 2: Set up a proportion.

$$\frac{\text{drug}}{\text{solution}} = \frac{\text{drug}}{\text{solution}}$$

$$\textit{Unknown} \quad \textit{Known}$$

$$\frac{15 \text{ gr}}{x\, \overline{\jmath}} = \frac{15 \text{ gr}}{1\, \overline{\jmath}}$$

$$15\, x = 15$$

$$x = \overline{\jmath}\, i$$

Example 2:
The physician ordered gr v of Tylenol (acetaminophen) elixir. On hand is a bottle labeled 120 mg/5 ml. How much medication should you give?

Step 1: Convert amount desired and solution on hand into a common unit.

$$\text{gr i} = 60 \text{ mg}$$

$$\text{gr v} = 300 \text{ mg}$$

Step 2: Set up a proportion according to the information given.

$$\frac{\text{drug}}{\text{solution}} = \frac{\text{drug}}{\text{solution}}$$

$$\frac{Unknown}{300 \text{ mg}} = \frac{Known}{120 \text{ mg}}$$
$$\frac{300 \text{ mg}}{x \text{ ml}} = \frac{120 \text{ mg}}{5 \text{ ml}}$$
$$120 \text{ x} = 1{,}500$$
$$x = 12.5 \text{ ml}$$

Solutions in vials or ampules
Ampules and vials of medication (in solution, crystals, or powder) are used for intradermal, subcutaneous, I.M., and I.V. injections.

Drugs already in solution
For drugs that are already in solution, simply calculate dosage the same way you do for oral solutions.
Example 1:
The physician ordered pentobarbital gr iss I.M. On hand is a multiple dose vial containing 40 mg/ml. How much medication should you give?

Step 1: Convert amount desired and solution on hand into a common unit.

$$\text{gr i} = 60 \text{ mg}$$
$$\text{gr iss} = 90 \text{ mg}$$

Step 2: Set up a proportion according to the information given.

$$\frac{\text{drug}}{\text{solution}} = \frac{\text{drug}}{\text{solution}}$$

$$\frac{Unknown}{\frac{90 \text{ mg}}{x \text{ ml}}} = \frac{Known}{\frac{40 \text{ mg}}{1 \text{ ml}}}$$

$$40 \text{ x} = 90$$
$$x = 2.25 \text{ ml}$$

Example 2:
The physician ordered Thorazine (chlorpromazine) 15 mg I.M. stat. On hand is a multiple dose vial containing 25 mg/ml. How much medication should you give your patient?

Step 1: No conversion necessary.

Step 2: Set up a proportion according to the information available.

$$\frac{\text{drug}}{\text{solution}} = \frac{\text{drug}}{\text{solution}}$$

$$\frac{Unknown}{\frac{15 \text{ mg}}{x \text{ ml}}} = \frac{Known}{\frac{25 \text{ mg}}{1 \text{ ml}}}$$

$$25 \text{ x} = 15$$
$$x = \frac{15}{25}$$
$$x = \text{⅗ ml or } 0.6 \text{ ml}$$

Drugs that require reconstitution
Certain medications that are given parenterally, such as some antibiotics, are unstable in solution and therefore are packaged in crystal or powder form. Directions for reconstituting are usually packaged with the medication; follow any specific directions included.

With multiple dose vials, if not otherwise specified, dissolve the medication in the amount of solution necessary to make 1 ml equal to the desired dose. Use this formula only when the amount of medication does not increase the amount of solution.

When the medication increases the amount of solution, follow the specific directions for the amount of diluent to be added. They will be packaged with the medication.
Example:
A vial contains 3 million units of aqueous penicillin G in dry powder. Your patient has an order for 300,000 units. How much sterile water would you add to the vial if specific directions have not been included by the manufacturer?

Set up a proportion with the information available.

$$\frac{\text{drug}}{\text{solution}} = \frac{\text{drug}}{\text{solution}}$$

$$\frac{Unknown}{\frac{3{,}000{,}000 \text{ units}}{x \text{ ml}}} = \frac{Known}{\frac{300{,}000 \text{ units}}{1 \text{ ml}}}$$

$$300{,}000 \text{ x} = 3{,}000{,}000$$

x = 10 ml added to the vial so that each ml contains 300,000 units

Generally, directions for adding the correct amount of solution to make a specific concentration will be included with the medication. For a drug like penicillin for injection, several concentrations can be produced from the same vial of powder by adding different quantities of solution.

Example:
Penicillin G sodium for injection can be reconstituted as follows:

Amount of diluent to be added	Concentration made
23 ml	200,000 units/ml
18 ml	250,000 units/ml
8 ml	500,000 units/ml
3 ml	1,000,000 units/ml

Insulin in a tuberculin syringe

Insulin is dispensed in different strengths indicating the number of units of insulin in 1 ml of solution. For example, U-40 has 40 units in every milliliter, and U-100 has 100 units in every milliliter.

The most accurate way to administer insulin is to use an insulin syringe calibrated in units per milliliter. Syringes are available in the scale U-100 as well as U-40. To draw up the correct dosage, use correlating insulin vials and syringes. When an insulin syringe is not available, you may use a tuberculin syringe. Since you know the strength of insulin you are using (for example, U-40 contains 40 units/ml), use the formula for calculating any other parenteral medication.

Example:
You have an order to give 20 units of U-40 insulin, but you do not have an insulin syringe. How much medication must be given?

Set up a proportion using the information available.

$$\frac{\text{units}}{\text{ml}} = \frac{\text{units}}{\text{ml}}$$

Unknown   *Known*

$$\frac{20 \text{ units}}{x \text{ ml}} = \frac{40 \text{ units}}{1 \text{ ml}}$$

$40 x = 20$

$x = 0.5 \text{ ml}$

Review Questions

1. How many milligrams are in 1 grain?

2. How many grains are in 1 gram?

3. How many micrograms are in 1 mg?

4. How many drops are in 1 teaspoon?

5. How many grains are in 0.4 mg?

6. How many milligrams are in 1/60 grain?

7. How many grams are in 7½ grains?

8. How many grains are in 150 mg?

9. How many grams would you give if the order is 15 mg of Valium?

10. How many milligrams of phenobarbital would you give if the order is 2 gr?

11. How many scored tablets of 100 mg each would you need to give 250 mg?

12. The physician orders 600 mg of drug to be given. The dosage form on hand is gr x tablets. How many tablets would you give?

13. The physician orders gr xv of drug to be given. If there are 7½ gr per 5 ml, how many teaspoons would you give?

14. If the physician has ordered 200,000 units of drug be given and the concentration of the drug on hand is 300,000 units per ml, how much would you draw up?

15. If you were asked to give 20 mg of a drug from a 10-ml vial containing 50 mg per ml, how much would you draw up?

16. If a vial contains 3 million units of an antibiotic in dry form, and you need to give 600,000 units, how much diluent would you add if specific directions have not been included by the manufacturer?

17. Using the same medication in the concentration you have prepared in question 16, how much would you draw up if the dose to be given were decreased to 300,000 units?

18. If you were asked to give 250 mg from a 10-ml vial labeled "0.5 g per ml," how much would you draw up?

19. To give 10 units of U-40 insulin in a tuberculin syringe, how much would you draw up?

20. To give 32 units of U-40 insulin in a tuberculin syringe, how much would you draw up?

Selected References

Dison, N. *Simplified Drugs and Solutions for Nurses, Including Arithmetic*, 8th ed. St. Louis: C.V. Mosby Co., 1983.

Drugs, 2nd ed. Nurse's Reference Library. Springhouse, Pa.: Springhouse Corp., 1984.

Keane, C.B., and Fletcher, S.M. *Drugs and Solutions: A Programmed Introduction*, 4th ed. Philadelphia: W.B. Saunders Co., 1980.

McHenry, R.W., ed. *Self-Teaching Tests in Arithmetic for Nurses*, 10th ed. St. Louis: C.V. Mosby Co., 1980.

Nursing87 Drug Handbook. Springhouse, Pa.: Springhouse Corp., 1987.

Richardson, L.I., and Richardson, J.K. *The Mathematics of Drugs and Solutions with Clinical Applications*. New York: McGraw-Hill Book Co., 1984.

Preparation and Administration Guidelines

Guidelines for preparing and administering medications and specific considerations in preparing oral and parenteral medications are covered in this chapter. Documentation is viewed as the final step in medication administration and is covered last.

General guidelines

- Administer no medication, not even a placebo, without a physician's order. Verbal orders should be taken only in emergencies, and then with extreme care to ensure accuracy. Such orders must follow established institutional policy.
- Avoid using the patient's own medications. Use them only if the physician writes an appropriate order on the chart and the pharmacy cannot obtain the drugs. All such drugs must first be identified by a pharmacist. If they cannot be identified, they must not be used. Most facilities also have a policy about this.
- Know why every drug you administer has been prescribed, its usual dosage range, its expected action, and its possible adverse reactions.
- When storing drugs, keep preparations designed only for external use separate from those designed for internal use. Insist that the pharmacist affix "external use only" labels on containers of topical medications. Make sure the pharmacist uses appropriate auxiliary labels on eye and ear medications.
- Keep narcotics and other controlled substances under double lock.
- Remember that names of different drugs may have similar spellings. Check each name very carefully. Never identify an item merely by its container, appearance, or customary shelf location. Check labels for expiration date. If a bottle has no label, return it to the pharmacy.
- Do not give medication that is discolored or in which a precipitate has formed unless the manufacturer's instructions indicate that doing so is not harmful. If in doubt, ask the pharmacist or check the manufacturer's directions.
- Always tightly replace the cap on any bottle of medication you open.
- Never leave desiccant capsules in a bottle. Discard them to avoid giving them to patients inadvertently.
- Never leave medications at a patient's bedside, except—on physician's orders—antacids, various lotions and ointments, nitroglycerin, and other medications that patients are permitted to self-administer. In these cases, make sure the patient understands proper use of the medication, and monitor carefully.

Preparing and administering medications

- Always wash your hands thoroughly before preparing or administering medications.
- Do not administer medications prepared by someone else. The nurse who administers the medication is responsible for errors.
- When preparing medications, guard against interruptions. If you have any doubt about a dose calculation or physical appearance or name of a drug, ask the pharmacist, check a proper drug reference, or double-check calculations with another nurse.

- Do not hold tablets or capsules in your hands.
- Administer medications as close as possible to the time prescribed. Be especially punctual when administering antibiotics, chemotherapeutic agents, and other drugs that must be maintained at a particular level in the blood.

If any medication is not given as scheduled, record the reason in the nurses' notes, and report it to the pharmacist.

- Check the name of the patient, his room number, and his bed number on his wristband. This is the only way to be certain of the patient's identity. Then address him by name.
- Tell the patient the name and purpose of the medication you are about to give. If the medication is new, take the time to explain what it is and why the physician ordered it.
- Always recheck the medication order when a patient expresses doubt or concern about the medication you are going to give him. There is *no* margin for error in administering drugs. Always go out of your way to make certain that you are giving the *right dose* of the *right medication* to the *right patient* at the *right time* by the *right route*.
- If a patient refuses to take his medication, try to find out why. In many cases, after you explain what the medication is and how it will help him, the patient will take the dose.
- If the patient still refuses, report this to the charge nurse and the physician and record the patient's reason for refusing the medication in the nurses' notes. Discard the medication, except in a unit dose system. In that case, return the medication in its wrapper or container, along with proper documentation, to the pharmacy.
- Always record the dose after giving medication to each patient to avoid errors of omission.

Special considerations with a unit dose system
- If you are using a unit dose system, administer one patient's medications at a time. Never enter a room with more than one patient's medications.
- Compare the dose on the label against the medication administration record.
- If you need more than one or two dosage units (tablets, capsules, or ampules) to pre-

---

MEDICATION IDENTIFICATION CHECKS

Before administering any drug, perform *three* identification checks. Check the name, dose, and route of administration on the label:
- when taking the drug container from the shelf or cart bin
- before pouring the medication
- after pouring the medication.

---

pare a single dose, question the order. Unless you are absolutely familiar with this need, check with a pharmacist before administering the dose. Something could be wrong. If large numbers of tablets or capsules are necessary, the pharmacist might be able to prepare a more convenient dosage form; for example, with the physician's approval, the pharmacist may dispense the oral solution of furosemide (Lasix).

Preparing oral medications

Pouring tablets and capsules
Preparing and administering oral medications requires clean, not sterile, technique. Wash your hands before pouring medications, and perform the three identification checks when removing tablets or capsules from stock bottles or cart bins.

To remove medication from a stock bottle, remove the lid and tap out the desired number of tablets or capsules into the lid. Then transfer the medication from the lid to a medication cup. Never return unwanted tablets or capsules to the stock bottle from the medication cup. This increases the possibility of returning a medication to the wrong bottle or contaminating the stock supply.

If the unit dose system is being used, do not remove drugs from packages until you are at the patient's bedside and he is ready to take the medication. Instead, place unopened packages in a medication cup after performing the three identification checks. These steps ensure the drug's identification and its returnability if it is refused.

ADMINISTERING MEDICATION TO AN ISOLATION PATIENT

- Review the isolation procedure for the specific type of isolation.
- Prepare yourself to enter the patient's room.
  In *reverse* isolation, the patient is to be protected. Wear a gown, mask, and gloves.
  In *strict* isolation, everyone entering the room is to be protected. Wear a gown, mask, and gloves.
  In *respiratory* isolation, everyone entering the room is to be protected from airborne bacteria inhaled into the lungs. Wear a mask.
- Carry the medication into the room in a medication cup. Do not bring a medication tray or cart into the room.
- If possible, use a disposable syringe to give an injection. When a cartridge injection system has to be used, the syringe should be kept in the room and must be cleaned properly before removing it from the room. Once removed from the room, it should be sterilized before reuse with other patients.
- If the patient is able, have him assume a comfortable position for taking the medication and ask him to pour his own glass of water. Assist him only if necessary.
- Give the patient the medication and remain with him until he has taken it.
- Offer information about the medication and answer any questions before leaving the room.
- Remove the gown, mask, and gloves according to institutional policy.
- Wash your hands using proper technique before leaving the room.

For any regimen that requires patient assessment before administering a drug, place the medication in a separate cup in case it must be withheld. For example, digoxin must be withheld if the patient's pulse rate is below 60 beats per minute.

Place sublingual and buccal medications in a separate cup so they will not be given orally by mistake.

Mixing medications with food or beverages
Sometimes a patient has difficulty swallowing medications or medications must be given through a gastrostomy or nasogastric tube. If the drug is unavailable in liquid form, a tablet may be crushed or a capsule opened and the medication mixed with a beverage or a small amount of soft food. However, check a drug reference or ask a pharmacist before doing this to be sure the drug's action will not be affected.

While most tablets can be crushed and mixed with food or beverages, *never* crush a sustained-release or enteric-coated tablet. The special coating on these tablets is designed to ensure proper absorption at the right time, in the right place. If you crush a sustained-release tablet, the entire dose is available for absorption all at once rather than over a period of hours. A drug overdose could result. Similarly, crushing an enteric-coated tablet destroys the drug's protective coating. As a result, the drug will dissolve in the stomach instead of in the small intestine, possibly causing gastric irritation or even vomiting.

Sustained-release *capsules* may be opened, but the contents must be mixed carefully since vigorous mixing can break up the beads that control the absorption rate of the active ingredients. Also, the patient should not chew more than necessary. (See *Drugs That May Not Be Crushed or Mixed Vigorously.*)

Tablets may be crushed by:
- using a mortar and pestle
- crushing between two paper medication cups with the pestle handle
- crushing the unit dose package with a hard object.

Wipe off the mortar and pestle before and after using them. Doing so prevents drug errors due to particles left on the equip-

DRUGS THAT MAY NOT BE CRUSHED OR MIXED VIGOROUSLY

Drug manufacturers may use these designations to indicate the sustained-release drug form:

Dura-Tabs	Gyrocaps	Spansules
Extentabs	Repetabs	Tembids
Gradumets	Sequels	

When attached to a drug name, these words and abbreviations indicate the sustained-release form:

Bd	LA	Span
CR	Plateau Cap	SR
Dur	SA	

Because of a peculiarity in their makeup, these drugs should not be mixed or crushed:

Azo-Mandelamine*	Povan Filmseals*
Depakote*	Pronestyl-SR*
Doraphyl*	Pyridium
Ery-Tab*	Ritalin SR
Eskalith CR*	Theoclear LA*
Inderal LA	Zorprin*
Mandelamine	
Micro-K Extencaps	
Nitrostat SR	
Norpace CR	

Do not crush enteric-coated and sustained-release tablets or vigorously mix sustained-release capsules. Here are some examples:

Aminodur Dura-Tabs*	E-Mycin	Procan SR*
Artane Sequels	Feosol Spansules*	Quibron-T/SR*
Azulfidine En-Tabs*	Indocin SR*	Quinaglute Dura-Tabs
Bayer Timed-Release Aspirin	Isordil Tembids	Quinidex Extentabs
	Kaon-Cl*	Slo-Phyllin Gyrocaps*
Chlor-Trimeton Repetabs*	Klotrix*	Slow-K
Combid Spansules	K-Tab*	Tedral SA
Compazine Spansules*	Modane	Theo-Dur
Desoxyn Gradumets*	Nicobid*	Theolair-SR*
Diamox Sequels	Nitro-Bid Plateau Caps*	Theophyl-SR*
Dimetane Extentabs	Nitrospan*	Thorazine Spansules*
Dimetapp Extentabs*	Ornade Spansules*	Trilafon Repetabs
Donnatal Extentabs	Pavabid Plateau Caps*	Valrelease*
Drixoral	Peritrate SA	
Dulcolax	Peritrate with phenobarbital SA	
Ecotrin		
Elixophyllin SR	Polaramine Repetabs	

*Not available in Canada.

ment. Also, remove as much of the crushed medication as possible from the equipment and include the particles in the dosage to ensure it is correct.

Crushed tablets or capsule contents are commonly mixed with a small amount of applesauce, ice cream, or pudding. Liquid medications are commonly mixed with juice, water, or soda. Food or beverages from the patient's meal tray, the unit refrigerator, or home may be used. Make sure the patient eats or drinks the *entire* mixture to ensure he receives the entire dose.

Measuring liquid medications
In a medication cup
Include the three identification checks with the following steps in this order:
- Uncap the bottle and place the cap topside down so the inside of the cap remains clean.
- Hold the medication cup at eye level and locate the correct marking.
- Hold the bottle so the label faces the palm of your hand to prevent dribbles from obscuring the label.

TYPES OF LIQUID MEDICATIONS AND NURSING CONSIDERATIONS

Type	Description	Nursing Considerations
Syrup	• A drug and preservative in a viscous, sugar/water solution, usually flavored	• When giving a syrup for a demulcent (soothing) effect, do not follow it with water. Tell the patient to sip the syrup slowly. • When giving a syrup for a systemic effect, you may dilute it. However, dilute only the dose being given. If you dilute the entire bottle, you may destroy the preservative and hasten contamination or decomposition. • Use caution when administering syrups to diabetic patients. Check with the pharmacist to see if a sugar-free syrup is available. • When giving syrups with other drugs, be sure to administer syrups *last*.
Suspension	• *Magma:* a thick, milky suspension of an insoluble (or partly soluble) inorganic drug, suspended in water • *Gel:* the same as magma but with smaller drug particles • *Emulsion:* droplets of fat or oil, suspended in water	• Always shake a suspension thoroughly before giving it. • If desired, you may dilute most suspensions with water before administration. However, do not dilute an *antacid* suspension, or it will not coat the stomach effectively.
Alcoholic solution	• *Elixir:* a clear mixture of a drug, alcohol, water, and sugar; sweet-tasting, but not as sweet or viscous as syrups (Alcohol concentration ranges from 8% to 78%.)	• Check the solution carefully. Never administer one that has precipitate at the bottom of the bottle. • If you want to dilute the solution, use only a small amount of water. More water could cause the drug to precipitate.

(continued)

TYPES OF LIQUID MEDICATIONS AND NURSING CONSIDERATIONS *(continued)*

Type	Description	Nursing Considerations
Alcoholic solution *(continued)*	• *Spirits:* a solution of volatile substances, for example, liquids, solids, or gases; the alcohol in the solution acts as a preservative and solvent; the solution is used primarily as a flavoring agent • *Tincture:* a solution of alcohol, or alcohol and water, with animal or vegetable products or chemical substances • *Fluidextract:* a bitter solution of vegetable drugs, usually sweetened with a syrup or flavoring; rarely prescribed, because fluidextracts are unusually potent as well as unpleasant tasting; the alcohol in the solution acts as a solvent or a preservative, or both	• Consult the pharmacist before you mix alcoholic solutions with liquids other than water. Mixing with other liquids may be contraindicated. • Follow administration with water, unless the solution is being given for cough relief. • Store the solution in an airtight container. Protect it from temperature extremes. Protect fluidextracts from light. • Use these solutions cautiously if your patient is an alcoholic. *Important:* Never give an alcoholic solution to a patient receiving Antabuse.
Reconstituted powders and tablets	• Solid drugs reconstituted with water (or another suitable liquid) and given to the patient in suspension or solution form	• Read the directions carefully before reconstituting powders and tablets. Do not use too much water with effervescent tablets or they will boil out of the glass. • Some powders will become gelatinous very quickly after you mix them. Administer them immediately after reconstitution. • Wait until effervescent tablets dissolve completely before you give them to a patient. Give without further dilution.

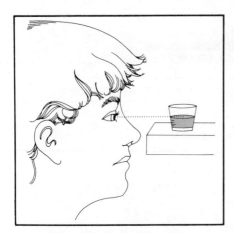

- Pour the desired amount into the cup.
- Recheck the dosage poured. Set the cup on a level surface and check it at eye level. Looking up or down at the medication level can give you an incorrect reading.
- Read the medication level at the *bottom* of the meniscus. If too much medication has been poured into the cup, discard the excess. Never return it to the bottle.
- Wipe the bottle lip with a damp paper towel, taking care not to touch the inside of the bottle.

If a medication is to be measured in *drops*, use a medicine dropper held at a 90° angle over the cup. This makes it easier to see and count each drop. Use only the dropper that comes with the medicine.

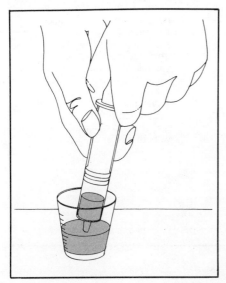

In a syringe
If a patient is unable to drink from a cup, a liquid medication can be measured and given with a syringe.
- Select a syringe based on the size of the dose.
- Pour the prescribed amount of medication into a medicine cup and withdraw the medicine from the cup with the syringe.
- Then hold the syringe upright at eye level with the needle up and read the measurement from the *top* edge of the rubber stopper. If you have withdrawn too much, squirt the excess into a sink or wastebasket. Do not return it to the bottle.

Preparing parenteral medications

Use of sterile technique
Sterile technique must be followed when preparing or administering medication for injection. Doing so prevents the introduction of a pathogen into body tissue, which

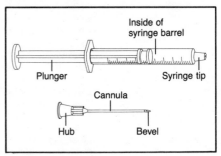

could cause local or systemic infection. The hub of the needle may be touched, but the needle cannula, the syringe plunger, the inside of the syringe barrel, and the syringe tip must remain sterile. If these areas become contaminated, the needle or syringe must be replaced.

Selecting a syringe
The size of the syringe is determined by the amount of solution to be injected. Syringes are available in 1-ml, 3-ml, 5-ml, 10-ml, 20-ml, and 50-ml sizes. The most commonly used syringe is the 3-ml size. Small doses of medication are most accurately measured in the 1-ml size. Insulin syringes calibrated in units instead of milliliters are also available to measure insulin.

CHOOSING THE RIGHT NEEDLE

Injection Route	Site	Common Needle Sizes	Standard Amount Injected
Intradermal	Skin	26G ⅜" (0.95 cm)	0.01 to 0.1 ml
Subcutaneous	Subcutaneous fat beneath layers of skin	25G to 27G ½" to 1" (1.27 to 2.54 cm)	0.5 to 2 ml
I.M.	Mid-deltoid	23G to 25G ⅝" to 1" (1.59 to 2.54 cm)	0.5 to 2 ml
	Gluteus medius (dorsogluteal)	20G to 23G 1½" to 3" (3.81 to 7.62 cm)	1 to 5 ml
	Gluteus medius and minimus (ventrogluteal)	20G to 23G 1½" to 3" (3.81 to 7.62 cm)	1 to 5 ml
	Vastus lateralis (preferred site for infants and children)	*Infants and children:* 22G to 25G ⅝" to 1" (1.59 to 2.54 cm) *Adults:* 20G to 23G 1½" (3.81 cm)	1 to 5 ml
	Rectus femoris (alternate site for infants)	22G to 25G ½" to 1" (1.27 to 2.54 cm)	1 to 3 ml
I.V.	Basilic and cephalic veins	25G ⅝" (1.59 cm) for slow injections; 19G to 23G 1" to 1½" (2.54 to 3.81 cm)	0.5 to 50 ml

Choosing the right needle

Needle choice is determined by injection site and type and amount of medication to be given. For intramuscular (I.M.) injections, muscle mass and amount of subcutaneous tissue covering the muscle are also factors. Select the shortest needle with the smallest gauge to minimize patient discomfort and facilitate medication administration.

Needle length is determined by the depth of the injection and the amount of subcutaneous tissue present. A 2" or 3" needle may be required to deliver medication into the gluteus medius muscle of an obese person, but a 1½" needle may reach the muscle mass in a slender person.

The gauge (width of the opening) of the needle is determined by the viscosity of the medication that must pass through it. The smaller the gauge number, the larger the needle opening. Large-diameter needles are reserved for injecting thick or oily medications (usually 20G) or for I.V. use (18G or 19G).

Using a prefilled syringe

When the unit dose medication system is being used, the pharmacist fills a syringe with the prescribed medication; it is then placed in the patient's cart bin. The prefilled syringe is labeled with the patient's name, room number, and contents. You must add the appropriate needle.

Filling a syringe

When filling a syringe, perform the three identification checks to minimize drug error. Read the label:
- as you select the medication
- before drawing it up
- after drawing it up.

Add 0.2 cc of air to the syringe for all I.M. injections. When the syringe is inverted during the injection, the air bubble rises to the plunger end of the syringe and follows the medication into the injection site. *The air clears the needle of medication and helps prevent leakage into the subcutaneous tissue following injection by creating an air block that reduces reflux (tracking) along the needle path.*

Cover the needle with its protective guard until the injection is to be given.

Withdrawing from an ampule

- Tap the top of the ampule with your fingernail to release any medication trapped there. This is important since ampules usually contain enough medication for only one dose.
- Wrap the neck of the ampule with a piece of gauze to protect your fingers from being cut.
- Hold the body of the ampule in one hand and the top between the thumb and finger of your other hand.
- With the ampule in an upright position, snap off the top. Inspect the solution for small particles of glass. Discard the solution if any are present.
- Insert the needle into the ampule, being careful not to touch the rim of the glass. Institutional policy may require the use of a filter needle.
- Withdraw the medication by pulling back on the plunger, and remove the needle without touching the rim.
- Discard any remaining medication since the sterility of the solution cannot be maintained.

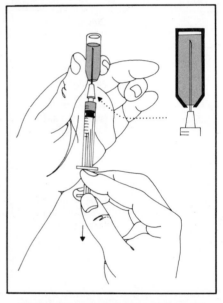

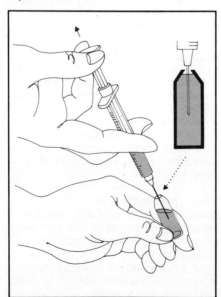

An ampule may also be inverted to withdraw medication. Place the needle inside it and then invert it, keeping the tip of the needle in solution at all times. If the tip does not remain in solution, medication will leave the container.

Withdrawing from a vial

- Clean the stopper with an alcohol sponge pad.
- Pull back on the syringe plunger until the amount of air in the barrel equals the exact amount of medication you want to withdraw from the vial.
- Insert the needle at an angle into the center of the vial stopper. This prevents coring, or the cutting away of pieces of rubber.

RECONSTITUTING POWDERED MEDICATION

To reconstitute a powdered medication you will need the medication, a vial of compatible diluent, an 18G needle and syringe, and an alcohol sponge. After you have assembled the equipment, remove the protective cap from the diluent vial and swab the stopper with alcohol. Then, follow these steps:

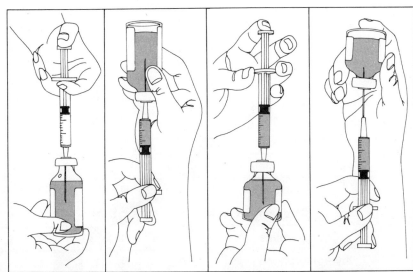

1. Inject air equal to the recommended amount of diluent into the vial, as shown here.

2. Then, draw up the recommended amount of diluent into the needle and syringe.

3. Swab the medication bottle's stopper, and inject the diluent into the bottle.

4. Mix the medication and diluent, then draw up the reconstituted medication.

Also, always use a small, thin needle (25G 1″) with a multidose vial. A small puncture reseals better, thereby reducing the risk of solution contamination.
• Inject the air. This creates pressure, which will make it easy to withdraw the medication. If no air is added to the vial, a vacuum is created and it will be hard or impossible to withdraw medication. If too much air is added to a vial, pressure inside the vial will increase and the solution will be forced into the syringe.
• Invert the vial and withdraw the medication.
• Remove the needle from the vial and check for excess air in the syringe. Remove excess air by pointing the needle up, tapping the side of the syringe if necessary, and pushing the plunger.

Reconstituting powdered medication
Some medications for parenteral use come in powdered or crystal form and must be reconstituted into a solution before being given. These medications must be dissolved in a correct diluent, such as sterile isotonic saline solution or bacteriostatic water. If the entire amount of medication in a vial is to be administered, add enough diluent to dissolve the medication—at least 1 to 2 ml. This amount will vary with the type and amount of medication contained in the vial or ampule. Directions for reconstituting are usually packaged with the medication; follow any specific directions included.

If several doses will be taken from the same vial, dissolve the medication in the amount of solution necessary to make 1 ml

COMPATIBILITY TABLE OF DRUGS COMBINED IN A SYRINGE

KEY
- **Y** Compatible
- **N** Not compatible
- **P** Provisionally compatible; use within 15 minutes of preparation
- **?** Conflicting reports on compatibility; mixing not recommended

(A blank space indicates no available data on compatibility.)

	atropine	butorphanol	chlorpromazine	codeine	diazepam	glycopyrrolate	hydromorphone	hydroxyzine	meperidine
atropine		P	P		N	Y	P	P	P
butorphanol	P		P		N	Y		Y	P
chlorpromazine	P	P			N	Y	P	P	P
codeine					N	Y		Y	
diazepam	N	N	N	N		N	N	N	N
glycopyrrolate	Y	Y	Y	Y	N		Y	Y	Y
hydromorphone	P		P		N	Y		P	
hydroxyzine	P	Y	P	Y	N	Y	P		P
meperidine	P	P	P		N	Y		P	
morphine	P	P	P		N	Y		P	N
nalbuphine	Y				N			Y	
pentobarbital	P	N	N	N	N	N	P	N	N
phenobarbital					N			N	
promethazine	P	Y	P		N	P	P	P	P
scopolamine	P	P	P		N	Y	P	P	P
secobarbital					N	N			
sodium bicarbonate					N	N			
thiopental			N		N	N			N

© 1987 by Springhouse Corporation

morphine	nalbuphine	pentobarbital	phenobarbital	promethazine	scopolamine	secobarbital	sodium bicarbonate	thiopental	
P	Y	P		P	P				atropine
P		N		Y	P				butorphanol
P		N		P	P			N	chlorpromazine
									codeine
N	N	N	N	N	N	N	N	N	diazepam
Y		N		Y	Y	N	N	N	glycopyrrolate
		P		P	P				hydromorphone
P	Y	N	N	P	P				hydroxyzine
N		N		P	P				meperidine
		?		?	P				morphine
		N		Y	Y				nalbuphine
?	N			N	P		Y	P	pentobarbital
									phenobarbital
?	Y	N			P			N	promethazine
P	Y	P		P				P	scopolamine
									secobarbital
		Y						N	sodium bicarbonate
N		P		N	P		N		thiopental

PREPARING CHEMOTHERAPEUTIC DRUGS FOR ADMINISTRATION

The following information is to protect the patient from a possible drug error that could be lethal and to protect you from possible long-term effects in handling cytotoxic agents.
- Verify the medication order on the cardex with the physician's order on the chart.
- Review the package insert regarding considerations in preparing the drug.
- Calculate the dose and have someone else check your results.
- Wear gloves and glasses or goggles while drawing up the medication. A gown can also be worn.
- Hold the vial so your hand is between the vial's stopper and your face in case the needle separates or the vial cracks.
- Using adhesive tape, label the syringe with the patient's name and room number and the drug's name and dose so it can be checked again before being given to the patient.

equal to the desired dose. Use this formula only when the amount of medication does not increase the amount of solution. When the medication increases the amount of solution, follow the directions packaged with the medication for the amount of diluent to be added.

Some medications are packaged by the manufacturer in "mix-o-vials," which contain the diluent in a sealed compartment within the neck of the vial. To make the solution, simply push the rubber stopper to remove the seal and then gently shake the vial.

After reconstituting a medication in a multidose vial, be sure you double-check the prescribed concentration, label it with the amount/ml as soon as it is prepared, and refrigerate the drug as required. Also, label the *date* and *time* that you reconstituted it and add your initials. If it is not labeled, you have no way of knowing the concentration or expiration date of the solution.

Combining drugs in a syringe
Combining two drugs in one syringe avoids the discomfort of two separate injections. Usually, drugs can be mixed in a syringe in one of three ways. They may be combined from two multidose vials, from one multidose vial and one ampule, or from two ampules. Such combinations are contraindicated when the combined doses exceed the amount of solution that can be absorbed from a single site or when the drugs are incompatible (see *Compatibility Table of Drugs Combined in a Syringe*, pp. 70 and 71).

Never combine two drugs if you are unsure of their compatibility. Although drug incompatibility often causes a visible reaction, such as clouding, bubbling, or precipitation, some incompatible combinations produce no visible reactions even though the chemical nature and action of the drugs are altered. Check appropriate references or with a pharmacist when you are unsure about specific compatibility. Never try to combine more than two drugs in one syringe.

Some medications are compatible for only a brief time after being combined and should be administered within 15 minutes after mixing. After this time, environmental factors—such as temperature, exposure to light, and humidity—may alter compatibility.

When using a *cartridge injection* system and a multidose vial, a separate needle and syringe are used to inject the air into the multidose vial. This prevents possible contamination of the multidose vial.

Mixing drugs from two multidose vials
- Using an alcohol sponge, wipe the rubber stopper on the first vial.
- Pull back the plunger until the volume of air drawn into the syringe equals the volume to be withdrawn from the vial.
- Insert the needle into the top of the vial, making sure that the bevel's tip does not touch the solution. Inject the air into the vial and withdraw the needle.

- Repeat the above steps for the second vial. Then, after injecting the air into the second vial, invert the vial, withdraw the prescribed dose, and then withdraw the needle.
- Wipe the rubber stopper of the first vial again and insert the needle, taking care not to depress the plunger. Doing so would contaminate the first vial with medication from the second vial.
- Invert the vial, withdraw the prescribed dose, and then withdraw the needle.

Mixing drugs from one multidose vial and one ampule

Withdraw the prescribed dose from the multidose vial first. Then withdraw the medication from the ampule. Doing so prevents contaminating the multidose vial with the medication from the ampule. Drugs from two ampules may be mixed in any order.

Preparing a cartridge-injection system

A cartridge-injection system, such as Tubex or Carpuject, is a convenient, easy-to-use method of injection that facilitates both accuracy and sterility. It consists of a metal or plastic cartridge holder syringe and a prefilled medication cartridge with needle attached. In this system the medication is premixed and premeasured, which saves time and helps ensure an exact dose. Because it is a closed system, the medication remains sealed in the cartridge until the injection is administered, maintaining sterility. Compatible drugs can be added to partially filled cartridges.

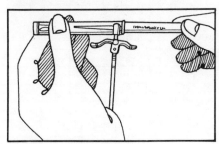

Loading a metal cartridge
- Hold the barrel of the syringe in one hand. With the other hand, pull back on the plunger rod and swing the handle down, so it hangs at a right angle to the barrel.
- Slide the cartridge, needle end first, into the barrel and turn it clockwise until you hear a click.
- Swing the plunger rod back in place and turn it clockwise until it is securely attached to the end of the cartridge.
- Reverse these steps to unload the cartridge.

Loading a plastic cartridge
- Grasp the barrel of the syringe, with the open side facing you, and pull back the plunger rod as far as possible.
- Disengage the locking screw by turning it counterclockwise.
- Insert the cartridge-needle unit—needle-end first—into the open side of the syringe.

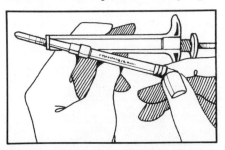

- Advance and engage the locking screw, and turn it clockwise beyond its initial resistance until it will no longer rotate.
- Advance the plunger rod and screw clockwise onto the threaded insert in the rubber plunger.

Preparing a ready injectable

A ready injectable—commercially premeasured medication packaged with a syringe and needle—allows for rapid drug administration in an emergency. Usually, preparing a ready injectable takes only 15 to 20 seconds. Other advantages include the reduced risk of breaking sterile technique during preparation and the easy identification of medication and dose.

If the medication is in a vial, remove the protector caps from the injector and vial. Then thread the vial into the injector and turn it until you meet resistance.

If the medication is in the syringe barrel, thread the rod into the plunger and turn it until you meet resistance.

Remove the needle guard and expel the air. Dilute the medication in an I.V. solution if required.

I.V. / DRUG COMPATIBILITY CHART

Key:
◢ = Compatible
■ = Incompatible
□ = Data unavailable
2,4,6,8,24 = Compatible only for the number of hours indicated
\ = Identical drug

	albumin	amikacin	aminophylline	amino acid injection	ampicillin	bretylium	calcium gluconate	carbenicillin	cefamandole	cefazolin	cefoxitin	cephalothin	chloramphenicol	cimetidine	clindamycin	corticotropin (ACTH)	dexamethasone	dextrose 5% in water	dextrose 5% in R.L.	dextrose 5% in 0.45% NSS	dextrose 5% in 0.9% NSS	diphenhydramine	dobutamine	dopamine	epinephrine	erythromycin (I.V.)	gentamicin	heparin sodium	hydrocortisone Na succinate	insulin (regular)
albumin	\																	◢	◢	◢	◢									
amikacin		\	8		■		24	8	■	8	■	■	24	24	24		■	24	24	24	24	24		■	24	■		■		
aminophylline		8	\	24	■		◢					■		■	■	■	◢	◢	◢	◢	◢	◢			■	◢	■	◢	◢	■
amino acid injection			24	\	12		24	24		24		24	■	24	24			◢	◢	◢	◢			24		24	24	24		24
ampicillin		■	■	■	\		■	■					■	◢	■			2	4	4	4			■		■	■	■	◢	
bretylium						\												◢	◢	◢	◢			◢						
calcium gluconate		24	◢	24	■		\	◢	■	■		■	◢		■	◢	◢	◢	◢	◢	◢	◢	■	24	■	◢	■	◢	◢	
carbenicillin		8	◢	24	■		◢	\		◢			■		24			◢	◢	◢	◢			24	■	■	■		24	
cefamandole		■					■		\									◢	◢	◢	◢						■			
cefazolin		8		24			■	◢		\			24	24			◢	◢	◢	◢	◢					■	■			
cefoxitin		■									\							◢	◢	◢	◢						■			
cephalothin		■	■	24			■					\	◢	24	24			◢	◢	◢	◢	■		6	■	■	■	8	24	8
chloramphenicol		24			■		◢	■		24		◢	\			◢	◢	◢	◢	◢	◢	◢		24		■	■	◢	◢	
cimetidine		24	■	24	◢		■			24		24		\	24	24		◢	◢	◢	◢					■	24			24
clindamycin		24	■	24				24				24		24	\			◢	◢	◢	◢						24	24	24	
corticotropin (ACTH)			■		■		◢						◢			\		◢	◢	◢	◢						■	24	24	
dexamethasone		■	■				◢			◢			◢				\	◢	◢	◢	◢	■					■	4	4	
dextrose 5% in water	◢	24	◢	◢	2	◢	◢	◢	◢	◢	◢	◢	◢	◢	◢	◢	◢	\				◢	◢	◢	◢	◢	◢	◢	◢	
dextrose 5% in R.L.	◢	24	◢	◢	4	◢	◢	◢	◢	◢	◢	◢	◢	◢	◢	◢	◢		\			◢	◢	◢	◢	◢	◢	◢	◢	
dextrose 5% in 0.45% NSS	◢	24	◢	◢	4	◢	◢	◢	◢	◢	◢	◢	◢	◢	◢	◢	◢			\		◢	◢	◢	◢	◢	◢	◢	◢	
dextrose 5% in 0.9% NSS	◢	24	◢	◢	4	◢	◢	◢	◢	◢	◢	◢	◢	◢	◢	◢	◢				\	◢	◢	◢	◢	◢	◢	◢	◢	
diphenhydramine		24	◢				◢					■	◢				■	◢	◢	◢	◢	\				24	■		■	
dobutamine							■											◢	◢	◢	◢		\	◢						
dopamine			■	24	■	◢	24	24				6	24					◢	◢	◢	◢		◢	\			6	24		
epinephrine		24	■				■	■				■	■					◢	◢	◢	◢				\		■			
erythromycin (I.V.)		■	◢	24	■		◢	■		■		■	■	■		◢		◢	◢	◢	◢	24				\	■	■	◢	
gentamicin		■	■	24	■		■	■	■	■	■	■	■	24	24	■	■	◢	◢	◢	◢	■		6	■	■	\	■	■	■
heparin sodium		■	◢	24	■		◢					8	◢		24	24	4	◢	◢	◢	◢			24		■	■	\	■	
hydrocortisone Na suc.			◢		◢		◢	24				24	◢		24	24	4	◢	◢	◢	◢	■		18		◢	■	■	\	8
insulin (regular)			■	24								8		24													■		8	\
isoproterenol			■	24			◢					◢						◢	◢	◢	◢						■	8		
kanamycin			◢	◢	■		■	■		■	24	■	◢		24	◢	◢	◢	◢	◢	◢	◢		24			■	■	■	
lactated Ringer's	◢		◢	◢	8	◢	◢	◢	◢	◢	◢	◢	◢	◢	◢	◢	■					◢	◢	◢	◢	◢	◢	◢	◢	
lidocaine			◢	24	■	◢	◢	◢	◢			■	◢				◢	◢	◢	◢	◢	◢		24	2	◢	◢	8	◢	■
metaraminol		24		24	■							◢	◢				■	◢	◢	◢	◢	■			◢	■	■	■	■	
methicillin		■	◢	24	■		◢					■	■			◢	◢	6	6	6	6	◢				◢	■	■	■	
methylprednisolone			6	24			■					■	◢		24			◢	◢	◢	◢	■		18			■	◢	4	■
mezlocillin		■																◢	◢	◢	◢						■			
moxalactam																		◢	◢	◢	◢									
multiple vitamin infusion				◢			◢			◢	24				24			◢	◢	◢	◢					■	■			
nafcillin			12		■								◢				◢	◢	◢	◢	◢	◢					■	◢	■	
netilmicin					■			■	■	■	■	■						◢	◢	◢	◢	◢							◢	
norepinephrine		24	■	24			◢					■				◢	◢	◢	◢	◢	◢						■	■	◢	
0.9% NSS	◢	24	◢	◢	8	◢	◢	◢	◢	◢	◢	◢	◢	◢	◢	◢	◢					◢	◢	◢	◢	◢	◢	◢	◢	◢
oxacillin		8	■	24	■					◢		■	■					◢	◢	◢	◢			24	■		■			
oxytocin										◢			◢					◢	◢	◢	◢						■			
penicillin G		8	■	24	■		◢			◢		■	◢	24	24	◢	◢	◢	◢	◢	◢	◢		6	■	◢	■	■	◢	■
phytonadione		24	■	24	■							■	◢				◢	◢	◢	◢	◢	◢			■		■	■		
piperacillin		■																◢	◢	◢	◢						■		◢	
polymyxin B		24			■			■		■		■	■					◢	■	■	■	◢				◢	■	■	◢	
potassium chloride		4	◢	24	◢	◢	◢	24		◢		◢	◢	24	24	◢	4	◢	◢	◢	◢			24		◢	■	◢	◢	◢
procainamide		■	◢			◢	◢						◢					◢				◢					■	◢	◢	■
sodium bicarbonate		24	◢			◢	■	24			24	◢	◢	◢	24	■		◢	◢	◢	◢		■	■	■	24	■		◢	■
tetracycline		8	■	24	■		■	■		■		■	■			◢	◢	◢	◢	◢	◢	◢		24	■	■	■	■	■	
thiamine																		◢	◢	◢	◢					■	■			
ticarcillin		■			■													◢	◢	◢	◢						■			
tobramycin							■	■	■	■	■	■			■			◢	◢	◢	◢						■	■		
vancomycin		24	■				■						■			◢	■	◢	◢	◢	◢	◢			■		■	■	■	
verapamil			◢			◢	◢											◢	◢	◢	◢									◢
vitamin B complex with C		24	■		■		◢	■		◢	24	◢	■	24	24	◢	4	◢	◢	◢	◢	◢			■	■	■	◢	◢	◢

Preparation and Administration Guidelines 75

	isoproterenol	kanamycin	lactated Ringer's	lidocaine	metaraminol	methicillin	methylprednisolone	mezlocillin	moxalactam	multiple vitamin infusion	nafcillin	netilmicin	norepinephrine	0.9% NSS	oxacillin	oxytocin	penicillin G	phytonadione	piperacillin	polymyxin B	potassium chloride	procainamide	sodium bicarbonate	tetracycline	thiamine	ticarcillin	tobramycin	vancomycin	verapamil	vitamin B complex with C	
							24								24	24	8		8	24		24	4		24	8			24	24	albumin
								6		12																					amikacin
24			24	24	24	24							24		24	24	24				24			24							aminophylline
																														amino acid injection
		8											8																	ampicillin
																														bretylium
																						24			24					calcium gluconate
																														carbenicillin
																														cefamandole
																														cefazolin
	24								24													24							24	cefoxitin
																														cephalothin
																24				24							24		24	chloramphenicol
	24				24			24								24				24		24							24	cimetidine
																														clindamycin
																						4							4	corticotropin (ACTH)
				6																										dexamethasone
				6																										dextrose 5% in water
				6																										dextrose 5% in R.L.
																														dextrose 5% in 0.45% NSS
				6																										dextrose 5% in 0.9% NSS
																														diphenhydramine
																														dobutamine
	24		24		18									24	6			24			24									dopamine
		2																												epinephrine
																					24									erythromycin (I.V.)
																														gentamicin
8		8																												heparin sodium
				4																										hydrocortisone Na suc.
																														insulin (regular)
																														isoproterenol
					6																									kanamycin
																														lactated Ringer's
																														lidocaine
	6												6																	metaraminol
																														methicillin
																														methylprednisolone
																														mezlocillin
																		4												moxalactam
																														multiple vitamin infusion
																														nafcillin
																														netilmicin
				6																										norepinephrine
																														0.9% NSS
																														oxacillin
																														oxytocin
					4																									penicillin G
																														phytonadione
																														piperacillin
																														polymyxin B
																														potassium chloride
																														procainamide
																														sodium bicarbonate
																														tetracycline
																														thiamine
																														ticarcillin
																														tobramycin
																														vancomycin
																														verapamil
																														vitamin B complex with C

Preparing admixtures

An *admixture* is an I.V. solution to which one or more compatible medications have been added. Admixtures are commonly administered through a secondary or piggyback line (see "Infusing a drug through a secondary line" in Chapter 8, Parenteral Administration of Medication, p. 105). Because the pharmacist has access to the most current information on drugs, admixtures should be prepared in the pharmacy.

However, if you are to prepare the admixture, sterile technique must be used. It is also necessary to establish compatibility of the solution with the drug. *Incompatibility* is an undesired physical or chemical reaction between a drug and a solution or another drug.

Physical incompatibility refers to any visible change in the solution after mixing, such as precipitation, altered color, gas formation, turbidity, or cloudiness. Such changes are produced by physical or chemical reactions involving the drug's pH, the solvent, and the container holding the admixture. *Chemical* incompatibility causes a drug to degrade to a therapeutically inactive or toxic product. This irreversible breakdown is not always visible.

General guidelines

Whenever possible, administer parenteral medications separately. To minimize incompatibilities, use a heparin lock to infuse multiple doses of a drug that is incompatible with other parenteral drugs.

If several incompatible drugs must be infused through the same I.V. line, clear the tubing between doses with a solution compatible with each drug. For example, you may have an order to administer phenytoin I.V. to a patient receiving an infusion of dextrose 5% in one-half normal saline solution ($D_5\frac{1}{2}$ NS); the two are incompatible. First stop the $D_5\frac{1}{2}$ NS, then clear the tubing with normal saline solution, administer the phenytoin, clear the tubing again with the normal saline solution, and finally restart the flow of $D_5\frac{1}{2}$ NS.

When medications must be administered concurrently or mixed in the same large-volume parenteral solution, refer to the *I.V./Drug Compatibility Chart,* pp. 74 and 75, and the following guidelines:

- Chemical analogs or families of drugs react similarly. If one drug in a class is incompatible with the desired solution, others in this class may be incompatible too.
- When preparing a drug, follow manufacturer's instructions meticulously because the preservatives used in some diluents may be incompatible with the drug. For example, bacteriostatic normal saline solution contains benzyl alcohol, which is incompatible with such a drug as chloramphenicol sodium succinate.
- When reconstituting I.V. drugs and inspecting for a precipitate, do not shake the container; rotate or swirl it instead. This action prevents air bubble entrapment and foaming, which impair accurate drug dose measurement in syringes and trigger air exclusion alarms when solutions are administered by infusion pump. Also, air bubbles may be mistaken for particles in the solution.
- When reconstituting a drug, thoroughly mix it before administering or adding it to a solution.
- Some drugs are adsorbed to (attracted to and retained on the surface of) glass and/or plastic I.V. containers and tubing. Check with the pharmacist regarding the type of I.V. container to use.
- When mixing drugs in a large-volume parenteral solution, add one drug at a time; then mix and examine the solution before adding other drugs. Thorough mixing before adding other drugs prevents layering. Also, avoid adding more than two drugs whenever possible.
- Chemical reactions depend on concentration. Minimize these reactions by adding the most concentrated or most soluble drug to the large-volume parenteral solution first.
- Some precipitates are too fine or too clear to be detected, or are the same color as the solution. When you swirl or rotate the container, inspect for a precipitate in good light against both a dark and light background.
- Watch for color changes in the membrane of any I.V. filter device, indicating drug incompatibility not visible in the solution. This reaction becomes visible as the drug is trapped and accumulates in the filter chamber.
- If you detect a physical change, such as a precipitate or discoloration, do not administer the admixture. Notify the pharmacist.

- Avoid administering intermittent medications along with total parenteral nutrition solutions by a central venous catheter. Doing so risks contamination and incompatibilities. Use a secondary line for these drugs.
- Avoid administering medications through the same peripheral venous sites used for amino acids and fat emulsions; instead, infuse them through a peripheral site not used for other drug therapy.
- Do not mix additives with blood or blood products.
- Avoid mixing drugs if no compatibility information is available. If you cannot find such information, consult the pharmacist.

Before adding medication
- Check the compatibility and dosage of the drug, diluent, and I.V. solution.
- Read the directions that come with the drug regarding mixing the drug in solution. If no directions are available, ask the pharmacist. Also, see "Standard Infusion/Piggyback List," in the appendix for information on specific drugs.
- Wash your hands.
- Verify that you have the correct drug by comparing its label with the order on the medication record. Read the label as you prepare the drug additive and again after you have added it to the solution.

- If the I.V. container is a *bottle*, remove the protective metal cap, leaving the rubber seal intact. This seal is sterile and does not need to be swabbed with alcohol for its first puncture. Drugs can be injected through it with a needle. When you are ready to connect the I.V. tubing, remove the seal. You should hear a pop that ensures the sterility of the container. The bottle top is sterile and does not need to be swabbed first.
- If the I.V. container is a *bag*, remove the protective cover on the injection port and swab the rubber-stoppered port.

Adding medication
Using a syringe and needle
When a *bottle* is being used, insert the needle through the rubber seal (center for nonvented bottles; administration set site for vented bottles). Inject the medication.

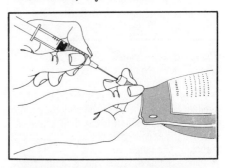

When a *bag* is being used, stabilize the injection port with one hand and insert the needle through the center of the rubber stopper with the other. Inject the medication and squeeze the injection port to empty it of medication.

Using a single-headed needle or pin
This device can be used only in an I.V. container with a vacuum present. The rubber seal on vented bottles must therefore remain in place. Also, because a vacuum must be present, this technique cannot be used to add a drug to an I.V. solution already hung. Since there is no way to control the amount of medication entering the I.V. container, the entire contents of the vial must be used.
- Remove the protective cap from the needle or pin on top of the drug vial.
- Invert the medication vial and insert the pin into the I.V. bottle's main port so the vacuum draws the drug into the bottle.

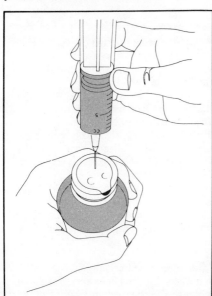

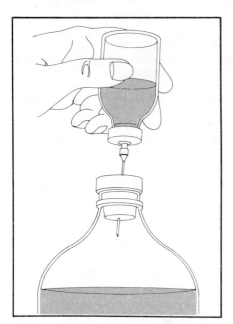

Using a double-headed needle or pin
This device also requires that a vacuum be present in the I.V. container.
• Remove the outside cover of the double-headed needle to expose the shorter needle.
• Insert this needle into the drug vial and remove the second half of the needle cover, exposing the longer needle.
• Invert the medication vial, and insert the longer needle into the center hole of the appropriate seal. The vacuum then draws the drug into the I.V. container.

Using a syringe with a filter needle
Filter needles are used to filter particulate matter from solutions drawn up from ampules and vials. Their use reduces the amount of particulate contamination in admixtures. Particulate matter includes glass, rubber, cotton and paper fibers, drug particles, molds, and metal.
• Place the filter needle on the syringe. Then wipe the ampule neck with an alcohol sponge, wrap it in a gauze pad, and snap off the neck, directing the force away from your body.
• Aspirate the ampule contents with the syringe. Then replace the filter needle or straw with a 25G 1" needle.
• Inject the drug into the I.V. container.

Using a transfer spike
A transfer spike can be used only in an I.V. container with a vacuum present. Therefore, it cannot be used once the solution is infusing or if the rubber seal on a vented bottle is removed.
• Remove the protective cover on the transfer spike.
• Invert the vial and center the spike over the rubber stopper or administration set site on a vented bottle.

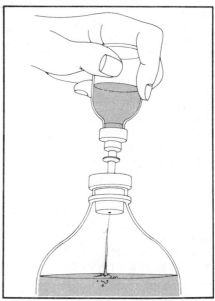

• Push the spike through the rubber stopper using a firm, downward motion. The vacuum will then draw the medication into the I.V. container.

Adding to a container already hung
To add a drug to an I.V. solution that has already been hung, always close the flow clamp to prevent delivering a bolus of the drug to the patient. Insert a syringe and needle into the injection site of a vented I.V. bottle or the injection port of an I.V. bag after wiping it with alcohol. Always invert the container several times to mix the solution thoroughly. Then open the flow clamp and adjust the flow rate.

After adding medication
• Recheck the drug dose and I.V. solution.
• Mix the solution well by shaking or in-

verting the container several times. If the solution is not mixed well, a lot of the medication will remain near the injection port and the patient could receive a bolus dose of medication. Also, if the drug has an oil or lipid base, as paraldehyde does, it will separate out of solution. Shake this type of solution every 15 to 30 minutes during the infusion.
• Examine the solution for precipitation, cloudiness, or discoloration. Discard it if you notice any of these.
• Connect an I.V. administration set to the container and prime the tubing.
• Fill out a medication label and place it on the back of the I.V. container. The label should include the patient's name and room number, type of I.V. solution, type and amount of medication added, and date and time of preparation.

Documenting medication given

Medication cardex
The first time you give a medication to a patient, enter your full signature, licensure status (SN, GN, RN, LPN), and identifying initials in the appropriate place on that patient's cardex.

Whenever you give a medication, record the dose as soon as possible to reduce the possibility that the patient will receive a double dose. Initial the cardex at the time and date the drug was given. Also, if a drug is ordered but not given, note this on the cardex, and chart the reason in the nurses' notes.

After giving an I.M. injection, record the site. Doing so will make proper site rotation easier.

Nurses' notes
Normally, medication administration is not documented in nurses' notes. However, there are the following exceptions.

When p.r.n. drugs are given
The date, time, and reason for the administration of p.r.n. drugs must be recorded. The patient's response or lack of response to the medication must also be recorded, as well as pertinent vital signs.

Example:
Date: 1/31 Time: 3 p.m. Complaining of severe incisional pain. Resp. 24. Demerol 75 mg I.M. given.
Signature, RN
Date: 1/31 Time: 3:30 p.m. States pain has lessened.
Signature, RN

When a drug is withheld
Sometimes drugs are withheld because of the patient's condition or laboratory test results. This must be recorded in the nurses' notes as well as on the medication cardex, and the charge nurse and physician must be notified. If a unit dose system is being used, notify the pharmacist.
Example:
Date: 2/5 Time: 10 a.m. Apical pulse 56. Digoxin 0.25 mg P.O. withheld. Dr. Harrison notified.
Signature, SN

When a drug is refused
If a patient refuses a medication, record it on the medication cardex and in the nurses' notes. When possible, the patient's own words should be recorded. Also, notify the charge nurse and the physician. Notify the pharmacist if a unit dose system is being used.
Example:
Date: 3/25 Time: 6 p.m. Pronestyl 250 mg P.O. refused. States "Makes me feel depressed." Dr. Lange notified.
Signature, RN

Review Questions

True or False
1. Medication cannot be given without a physician's order.

2. Medications can be left at the patient's bedside.

3. If a nurse gives a medication prepared by another nurse, the nurse who prepared the medication is responsible for any errors.

4. A nurse may hold tablets or capsules.

5. Asking the name of the patient is a safe way to correctly identify him before giving a medication.

6. If a patient expresses doubt about the medication you are about to give, the medication should be rechecked.

7. Remove medication from unit dose packages when you are at the patient's bedside.

8. Unused medication may be returned to a stock bottle.

9. Sustained-release and enteric-coated tablets may be crushed.

10. Read the bottom of the meniscus when checking the amount of liquid medication in a medication cup.

11. The larger the needle gauge, the smaller the needle opening.

12. A common needle size for an I.M. injection is 22G 1½".

13. Add 0.2 cc of air to the syringe for an I.M. injection.

14. The purpose of wrapping the neck of an ampule with gauze before opening it is to maintain sterility of the solution.

15. Air must be added to a vial before medication can be withdrawn.

16. If a drug is added to a solution and a precipitate forms, the solution may be administered.

17. Chemical incompatibility reactions are not always visible, so it is necessary to check a compatibility chart or question the pharmacist before mixing a drug in a solution or with another drug.

18. Whenever possible, administer I.V. medications separately.

19. Shaking a container is the best way to thoroughly mix a drug in solution.

20. Always read manufacturer's instructions before reconstituting a drug.

21. When adding two drugs to an I.V. solution, add one at a time, mix each thoroughly, and examine the solution after each addition.

Brief Response:

22. State the three identification checks that are performed to minimize the chance of drug error.

23. Which part(s) of the syringe must remain sterile?

24. What information should be on the label of an admixture?

25. Define incompatibility as it pertains to drugs and I.V. solutions.

26. What are some of the measures a nurse can take to protect herself when preparing cytotoxic medications for administration?

27. For the patient's safety, what are some of the actions a nurse can take to ensure a cytotoxic medication has been properly prepared?

Multiple Choice (one best answer)

28. Which of the following are factors in needle selection for an injection?
   1. Depth of the injection
   2. Type of medication to be given
   3. Viscosity of the medication
   4. Amount of subcutaneous tissue present
   A. 1 and 2
   B. 1, 2, and 3
   C. 1, 2, 3, and 4

29. When do you record that a medication was given?
   A. Before going into the patient's room
   B. Immediately after leaving the patient's room
   C. When all the medications have been given

30. When reconstituting medication in a multidose vial, dissolve the medication in the amount of solution necessary to make 1 ml:
   A. Less than the desired dose
   B. Equal to the desired dose
   C. Greater than the desired dose

31. What information should be put on the label of a multidose vial after the medication has been reconstituted?
    A. Concentration (amt/ml)
    B. Date of preparation
    C. Time of preparation
    D. All of the above

32. When combining two drugs in the same syringe, which medication is drawn up first?
    A. Medication in the multidose vial
    B. Medication in the ampule

33. What is the most important consideration when combining two drugs in the same syringe?
    A. Whether or not they will fit
    B. Drawing up the appropriate one first
    C. Compatibility of the two drugs
    D. Not contaminating a multidose vial

34. Which of the following are nursing concerns when preparing an admixture?
    1. Maintaining sterile technique
    2. Preventing incompatibilities
    3. Following manufacturer's instructions for mixing the drug
    4. Mixing the drug well
    5. Labeling the I.V. container properly
    A. 1 and 2
    B. 1, 2, and 3
    C. 1, 2, 3, and 4
    D. 1, 2, 3, 4, and 5

35. If you are going to administer a drug through an injection port in an I.V. line and the drug is not compatible with the I.V. solution, you should:
    A. Not give the drug intravenously
    B. Give the drug very slowly
    C. Give the drug very quickly
    D. Flush the tubing with a solution compatible with the drug before and after giving it

36. Which of the following are true regarding giving medications to a patient in isolation?
    1. The isolation procedure for the specific type of isolation must be followed.
    2. The medication cart or tray must not enter the room.
    3. Nondisposable syringes must be left in the room.
    4. You must wash your hands before leaving the room.
    A. 1 and 2
    B. 1 and 3
    C. 2, 3, and 4
    D. 1, 2, 3, and 4

Selected References

Drug Interactions. Nursing Now Series. Springhouse, Pa.: Springhouse Corp., 1984.
Drugs, 2nd ed. Nurse's Reference Library. Springhouse, Pa.: Springhouse Corp., 1984.
Giving Medications. Nursing Photobook Series. Springhouse, Pa.: Springhouse Corp., 1982.
Lerman, F., and Weinbert, R. *Drug Interactions Index.* Oradell, N.J.: Medical Economics Books, 1982.
Motz-Harding, E., and Good, F. "The Right Solution—Mixing I.V. Drugs Thoroughly," *Nursing85* 15(2):62-64, February 1985.
Nursing87 Drug Handbook. Springhouse, Pa.: Springhouse Corp., 1987.
Nursing87 MediQuik Cards. Springhouse, Pa.: Springhouse Corp., 1987.
Procedures. Nurse's Reference Library. Springhouse, Pa.: Springhouse Corp., 1983.

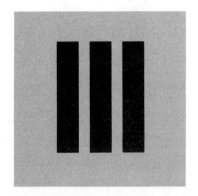

Medication Administration Procedures

7 Administering Oral Medications 84

8 Parenteral Administration of Medication 92

9 Application of Medication to the Eye, Ear, Nose, and Throat 128

10 Topical Application of Medication 138

11 Inhalation Administration of Medication 159

Administering Oral Medications

Administering oral medication is one of the most commonly performed nursing procedures. This method relies on gastrointestinal absorption and includes giving medication not only by mouth, but also through a nasogastric tube or gastrostomy tube. This chapter discusses how to achieve safe and effective medication administration by these three routes.

Oral administration of drugs

Because oral administration of drugs is generally safest, most convenient, and least expensive, most drugs are commonly administered by this route. Drugs for oral administration are available in many different forms: tablets, enteric-coated tablets, capsules, caplets, syrups, elixirs, oils, liquids, suspensions, powders, and granules. Some require special preparation before administration, such as mixing with juice to make them more palatable. Oils, powders, and granules most often require such preparation. (See Chapter 6, Preparation and Administration Guidelines.)

Oral drugs are sometimes prescribed in higher dosages than their parenteral equivalents because after absorption through the gastrointestinal system, they are immediately broken down by the liver before they reach the systemic circulation. Nausea, vomiting, inability to swallow, decreased consciousness, and unconsciousness may contraindicate oral administration.

Equipment and materials

You will need the patient's medication record and chart, the prescribed medication, and a medication cup. You may need an appropriate vehicle (jelly or applesauce) for crushed pills (a common practice in oral administration to children or the elderly), a liquid (juice, water, or milk), and a straw or a syringe (for administering unpleasant-tasting liquids orally).

Steps
- Confirm the identity of the patient by checking the name, room number, and bed number on his wristband.
- Wash your hands.
- Give the patient his medication and, as needed, an appropriate liquid or vehicle to aid swallowing, minimize side effects, or promote absorption.
- Stay with the patient until he has swallowed the drug. If he seems confused or disoriented, check his mouth to make sure he has swallowed it.
- If you are giving a liquid medication through a syringe, place the patient in an upright or high Fowler's position. To minimize aspiration risk, place the syringe tip in the pocket between the cheek and the second molar, and instill the medication slowly. Then discard the syringe.
- If you are using a medication tray instead of a cart, turn over the patient's medication card to signify that the medication was given.
- Document that the medication was given on the medication cardex.
- If the patient refuses a drug, document the refusal and his reason in the nurses' notes and notify the charge nurse and the patient's physician, as needed. Also note if a drug was omitted or withheld for other reasons, such as radiology or laboratory tests.

Nursing considerations
- Verify the order on the patient's medication record by checking it against the physician's order if you are uncertain of a medication or its dose.

- Make sure you have a written order for every medication given. Verbal orders should be signed by the physician within the specified time. (Hospitals usually require a signature within 24 hours; long-term care facilities, within 48 hours.)
- Never give a medication prepared by someone else.
- Never have your medication cart or tray out of your sight: *This prevents anyone from rearranging the medications or taking one without your knowledge.*
- Never return unused medications to stock containers. Instead, dispose of them and notify the pharmacy. Keep in mind that the disposal of any narcotic drug must be co-signed by another nurse, as mandated by law.
- If the patient has questions about his medication, the dose, or the frequency, check his medication record again. If the medication is correct, reassure him. Make sure you tell him about any changes in his medication or dosage. Instruct him, as appropriate, about possible side effects. Ask him to report any change that he feels may be a side effect.
- To avoid damaging or staining the patient's teeth, give acid or iron preparations through a straw. Also, suggest that the patient remove his dentures if appropriate.
- Give cough medicines and other syrups last and undiluted. When giving a syrup for a demulcent (soothing) effect, do not follow it with water. Do not dilute antacids or any other medication that is labeled not to be diluted.
- Follow administration of an alcoholic solution, such as an elixir or tincture, with water, unless it is given for cough relief.
- If the patient vomits after receiving his medication, readminister according to the physician's order. Whether or not to readminister depends on several factors, such as the type of medication, the elapsed time between administration and vomiting, the reason for the vomiting, and the condition (status) of the patient.

Unpleasant taste
The following techniques may help the patient tolerate unpleasant-tasting medications.
- Have the patient take an unpleasant-tasting liquid through a straw. Because the liquid contacts fewer taste buds, it is usually more palatable. As an alternative, disguise the taste by diluting the medication with water, juice, or Coke syrup. But first, make sure the medication is compatible with the other liquid.
- Unpalatable liquid medications may be given with a syringe. Bypass the patient's taste buds by instilling the medication into the pocket between his cheek and second molar.
- Ask the patient to suck ice chips to numb his taste buds before he takes unpalatable medication. Or pour liquid medication over ice and give it through a straw. Avoid this method if you are giving a small dose, however, because it may affect accuracy.
- If the medication is oily, chill it first. Store oily medications in a refrigerator, unless contraindicated.
- Suggest that the patient hold his nose as he swallows if the medication has an unpleasant taste.
- Minimize a bitter aftertaste by offering the patient hard candy or chewing gum after the medication. Or suggest that he gargle or rinse his mouth with water or mouthwash.

Difficulty swallowing
The following techniques may help the patient who has difficulty swallowing capsules or tablets.
- If the patient has trouble swallowing a capsule, suggest that he place it in his mouth with a small amount of water and then tilt his head forward and swallow. Because the capsule is lighter than water, it will float back toward the throat, where it can be swallowed easily.
- If a patient cannot swallow a whole tablet or capsule, ask the pharmacist if the drug is available in liquid form or if it can be administered by another route. If not, ask him if you can crush the tablet or open the capsule and mix it with food. Remember to contact the physician for an order to change the route of administration when necessary.

Administering medication through a nasogastric tube

Besides providing an alternative means of nourishment, the nasogastric tube allows direct instillation of medication into the gastrointestinal system of patients who

HOW TO INSTILL MEDICATION THROUGH A NASOGASTRIC TUBE

With the patient in Fowler's or semi-Fowler's position (as shown), hold the tube slightly above the level of the patient's nose. Tilt the tube slightly to prevent air from entering. Then, slowly pour the medication into the syringe.

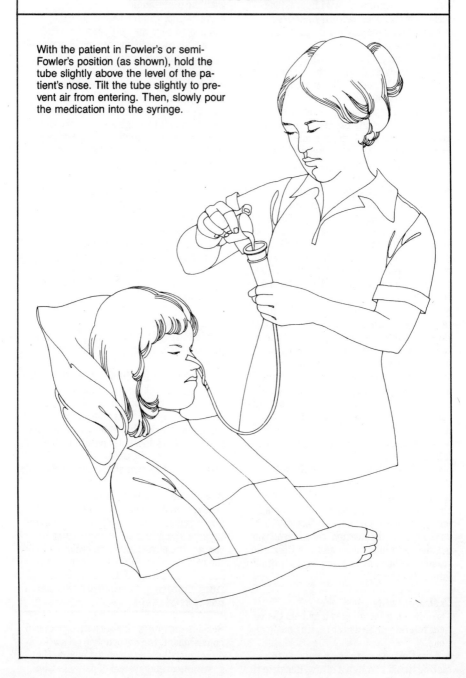

cannot ingest it orally. This is a safe and relatively simple procedure. Before instillation, however, the patency and position of the tube must be carefully checked. The procedure is contraindicated if the tube is obstructed or improperly positioned, or if the patient is vomiting around the tube or has absent bowel sounds.

Equipment and materials
You will need the prescribed medication, a towel or linen-saver pad, a 50- or 60-ml piston type catheter-tipped syringe, two 4" × 4" gauze sponges, a stethoscope, diluting liquid (such as juice, water, or nutritional supplement), a cup for mixing medication and fluids, a spoon, 50 ml of water, a rubber band, and a clamp (if not already attached to the tube).

Preparation
Gather necessary equipment and materials for use at the patient's bedside. Liquids should be at room temperature. *Administering cold liquid through the nasogastric tube can cause abdominal cramping.* Although this is not a sterile procedure, make sure the cups, syringe, spoon, and gauze are clean. If the prescribed medication is in tablet form, crush the tablets to ready them for mixing with the diluting liquid. Take the medication and equipment to the patient's bedside.

Steps
- Confirm the identity of the patient by checking his name, room number, and bed number on his wristband.
- Explain the procedure to him, if necessary, and provide privacy.
- Wash your hands.
- Unpin the tube from the patient's gown and remove any dressing at the end of the tube. To avoid soiling the sheets during the procedure, fold them back to the patient's waist and drape his chest with the towel or linen-saver pad.
- Elevate the head of the bed so the patient is in Fowler's or semi-Fowler's position.
- After removing the clamp from the tube, take the syringe and create a 10-cc air space in its chamber. Then attach the syringe to the end of the tube.
- Auscultate the patient's abdomen about 3" (8 cm) below the sternum with the stethoscope. Then gently instill the 10 cc of air into the tube. You should hear the air bubble entering the stomach. If you hear this sound, gently draw back on the piston of the syringe. The appearance of gastric contents confirms that the tube is patent and in the stomach. If no gastric contents appear when you draw back on the piston of the syringe, the tube may have risen into the patient's esophagus. In this case you will have to advance it before proceeding.
- If you meet resistance in attempting to aspirate stomach contents, stop the procedure. Resistance may indicate a nonpatent tube or improper tube placement. If the tube seems to be in the stomach, resistance probably means the tube is lying against the stomach wall. To relieve resistance, withdraw the tube slightly.
- After you have established tube patency and correct positioning, replace the clamp on the tube, detach the syringe, and lay the end of the tube on the 4" × 4" gauze sponge.
- Mix the crushed tablets with the diluting liquid. If the medication is in capsule form, open the capsules and empty their contents into the liquid. Pour liquid medications directly into the diluting liquid. Stir well with the spoon. (If the medication was in tablet form, make sure the particles are small enough to pass through the eyes at the distal end of the tube.)
- Reattach the syringe, without the piston, to the end of the tube, and remove the clamp.
- Holding the tube at a level slightly above the patient's nose, pour 30 ml of the diluted medication into the syringe barrel. To prevent air from entering the patient's stomach, hold the tube at a slight angle. If necessary, raise the tube slightly higher to increase the flow rate.
- If the medication flows smoothly, slowly add more until the entire dose has been given. To prevent air from entering the patient's stomach, add more medication before the syringe empties completely.
- If the medication does not flow properly, do not force it. It may be too thick to flow through the tube. If so, dilute it with water. If you suspect tube placement is inhibiting flow, stop the procedure and reevaluate placement.

- Watch the patient's reaction throughout the instillation. If he shows any sign of discomfort, stop the procedure immediately.
- As the last of the medication flows out of the syringe, start to irrigate the tube by adding the 50 ml of water. Irrigation clears medication from the sides of the tube and from the distal end, reducing the risk of clogging.
- When the water stops flowing, quickly clamp the tube. Detach the syringe from the tube and dispose of it properly.
- Cover the end of the tube with the other 4" × 4" sponge and secure it with the rubber band.
- Repin the nasogastric tube to the patient's gown.
- Remove the towel or linen-saver pad and reposition bed linens.
- Leave the patient in Fowler's or semi-Fowler's position for at least 30 minutes after the procedure *to facilitate the downward flow of medication into his stomach and to prevent reflux into the esophagus.*
- Document on the medication cardex that the medication was given.
- Note the amount of fluid instilled on the intake and output sheet.

Nursing considerations
- To prevent instillation of too much fluid (more than 400 ml of liquid at one time for an adult), plan the drug instillation, if possible, so it does not coincide with the patient's regular tube feeding. When you must schedule both simultaneously, give the medication first to ensure that the patient receives prescribed drug therapy even if he cannot tolerate an entire feeding.
- Do not administer oily medications and enteric-coated or sustained-release tablets through a nasogastric tube. Oily medications cling to the sides of the tube and resist mixing with the irrigating solution. Crushing enteric-coated or sustained-release tablets destroys their intended effect.
- If the patient complains of nausea, leave the tube unclamped (but covered) until the feeling subsides.
- If the patient is uncomfortable sitting in Fowler's or semi-Fowler's position, place him on his *right* side with the head of the bed slightly elevated. This will facilitate gastric emptying and discourage regurgitation.
- If the patient is receiving medications such as antacids that should remain in the stomach longer, position him on his *left* side with the head of the bed slightly elevated to discourage gastric emptying.
- If possible, teach the patient who requires long-term treatment to instill medication through his nasogastric tube. Have him observe the procedure several times before allowing him to try it. Stay with him when he performs the procedure the first few times so you can answer any questions. Provide needed assistance and give him positive reinforcement.

Administering medication through a gastrostomy tube

A gastrostomy tube provides a means for long-term administration of nutrients and medications to patients who cannot ingest them orally. The tube is surgically inserted directly into the stomach and eliminates the risk of fluid aspiration into the lungs, which is a constant danger with a nasogastric tube. Before medication is instilled through a gastrostomy tube, the tube should be tested for patency and the fluids should be warmed or cooled to room temperature. This procedure is contraindicated in patients with absent bowel sounds or an obstructed tube.

Equipment and materials
You will need the patient's medication record and chart (and intake and output sheet), the prescribed medication, a diluting liquid (such as juice, water, or a nutritional supplement), a spoon, a towel or linen-saver pad, a catheter-tipped syringe or tube-feeding funnel, water (at least 100 ml), a cup for mixing medication and fluid, four 4" × 4" gauze sponges, a rubber band, tape, and a clamp if not already attached to the tube.

Preparation
Make sure all liquids are at room temperature. *Pouring cold liquid into the tube can cause abdominal cramping.* Take all equipment to the patient's bedside. This is not a sterile procedure, but make sure the cups, syringe or funnel, spoon, and gauze are clean. If the prescribed medication is in tablet form, crush the tablets to ready them for mixing with the diluting liquid.

COMPARING NASOGASTRIC AND GASTROSTOMY TUBES

Chances are you will never use a nasogastric or gastrostomy tube just to give medications. But if you use a tube to feed your patient, you can use it to give oral medications, too. In either case, you will need to be familiar not only with the procedure for administering medications through these tubes, but also with the tubes themselves. Below you will find key points to remember about nasogastric and gastrostomy tubes.

Nasogastric tube

- Small-diameter, pliable plastic or rubber tube
- Tube is measured, then threaded through the nose into the esophagus and into the stomach
- Provides direct route for delivery of medication and feedings to the stomach when the patient cannot tolerate them orally
- May be inserted by a nurse
- Taped in position
- Short-term use
- May require frequent replacement due to obstruction of the tube's lumen or displacement of tube

Gastrostomy tube

- Pliable plastic or rubber tube
- Inserted through a small surgical opening into the stomach
- Provides the most direct route for delivery of medications and feedings to the stomach when the patient cannot tolerate them orally
- Must be inserted by a physician
- Held in position with sutures
- Long-term or permanent use, or when nasogastric intubation is contraindicated
- Easy to maintain

Steps
- Confirm the identity of the patient by checking the name, room number, and bed number on his wristband.
- After closing the door or drawing the curtain to ensure privacy, explain the procedure to him.
- Wash your hands.
- To avoid soiling the sheets during the procedure, fold them below the gastrostomy tube and drape the patient's chest with the towel or linen-saver pad.
- To facilitate digestion and prevent fluid reflux into the esophagus, elevate the head of the bed before instilling any medication.
- Remove the dressing that covers the tube. Then remove the dressing at the tip of the tube and attach the syringe or funnel to the tip.
- Release the clamp and instill about 10 ml of water into the tube through the syringe to check for patency. If the water flows in easily, the tube is patent. If it flows in slowly, raise the syringe or funnel to increase pressure. If the water still does not flow properly, stop the procedure and notify the physician.
- After you have established tube patency and correct positioning, replace the clamp on the tube, detach the syringe, and place the end of the tube on a clean 4" × 4" gauze sponge.
- Mix the medication with the appropriate amount of diluting liquid (usually 30 ml) and stir with the spoon. If the medication is in capsule form, open the capsules and empty their contents into the liquid. Pour liquid medications directly into the diluting liquid. Stir well. (If the medication was in tablet form, make sure the particles are small enough to pass through the eyes at the end of the tube.)
- Reattach the syringe, without the piston, and remove the clamp.
- Pour the medication into the syringe or funnel 30 ml at a time. Tilt the tube to allow air to escape as the fluid flows downward.
- After the medication drains through the syringe or funnel, pour in about 30 ml of water to irrigate the tube.
- Tighten the clamp, then place one 4" × 4" gauze sponge on the end of the tube and secure it with the rubber band.
- Cover the tube with the other two 4" × 4" gauze sponges and secure them firmly with tape.
- Remove the towel or linen-saver pad and reposition the bed linens.
- Keep the head of the bed elevated for at least 30 minutes after the procedure to aid digestion.
- Document that the medication was given on the medication cardex.
- Record the fluid instilled on the intake and output sheet.

Nursing considerations
- Sometimes Montgomery straps or an abdominal binder, applied gently, are used *to hold the tube in place and prevent accidental dislodging.*
- Before pouring medication into the tube, gently lift the dressings around the tube to assess the skin for irritation caused by gastric secretions. Report any redness or irritation to the physician.
- To prevent instillation of too much fluid (more than 400 ml of liquid at one time for an adult), plan the drug instillation so it does not coincide with the patient's scheduled tube feeding. When both must be scheduled simultaneously, give the medication first to ensure that the patient receives prescribed drug therapy even if he cannot tolerate an entire feeding.
- Do not give oily medications and enteric-coated or sustained-release tablets through a gastrostomy tube. Oily medications cling to the sides of the tube and resist mixing with the irrigating solution. Crushing enteric-coated or sustained-release tablets destroys their intended effect.
- If the patient complains of nausea, leave the tube unclamped, but covered, until the feeling subsides.
- If the patient is uncomfortable sitting up, position him on his *right* side with the head of the bed slightly elevated. This will facilitate gastric emptying.
- If the patient is receiving medications such as antacids that should remain in the stomach longer, position him on his *left* side with the head of the bed slightly elevated to discourage gastric emptying.
- If possible, teach the patient who requires long-term treatment to instill medication through his gastrostomy tube. Have him observe the procedure several times before al-

lowing him to try it. Stay with him when he performs the procedure the first few times so you can answer any questions. Provide needed assistance and give him positive reinforcement.

Review Questions

1. Where is the syringe placed in the patient's mouth when administering a liquid medication orally? Why?

2. How should acid or iron preparations be administered? Why?

3. How can unpleasant-tasting medications be made more palatable? Name five ways.

4. How do you check for patency and proper positioning of a nasogastric tube?

5. How much of the diluted medication is poured into the syringe at one time during the instillation through a nasogastric or gastrostomy tube?

6. How is the flow rate of medication through the nasogastric or gastrostomy tube regulated?

7. How do you check for patency of a gastrostomy tube?

8. Why should nasogastric and gastrostomy tubes be irrigated after medication instillation? How much water should be used for irrigation?

9. How can the flow of medication be facilitated through the gastrointestinal tract?

10. Why should liquids be at room temperature for instillation through a nasogastric or gastrostomy tube?

11. Name some contraindications for administering oral medications:
   A. By mouth
   B. Through a nasogastric tube
   C. Through a gastrostomy tube

Selected References

Procedures. Nurse's Reference Library. Springhouse, Pa.: Springhouse Corp., 1983.

Rodman, M. *Clinical Pharmacology in Nursing,* 2nd ed. Philadelphia: J.B. Lippincott Co., 1984.

Wieck, L., et al. *Illustrated Manual of Nursing Techniques,* 3rd ed. Philadelphia: J.B. Lippincott Co., 1986.

Parenteral Administration of Medication

The term *parenteral*, although it means any route other than enteral, or gastrointestinal, is ordinarily used to refer to methods of giving drugs by *injection*. This chapter covers the most common procedures for parenteral administration of medications. Less common procedures are listed in *Less Common Parenteral Routes of Administration*.

INTRADERMAL

Giving an intradermal injection

Intradermal injections are given into the outer layers of the skin in very small amounts, usually 0.5 ml or less. They are used primarily for diagnostic purposes, as in allergy or tuberculin testing. There is very little systemic absorption of intradermally injected agents, so this type of injection is used primarily to produce a local effect. A tuberculin syringe with a 26G or 27G needle (½" to ⅝") is generally used. The ventral forearm is the most commonly used site because of its easy accessibility and lack of hair. In extensive allergy testing, the outer aspect of the upper arms and the area of the back between the scapulae are used (see *Intradermal Injection Sites*).

Equipment and materials
You will need a prepared agent in a syringe with an appropriate needle and alcohol sponges.

Steps
• Confirm the identity of the patient by checking his name, room number, and bed number on his wristband.
• Tell him where you will be giving the injection(s).
• Instruct the patient to sit up and to extend his arm and support it on a flat surface, with the ventral forearm exposed.
• With an alcohol sponge, cleanse the surface of the ventral forearm about 2 or 3 fingerbreadths distal to the antecubital space. You may also cleanse the area with acetone to remove skin oils that may interfere with test results. Be sure the test site you have chosen is free of hair or blemishes. Allow the skin to dry completely before administering the injection.
• While holding the patient's forearm in your hand, stretch the skin taut with your thumb.
• With your free hand, hold the needle at a 15° angle to the patient's arm, with its bevel up.

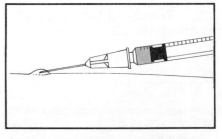

• Insert the needle about ⅛" below the epidermis at sites 2" (5 cm) apart. Stop when the needle bevel is under the skin, and inject the antigen slowly. You should feel some resistance as you do this, and a wheal should form as you inject the antigen. If no

LESS COMMON PARENTERAL ROUTES OF ADMINISTRATION

Intraamniotic—into the amniotic sac
Intracardiac—into the heart
Intradiskal—into the vertebral disk
Intralesional—into a lesion
Intraocular—into the eye
Intraperitoneal—into the peritoneal cavity
Intrapleural—into the pleural space of the lungs
Intraspinal—into the spinal cord

wheal forms, you have injected the antigen too deeply; withdraw the needle and administer another test dose at least 2" (5 cm) from the first site.
• Withdraw the needle at the same angle at which it was inserted. *Do not rub the site.* This could cause irritation in the underlying tissue, which may affect test results.
• Circle each test site with a marking pen, and label each site according to the recall antigen given. Instruct the patient to refrain from washing off the circles until the test is completed.
• Dispose of needles and syringes according to institutional policy.
• Document which agents were given on the patient's chart or medication cardex.
• Assess the patient's response to the skin testing in 24 to 48 hours.

Nursing considerations
In patients hypersensitive to the test antigens, a severe anaphylactic response can result. This requires immediate epinephrine injection and other emergency resuscitation procedures. Be especially alert after giving a test dose of penicillin or tetanus antitoxin.

SUBCUTANEOUS
Giving a subcutaneous injection

Injection into the adipose tissues (fatty layer) beneath the skin delivers a drug into the bloodstream more rapidly than oral administration and allows slower, more sustained drug administration than intramus-

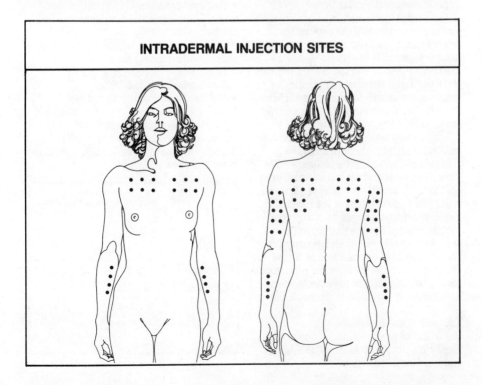

INTRADERMAL INJECTION SITES

GUIDELINES FOR INSULIN AND HEPARIN INJECTIONS

Insulin
- To establish more consistent blood levels, rotate insulin injection sites within anatomic regions. Absorption varies from one region to another. Preferred insulin injection sites are the arms, abdomen, thighs, and buttocks.
- Make sure the type of insulin, dose, and syringe are correct.
- When combining insulins in a syringe, make sure they are compatible. Regular insulin can be mixed with *all* types. Prompt insulin zinc suspension (Semilente) *cannot* be mixed with NPH insulin. Follow institutional policy as to which insulin to draw up first.
- Before drawing up insulin suspension, gently roll and invert the bottle to ensure even drug particle distribution. *Do not shake the bottle, because this can cause foam or bubbles to develop, changing the potency and altering the dose.*

Heparin
- The preferred site for heparin injections is the lower abdominal fat pad, 2" (5 cm) beneath the umbilicus, from iliac crest to crest. Injecting heparin into this area, which is not involved in muscular activity, reduces the risk of local capillary bleeding. Always rotate the sites from one side to the other.
- Do not administer any injections within 2" of a scar, a bruise, or the umbilicus.
- Do not aspirate to check for blood return *because this may cause bleeding into the tissues at the site.*
- Do not rub or massage the site after the injection. Rubbing can cause localized minute hemorrhages or bruises.
- If the patient bruises easily, apply ice to the site for the first 5 minutes after the injection to minimize local hemorrhage.

---

cular injection. It also causes minimal tissue trauma and carries little risk of striking large blood vessels and nerves. Absorbed mainly through the capillaries, drugs recommended for subcutaneous injection are nonirritating aqueous solutions and suspensions contained in fluid volumes of 0.5 to 2.0 ml. Heparin and insulin, for example, are usually administered subcutaneously. (See *Guidelines for Insulin and Heparin Injections.*)

Drugs and solutions for subcutaneous injection are injected through a relatively short needle, using sterile technique. The most common subcutaneous injection sites are the outer aspects of the upper arm, anterior thigh, loose tissue of the lower abdomen, buttocks, and upper back. Injection is contraindicated in sites that are inflamed or edematous. Do not administer any injections within 2" (5 cm) of a scar, a bruise, or the umbilicus. Subcutaneous injections may also be contraindicated in patients who have impaired coagulation mechanisms.

Equipment and materials
You will need prepared medication in a syringe with an appropriate needle attached and two alcohol sponges.

Steps
- Confirm the identity of the patient by checking the name, room number, and bed number on his wristband.
- Tell him where you will be giving the injection, and provide privacy.
- Select an appropriate injection site (see *Subcutaneous Injection Sites*).
- Rotate sites according to a planned schedule for patients who require repeated injections. Use different areas of the body, unless contraindicated by the specific drug. Heparin, for example, can be injected only in certain sites.

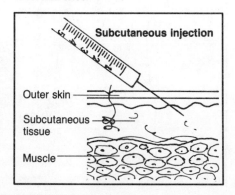

SUBCUTANEOUS INJECTION SITES

Subcutaneous injection sites (shown by dotted areas) include the fat pads on the abdomen, upper hips, upper back, and lateral upper arms and thighs. For subcutaneous injections administered regularly, rotate sites. Choose one injection site in one area, move to a corresponding injection site in the next area, and so on. When returning to an area, choose a new site in that area.

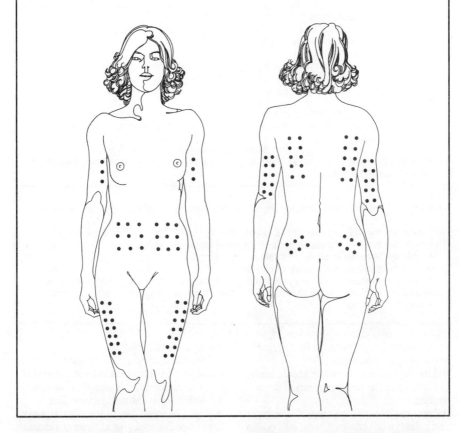

- Position and drape the patient.
- Cleanse the injection site with a sterile alcohol sponge, beginning at the center of the site and moving outward in a circular motion. Allow the skin to dry, so alcohol is not introduced into subcutaneous tissues as the needle is inserted. (This precaution avoids a stinging sensation.)
- Remove the protective needle cover.
- With your nondominant hand, pinch the skin around the injection site and elevate the subcutaneous tissue, forming a fat fold.
- Tell the patient he will feel a prick when you insert the needle. Then, as you say this, insert the needle quickly and in one motion.
- Inject the needle with the bevel up at a 45° angle (see illustration *Subcutaneous injection*). If a fat fold is more than 1", the needle may be injected at a 90° angle.
- Release the patient's skin to avoid injecting into compressed tissue and irritating nerve fibers.
- Pull back on the plunger slightly. If no blood is aspirated, begin injecting the drug slowly. If blood appears on aspiration, with-

SUBCUTANEOUS INFUSION OF MEDICATION

Occasionally, medications such as deferoxamine mesylate (Desferal), morphine, or chemotherapeutic drugs are given by subcutaneous infusion rather than the I.M. or I.V. route. The procedure is often taught to patients for self-administration of medication at home. Medication is administered over a specified period of time and is absorbed through the capillaries. This procedure is similar to *hypodermoclysis,* which is the subcutaneous infusion of I.V. fluids.

Equipment and materials
- Prescribed medication in a syringe or added to prescribed I.V. solution
- 25G or 27G butterfly with ⅝" needle
- Alcohol sponge
- Infusion pump with alarm or pump with battery and belt for home use
- Adhesive bandage or transparent occlusive dressing

Preparation
- Prime the I.V. tubing and needle if the medication is in I.V. solution.
- Attach the butterfly to the syringe if the medication is in a syringe, and prime the butterfly needle.
- Set up the infusion pump system according to manufacturer's instructions.
- If a pump with a belt is being used, attach the pump to the belt and have the patient put it around his waist.

Steps
- Wipe the insertion site (usually the abdomen) with an alcohol sponge, and allow the skin to dry.
- Pinch up the skin and insert the needle at a 15° to 45° angle with the bevel up (down for Desferal). Advance the entire needle under the skin.
- Tape the butterfly in place and secure the tubing.
- Start the infusion at the prescribed rate.
- Check the infusion rate frequently and adjust it according to the patient's ability to absorb the fluid. Too much pressure within the tissue can impair circulation and result in tissue sloughing.

draw the needle, prepare another syringe, and repeat the procedure.
- After injection, remove the needle gently but quickly at the same angle used for insertion.
- Cover the site with an alcohol sponge, and massage the site gently (unless contraindicated) to distribute the drug and facilitate absorption.
- Remove the sponge, and check the injection site for bleeding.
- Replace the needle cover, being careful not to stick yourself with the contaminated needle.
- Dispose of needles and syringes according to institutional policy.
- Document the medication given on the medication cardex.
- Continue to assess the patient's response to drug therapy.

Nursing considerations
- Concentrated or irritating solutions may cause sterile abscesses to form. A natural immune response, this complication can be minimized by rotating injection sites.
- Repeated injections to the same site can cause lipodystrophy, or atrophy of subcutaneous fat. This complication can also be minimized by rotating injection sites.
- Occasionally, a medication is given by subcutaneous *infusion* rather than injection. (See *Subcutaneous Infusion of Medication.*)
- Insulin infusion pumps are now in general clinical use for the control of diabetes. The pump eliminates the need for multiple injections in diabetics whose blood sugar is difficult to control (see *Use of an Insulin Infusion Pump*).

USE OF AN INSULIN INFUSION PUMP

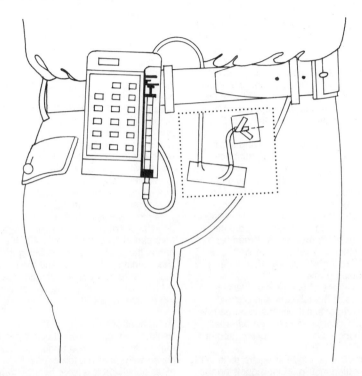

Continuous subcutaneous insulin infusion (CSII) pumps are small, lightweight, and fit nicely on a belt or in a pocket. They are made of high-impact plastic and basically consist of a syringe (to hold the insulin), a syringe plunger, and a mechanism to drive the plunger. When the plunger is depressed, insulin flows from the syringe, through tubing, and into the body tissue through a needle inserted subcutaneously.

The patient wears the pump continuously but may remove it and cap the needle for any activities that might damage the pump, such as swimming, bathing, or contact sports. He may remove it for sexual activity if he wishes. As long as he does not leave it off for more than an hour at a time, he need not administer additional insulin when he reattaches it.

CSII pumps are powered by disposable or rechargeable batteries. Most rechargeable batteries last about 24 hours and require 16 hours to recharge fully. The patient recharges one set of batteries while a second set powers the pump. A third set of batteries and an extra recharger are kept in case the batteries discharge accidentally.

Most pumps have alarms that warn the patient of various problems, such as run-down batteries, a blocked needle or tubing, or a runaway (a malfunction that causes the plunger driver to deliver insulin uncontrollably).

Routine Pump Care
The patient using an insulin infusion pump must develop a regular routine of pump care. This includes monitoring blood glucose levels, charging and changing the batteries, and changing the syringe tubing, needle, and insertion site.

Blood glucose levels should be checked 2 hours before or 2 hours after each meal every day, and at 3 a.m. once a week. If blood glucose levels ever ex-

(continued)

USE OF AN INSULIN INFUSION PUMP (continued)

ceed 200 mg/dl, the patient should immediately test his urine for ketone bodies. If they are present, he may need additional insulin and increased fluids. He should monitor his blood glucose level every 2 hours until it returns to normal and his urine is free of ketone bodies. He should call the diabetes nurse specialist or his physician if his blood glucose level has not returned to normal within 6 to 8 hours.

Since the patient is receiving a constant infusion of insulin, he must eat snacks to keep his blood glucose levels within 80 to 140 mg/dl. He should administer a bolus infusion before breakfast, lunch, and dinner.

Because he sets the time of his premeal boluses, the patient has greater flexibility in his mealtimes. When his blood glucose levels remain stable, he can delay a meal, but he should eat a snack during this time.

Many types of pumps are available. Because of the difference in pumps, manufacturer's instructions must be followed to charge and change batteries and change the syringe, tubing, and needle.

Some earlier models require dilution of rapid-acting insulin. Most models on the market today do not. The patient simply fills the syringe with enough rapid-acting insulin for 1 day and places it in the pump. Besides being easier to use, undiluted insulin seems to reduce the incidence of abscesses at the insertion site and to increase insulin absorption. If the patient is using a model that does require diluted insulin, insulin diluent or normal saline is used in an amount determined by the physician.

To prevent skin irritation, the patient should change the needle and insertion site every 1½ days (according to American Diabetes Association policy). He must prepare the site by washing it with soap and water, then applying alcohol or povidone-iodine. A skin barrier, similar to those used in ostomy care, helps protect the skin from the tape used to secure the needle.

The most commonly used insertion site—and the one providing the best insulin absorption—is the abdomen. To prevent irritation there, the patient should be careful not to insert the needle horizontally, too shallowly, or at the waistline. A man may have to shave the site, as well. The patient inserts the needle subcutaneously at a 30° to 60° angle and tapes it in place. He covers the needle and a small loop of tubing made near it with a 1¼" × 2" (3- × 5-cm) piece of polyurethane dressing. (He can cover just the needle with the dressing and tape the loop separately.) The patient can frequently check the site through this dressing for redness and leakage.

Another possible problem at the insertion site is abscess formation. The patient can prevent this by washing his hands thoroughly before touching the site, bathing before changing the needle, making sure he does not contaminate the solution while diluting it, and changing the needle frequently.

Complications

Besides skin irritation and abscess formation, insulin infusion pumps are associated with other complications. Probably most significant is severe hypoglycemia resulting from insulin excess, increased activity, or delayed food consumption. To prevent this, the patient must eat meals and snacks on time.

After a patient has worn an insulin infusion pump for a while, the usual symptoms of hypoglycemia can change from those of a sympathetic nervous system response (sweating, rapid heart rate, and hunger) to those of a central nervous system response (confusion and loss of consciousness). This happens because the constant infusion of insulin by the pump eliminates the sudden drop in blood glucose level that produces a sympathetic response. The patient or a family member should notify the physician if blood glucose levels are persistently below 60 mg/dl. Also, a family member should be taught how to inject glucagon in case the patient loses consciousness.

(continued)

USE OF AN INSULIN INFUSION PUMP (continued)

Two other possible complications that can occur with an insulin pump are ketoacidosis and hyperglycemia. These can result from lack of insulin caused by leakage around the needle, obstruction of the needle, mechanical failure, or disconnection of the tubing from the syringe. They can be prevented by observing the site carefully, checking operation of the pump frequently, and responding immediately to high blood glucose levels and ketone bodies in the urine.

The CSII pump is an alternative to conventional insulin injection therapy in the control of diabetes mellitus. This type of pump delivers insulin in small (basal) doses every few minutes and large (bolus) doses as manually set by the patient, usually one-half hour before meals. Approximately half the daily insulin dose is given in basal doses and half in bolus doses.

Instruction on the use of this pump and stabilization of blood glucose levels requires hospitalization. Patients selected to use the pump must be highly motivated to improve glucose control, willing to work closely with health care providers, willing to assume significant responsibility for their daily care, able to self-monitor blood glucose levels, and able to understand and demonstrate the use of the pump.

Some models of the CSII pump offer the following features:

- multiple basal rates
- meal bolus
- meal bolus delay
- dose limit protection
- programmable automatic shutdown and alarm
- hold for stopping insulin delivery
- alarms
- accumulated dose readout
- keyboard lockout
- function code review
- timer for self-monitoring of glucose

INTRAMUSCULAR

Giving an intramuscular injection

Intramuscular (I.M.) injections deposit medication deep into muscle tissue, where a large network of blood vessels can absorb it readily. The rate of drug absorption from this route of administration is more rapid than from the subcutaneous route, but slower than from the I.V. route. The needle used is longer and of smaller gauge than that used in subcutaneous injections, and larger volumes of medication (up to 5 ml in appropriate sites) may be given I.M. This route of administration is an alternative route for patients who cannot take medication orally and for drugs that are changed by digestive juices. And because muscle tissue has few sensory nerves, I.M. injection allows less painful administration of irritating drugs.

The site for an I.M. injection must be chosen carefully, taking into account the patient's general physical status and the type and amount of medication to be injected. Insertion of a needle into a nerve can cause permanent or partial paralysis of the nerve, and insertion of a needle into a blood vessel can result in I.V. rather than I.M. administration of the drug or in bleeding from the vessel.

I.M. injections should not be administered at inflamed, edematous, or irritated sites or at those containing moles, birthmarks, scar tissue, or other lesions. I.M. injections also may be contraindicated in patients with impaired coagulation mechanisms, with occlusive peripheral vascular disease, or in shock; these conditions impair peripheral absorption. I.M. injections require sterile technique to prevent intro-

I.M. INJECTION SITES

1. Deltoid muscle

Because this muscle is small, this injection site is used only when small doses of medication are administered or when other injection sites are inaccessible because of casts, dressings, the patient's inability to change positions, or other obstructions. Avoid inserting the needle into the radial nerve, which would result in permanent or partial paralysis of the arm. The patient may stand, sit, or lie down. To relax the muscle, he should have his arm at his side with the elbow flexed.

Locate the densest area of muscle and avoid major nerves and blood vessels by finding the lower edge of the acromial process and the point on the lateral arm in line with the axilla. Insert the needle 1" to 2" (2.5 to 5 cm) below the acromial process, usually 2 to 3 fingerbreadths.

Standard ml injected: 0.5 (range 0.5 to 2 ml).

2. Dorsogluteal site (gluteus medius)

This is the most popular I.M. injection site in adults. However, it can also be a dangerous site, because insertion of a needle into the sciatic nerve can cause permanent or partial paralysis of the involved leg. To relax the gluteal muscle, the patient should lie down with his toes pointed in, or lie on his side with the knee and hip of his upper leg flexed and anterior to the lower leg.

To locate the injection site, palpate the posterior superior iliac spine and the greater trochanter of the femur. Draw an imaginary line between these two bony prominences. Restrict injections to the area above and outside the imaginary line.

Another method is to visually divide the buttocks into quadrants and inject the outer upper quadrant, about 2" to 3" (5 to 7.5 cm) below the iliac crest.

Standard ml injected: 2 to 4 (range 1 to 5 ml).

3. Ventrogluteal site (gluteus medius and gluteus minimus)

The muscles of this site are situated deep and away from major nerves and blood vessels. This site is therefore safe

(continued)

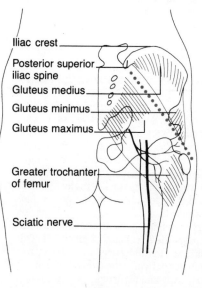

I.M. INJECTION SITES (continued)

to use in emaciated patients, infants, and children. The patient may lie on his side, back, or abdomen. To relax the involved muscles, he should flex his hip and knee.

First, locate the greater trochanter of the femur with the heel of your hand. Then, spread your index and middle fingers to form a V from the anterior superior iliac spine to the farthest point you can reach along the iliac crest. Insert the needle into the area between your two fingers. Remove your hand before inserting the needle.

Standard ml injected: 1 to 4 (range 1 to 5 ml).

4. Vastus lateralis muscle

This muscle is used most often for infants and children, because it is usually the best-developed muscle of those available for injection and because it contains no major nerves or blood vessels. The patient should lie down for the injection. He should relax the muscle by slightly flexing his knee.

Use the lateral muscle of the quadriceps group, along that length of the muscle from a handbreadth below the greater trochanter to a handbreadth above the knee. Insert the needle into the middle third of the muscle on a plane parallel to the surface on which the patient is lying. To be sure the medication is given into the muscle, grasp the muscle between your thumb and index finger before inserting the needle.

Standard ml injected: 1 to 4 (range 1 to 5 ml; 1 to 3 ml for infants).

5. Rectus femoris muscle

This site is rarely used by nurses because many patients complain of discomfort when it is used for injections. It is, however, used by patients for self-injection, because of its accessibility. Have the patient lie down, or have him sit if he is learning self-injection.

Grasp the muscle between your thumb and index finger (to avoid striking the femur), and inject the needle into the middle third of the front of the thigh.

Standard ml injected: 1 to 2 (range 1 to 3 ml).

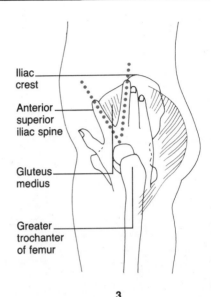

3

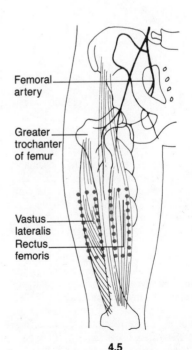

4,5

ducing a pathogen into the tissue, which could cause an infection.

Equipment and materials
You will need prepared medication in a syringe with an appropriate needle attached and two alcohol sponges.

Steps
• Confirm the identity of the patient by checking the name, room number, and bed number on his wristband.
• Tell him where you will be giving the injection. Provide privacy, and position and drape him appropriately. Make sure that the area is well exposed and that lighting is adequate.
• Loosen the protective needle cover, but do not remove it.
• Locate the injection site (see *I.M. Injection Sites*, pp. 100 and 101) and cleanse the skin with an alcohol sponge (see illustration).

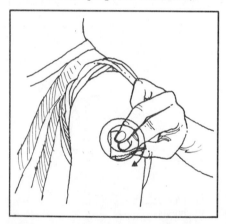

• Move the sponge outward in a circular motion, to a circumference of about 2" (5 cm) from the injection site. Allow the skin to dry, so that alcohol is not introduced into the subcutaneous tissue as the needle is inserted. (This precaution prevents pain or burning.)
• Remove the protective needle cover.
• With the thumb and index finger of your nondominant hand, press down and stretch the skin of the injection site. This reduces the thickness of subcutaneous tissue that must be pierced to reach the muscle. This is required with an obese patient. If the patient is emaciated, raise the underlying muscle mass by pinching the tissue between the thumb and index finger.

• Position the syringe at a 90° angle to the skin surface, with the needle a couple of inches from the skin. Tell the patient that he will feel a prick as you insert the needle. Then, as you say this, quickly and firmly thrust the needle through the skin and subcutaneous tissue, deep into the muscle.
• Hold the syringe with your nondominant hand, if desired. Pull back slightly on the plunger with your dominant hand. If no blood is aspirated, place your thumb on the plunger rod and *slowly* inject the medication into the muscle. A slow, steady injection rate allows the muscle to distend gradually and accept the medication under minimal pressure. You should feel little or no resistance against the force of the injection. The air bubble added to the syringe when it was prepared should follow the medication into the injection site to create an air block and prevent tracking of the medication back into subcutaneous tissue.
• If blood appears in the syringe on aspiration, the needle is in a blood vessel. If this occurs, withdraw the needle, prepare another injection with new equipment, and inject another site. Do not inject the bloody solution.
• After the injection, gently but rapidly remove the needle at a 90° angle.
• Cover the injection site immediately with a new alcohol sponge, apply gentle pressure, and unless contraindicated, massage the muscle to help distribute the drug and promote absorption.
• Remove the alcohol sponge and inspect the injection site for signs of active bleeding. If bleeding continues, apply pressure to the site.
• Replace the needle cover, being careful not to stick yourself with the contaminated needle.
• Discard needles and syringes according to institutional policies.
• Document that the medication was given on the medication cardex, and note the injection site.
• Continue to assess the patient's response to drug therapy.

Nursing considerations
• Try to minimize the pain of injections by following the suggestions in *Reducing the Pain of I.M. Injections.*

REDUCING THE PAIN OF I.M. INJECTIONS

You can reduce the pain of I.M. injections by following these tips.
- *Encourage the patient to relax the muscle.* Injections into tense muscles cause more pain and bleeding than injections into relaxed muscles. (Give injections into the gluteal muscles while the patient lies face down with his toes pointed in, or on his side with the knee and hip of the upper leg flexed and anterior to the lower leg.)
- *Avoid extra-sensitive areas.* When you choose the injection site, roll the muscle mass under your fingers and look for twitching. This indicates an extra-sensitive "trigger" area. Injections in this area may cause referred pain or a sharp pain as if the nerve were hit.
- *Wait until the skin antiseptic is dry.* If the antiseptic is still wet, it clings to the needle, creating pain when it reaches the sensory nerves of the subcutaneous tissues.
- *Always use a new needle.* The point and bevel of the needle can be dulled when they pass through the rubber stoppers in vials. Unless you change the needle, the dulled or rough edge that results causes more friction and pain during injection. Changing the needle also removes another source of pain—irritating medication that adheres to the outside of the needle when you draw the medication out of the vial.
- *Draw about 0.2 cc of air into the syringe.* This clears the needle bore of medication, which could leak out through the needle before or during insertion. When the needle is inverted for the injection, the air bubble rises to the plunger end of the syringe. Injecting this harmless air bubble reduces "tracking"—the leakage of medication from the needle injection path.
- *Dart the needle in rapidly and withdraw it rapidly to minimize puncture pain.*
- *Aspirate to be sure the needle is not in a blood vessel.* Then, inject the medication slowly to allow it to spread into the tissue under less pressure.
- *Unless contraindicated, massage the relaxed muscle to distribute the medication better and increase its absorption.* This will reduce the pain caused by tissue stretching from a large-volume injection. (Physical exercise of the injected muscle serves the same purpose.)
- *If the patient has experienced pain or emotional trauma from repeated injections, consider numbing the area before cleansing it by holding ice on it for several seconds.*

- Never use the gluteal muscles, which develop from walking, as the injection site for children under age 3 or for those who have been walking for less than a year.
- Keep a rotation record of all available injection sites, divided into body areas, for patients who require repeated injections.
- Rotate from a site in the first area to a site in each of the other areas. Then return to a site in the first area that is at least 1" (2.5 cm) away from the previous injection site used in that area. Failure to rotate sites in patients who require repeated injections can lead to deposits of unabsorbed drugs. Such deposits can reduce the desired pharmacologic effect and may lead to abscess formation or tissue fibrosis.
- If you must inject more than 5 ml of solution, divide the solution and inject it at two separate sites unless the gluteal muscles and vastus lateralis are well developed.
- I.M. injections can traumatize local muscle cells, causing elevated serum levels of enzymes (creatine phosphokinase [CPK]) that can be confused with the elevated enzymes resulting from damage to cardiac muscle, as in myocardial infarction. To differentiate between skeletal and cardiac muscle damage, diagnostic tests for suspected myocardial infarction must identify the isoenzyme of CPK specific to cardiac muscle (CPK-MB/CPK$_2$) and must include tests for lactic dehydrogenase (LDH) and serum glutamic-oxaloacetic transaminase (SGOT).
- Oral or I.V. routes are preferred for administration of drugs that are poorly ab-

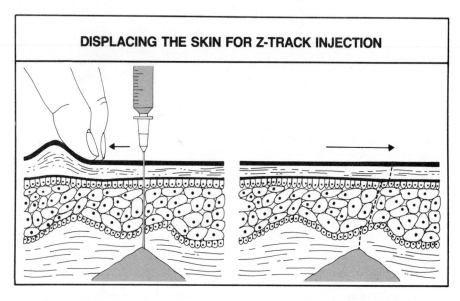

DISPLACING THE SKIN FOR Z-TRACK INJECTION

sorbed by muscle tissue, such as phenytoin, digoxin, chlordiazepoxide, diazepam, and haloperidol.

Giving a Z-track injection

The Z-track method of I.M. injection prevents leakage (tracking) of medication back into subcutaneous tissue after the injection is given. It is used with certain drugs—primarily iron preparations, such as iron dextran—that irritate or discolor subcutaneous tissue. Lateral displacement of the skin before injection helps seal the drug in the muscle after the skin is released. This procedure requires careful attention to technique, because leakage into subcutaneous tissue can cause patient discomfort or may permanently stain tissue if an iron preparation is being given. This type of injection is given only in the outer upper quadrant of the buttocks.

Equipment and materials
You will need two 20G needles at least 2" long, prescribed medication, a 3- to 5-ml syringe, and two sterile alcohol sponges.

Preparation
Attach one needle to the syringe, and draw up the prescribed medication. Then, draw 0.2 to 0.5 cc of air (depending on institutional policy) into the syringe. Remove the first needle, and attach the second to prevent introduction of medication from the outside of the first needle into subcutaneous tissue.

Steps
- Confirm the identity of the patient by checking the name, room number, and bed number on his wristband.
- Tell him where you will be giving the injection, and provide privacy.
- Have him lie in the prone or lateral position.
- Cleanse an area on the outer upper quadrant of the buttock with a sterile alcohol sponge.
- Displace the skin laterally by pulling it about ½" (1 cm) away from the injection site. (See *Displacing the Skin for Z-Track Injection.*)
- Insert the needle into the muscle at a 90° angle.
- Pull back on the plunger slightly. If no blood is aspirated, inject the drug slowly, followed by the air, which helps clear the needle and prevents tracking of the medication through subcutaneous tissue.
- Encourage the patient to walk or to move about in bed to facilitate absorption from the injection site.

- Discard the needles and syringe according to institutional policy.
- Document that the medication was given on the medication cardex.
- Continue to assess the patient's response to drug therapy.

Nursing considerations
- Never inject more than 5 ml into a single site using the Z-track method.
- Alternate gluteal sites for repeated injections.
- If the patient is on bed rest, encourage active range-of-motion exercises or perform passive range-of-motion exercises to facilitate absorption from the injection site.

INTRAVENOUS

Infusing a drug through a primary line

A primary line consists of a bottle or bag of I.V. solution and an administration set connected to an I.V. catheter or needle in the patient. Medication may be added to the solution, and the primary line may be used for continuous drug infusion. An I.V. pump or controller is useful in maintaining a constant infusion rate.

Equipment and materials
You will need prescribed medication in the I.V. solution, an administration set attached to the I.V. container and primed, and an I.V. pole.

If an infusion control device is indicated, attach it to the I.V. pole and thread the administration tubing through it according to the manufacturer's instructions.

Steps
- Confirm the identity of the patient by checking the name, room number, and bed number on his wristband.
- Explain the procedure to him.
- Wash your hands and perform the venipuncture (see "Inserting a peripheral line," p. 195).
- Remove the protective cap at the end of the administration tubing, and attach the tubing to the I.V. catheter or needle using sterile technique.
- Begin the infusion at the determined flow rate.
- Document the time the infusion began on the medication cardex.
- In the nurses' notes record venipuncture site, type and amount of medication, type and amount of I.V. solution hung, rate of infusion, and time the infusion began.
- When the contents of the I.V. container have been infused, or at the end of the shift, record the total amount of solution infused with the medication on the intake and output sheet.
- Continue to assess the patient's response to drug therapy.

Nursing considerations
During drug infusion, monitor the venipuncture site for signs of infiltration. Some drugs cause minor-to-severe tissue damage upon infiltration. Also, if infiltration occurs, the patient does not receive the prescribed amount of I.V. medication. The I.V. infusion should be stopped and started at another site.

Infusing a drug through a secondary line

A secondary I.V. line is a complete I.V. set—container, tubing, and needle—connected to the injection port of a primary line. It can be used for continuous or intermittent drug infusion. When used continuously, a secondary I.V. line permits drug infusion and titration while the primary line maintains a constant total infusion rate. When used intermittently, it is commonly called a piggyback set. The primary line maintains venous access between drug doses. Antibiotics are most commonly administered by intermittent (piggyback) infusion. A true piggyback system consists of a small infusion container for the intermittent drug, hung higher than the primary I.V. container. (See *Piggyback Set*, p. 106.)

I.V. pumps may be used to maintain constant infusion rates, especially with a drug such as lidocaine. A pump allows more accurate control of drug dosage and helps maintain venous access since the drug is delivered under sufficient pressure to prevent clot formation in the I.V. cannula.

A secondary I.V. line should not be connected to a hyperalimentation line because of the risk of contamination.

PIGGYBACK SET

A piggyback set—used solely for intermittent drug infusion—includes a small I.V. container, short tubing, and usually a macrodrip system. It connects into a primary line's upper Y-port (piggyback port). For the set to work, you must use an extension hook to position the primary I.V. container below the piggyback container, as shown.

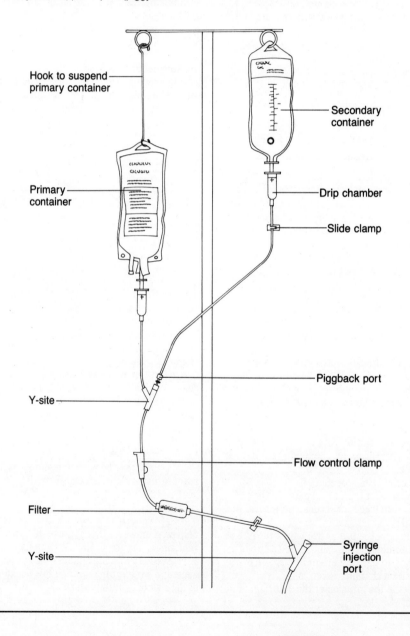

TAPING AN I.V. CONNECTION

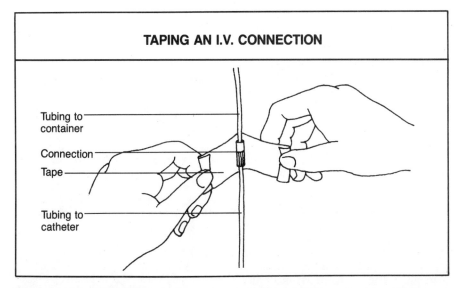

Tubing to container
Connection
Tape
Tubing to catheter

Equipment and materials
You will need prescribed I.V. medication in a prescribed I.V. solution, an administration set attached to the I.V. container and primed, a 22G 1" needle attached to the tubing and primed, alcohol sponges, 1" adhesive tape, and an extension hook for the piggyback set.

For intermittent infusion, the primary line often has a piggyback port with a backcheck valve, which stops the flow from the primary line during drug infusion and returns to the primary flow after infusion. A volume-control set can also be used with an intermittent infusion line (see *Volume-Control Sets*, p. 109).

See if the primary line has a secondary injection port. If it does not, and the medications will be given regularly, replace the I.V. set with one that has a secondary injection port. Repeated punctures of injection ports can cause an imperfect seal, resulting in leakage or contamination.

Steps
• Confirm the identity of the patient by checking the name, room number, and bed number on his wristband.
• Check the line for patency, and check the venipuncture site for infiltration, phlebitis, or infection.

• If the drug is incompatible with the primary I.V. solution, replace the solution with normal saline solution (unless contraindicated) and flush the line before starting the drug infusion. Many institutional protocols require removing the primary (incompatible) I.V. solution and inserting a sterile I.V. plug into the container until you are ready to rehang it. This will maintain sterility of the solution and prevent someone else from inadvertently restarting the incompatible solution before the line is flushed with normal saline solution.
• Hang the secondary container and select the injection port. The piggyback port is generally used for intermittent infusions, while the secondary port is generally used for simultaneous infusion with the primary solution.
• Wipe the injection port of the primary line with an alcohol sponge.
• Insert the needle from the secondary line into the injection port and tape it securely to the primary line (see *Taping an I.V. Connection*).
• *To run the secondary container solely,* lower the primary container with an extension hook. *To run both containers simultaneously,* place them at the same height.
• Open the clamp and adjust the drip rate. *For continuous infusion,* set the secondary solution to the desired drip rate and adjust

the primary solution to achieve the desired total infusion rate. *For intermittent infusion,* set the secondary solution to the desired drip rate, leaving the primary drip rate as required upon completion of the secondary infusion.
• Document that the medication was given on the medication cardex.
• When the I.V. containers are empty, or at the end of the shift, record the total amount of solution infused on the intake and output sheet.
• Continue to assess the patient's response to drug therapy.

Nursing considerations
• If institutional policy allows, use a pump for drug infusion, since it allows for more accurate control of drug dosage. Put a time tape on the secondary container to help prevent use of an inaccurate administration rate.
• If the secondary solution tubing will be reused, close the clamp on the tubing and follow institutional policy: either remove the needle and replace it with a new one, or leave it securely taped in the injection port and label it with the time and date it was first used. In this case, also leave the empty container in place until you replace it at the prescribed time. When reusing secondary tubing, change it according to institutional policy (usually every 24 to 48 hours).
• If the secondary tubing will not be reused, discard it appropriately with the I.V. container.

Using a volume-control set

A volume-control set—an I.V. line with a chamber—delivers precise amounts of fluid and shuts off when the fluid is gone, preventing air from entering the I.V. line. This device is attached to the I.V. solution container. It is useful for continuous infusion of fluids or medication to children or for intermittent infusion of medication to adults already receiving I.V. therapy. However, I.V. pumps and controllers are currently taking over this function.
 Although various models of volume-control sets are available (see *Volume-Control Sets*), each set consists of a graduated chamber (120 to 250 ml), with a spike and filtered air line on top and administration tubing underneath. Inspect a set for defects before using it.

Equipment and materials
For use in a primary line, you will need I.V. solution, a volume-control set, an I.V. pole, prepared medication in a syringe with a 20G or 22G 1" needle attached, and an alcohol sponge.
 For use in a secondary line, you will need I.V. solution, a volume-control set, a 20G or 22G 1" needle and adhesive tape (for piggybacking), prepared medication in a syringe with a 20G or 22G 1" needle attached, and alcohol sponges.

Preparation
Wash your hands and remove the volume-control set from its box. Close all clamps. Remove the guard from the volume-control set spike, insert the spike into the I.V. solution container, and hang the container on the I.V. pole. (If desired, spike a new solution bag after hanging it.) Open the air vent clamp; then, open the lower clamp on the I.V. tubing and slide it upward until it is positioned slightly below the drip chamber. Next, close the clamp.
 If you are using a volume-control set with a hinged latex valve or floating latex diaphragm, open the upper clamp until the fluid chamber fills with about 30 ml of solution. Then close the clamp and carefully squeeze the drip chamber until it is half full.
 If you are using a volume-control set with a membrane filter, open the upper clamp until the fluid chamber fills with about 30 ml of solution; then close the clamp. Open the lower clamp and squeeze the drip chamber flat with two fingers of your opposite hand. *If you squeeze the drip chamber with the lower clamp closed, you will damage the membrane filter.* Keeping the drip chamber flat, close the lower clamp. Now, release and reshape the drip chamber so it fills halfway.
 Open the lower clamp, prime the tubing, and close the clamp. *To use in a primary line,* insert the adapter into the catheter or needle hub. *To use in a secondary line,* attach a 20G or 22G 1" needle to the adapter on the volume-control set. Wipe the injec-

VOLUME-CONTROL SETS

Because of differences in their structures, the three types of volume-control sets—the membrane filter, the hinged latex valve, and the floating latex diaphragm—have different air lock mechanisms.

The membrane filter, shown in the device at left, is rigid and remains stationary at the bottom of the fluid chamber.

As long as the filter stays wet, it prevents air from entering the drip chamber. The hinged latex valve, shown in the center device, and the floating latex diaphragm, shown in the device at right, rise when the fluid chamber is full and fall to cover the opening in the bottom of the chamber when it is empty, preventing air from entering the drip chamber.

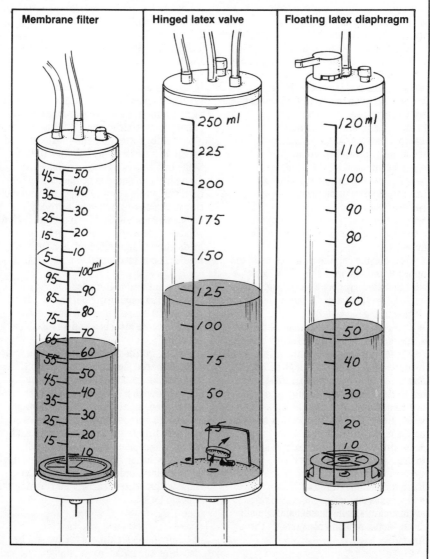

tion port of the primary tubing with an alcohol sponge, and insert the needle. Then tape the connection.

Steps
• Before adding medication to the volume-control set, confirm the identity of the patient by checking his name, room number, and bed number on his wristband.
• Check the line for patency, and check the venipuncture site for infiltration, phlebitis, or infection.
• To add medication to the chamber, wipe the injection port on the volume-control set with an alcohol sponge, and inject the medication. Place a label on the chamber indicating the drug, the dose, and the time and date. Do not write directly on the chamber with ink (the plastic absorbs ink), and do not place the label over the numbers.
• Open the upper clamp, fill the fluid chamber with the prescribed amount of solution to dilute the medication, and close the clamp. Gently rotate the chamber to mix the medication and solution.
• If present, turn off the primary solution, or set a low drip rate to maintain an open line after the solution in the secondary line has been infused.
• Open the lower clamp on the volume-control set, and adjust the drip rate as ordered.
• After completing the infusion, open the upper clamp and let 10 ml of I.V. solution flow into the chamber and through the tubing to flush them and deliver all of the medication to the patient.
• If you are using the volume-control set in a *secondary I.V. line*, close the lower clamp and reset the flow rate on the primary line. If you are using the set in a *primary I.V. line*, close the lower clamp, refill the chamber to the prescribed amount, and begin the infusion again.
• Document that the medication was given on the medication cardex.
• Continue to assess the patient's response to drug therapy.

Nursing considerations
• If you are using a membrane filter set, avoid administering suspensions, emulsions, blood, or blood components through it.

• If you are using a latex diaphragm set, the diaphragm may stick after repeated use. If it does, close the air vent and upper clamp, invert the drip chamber, and squeeze it. If the diaphragm opens, reopen the clamp and continue to use the set; if not, replace the set.
• If the drip chamber of a hinged latex valve or floating latex diaphragm set overfills, immediately close the upper clamp and air vent, invert the chamber, and squeeze the excess fluid from the drip chamber back into the graduated chamber.
• Change the volume-control set according to institutional policy.

Infusing a drug through a heparin lock

Infusing a drug through a heparin lock (also known as an intermittent infusion device) eliminates the need for multiple venipunctures or continuous I.V. infusion. It allows intermittent administration of medication by infusion or by I.V. push injection. Some institutional policies require that a dilute heparin solution be injected as the final step in this procedure, to prevent clotting in the device. When this is done, the device must be flushed with normal saline solution before and after the prescribed medication is administered, in case the medication is incompatible with heparin.

Equipment and materials
For I.V. push administration, you will need prepared medication in a syringe with a 22G 1" needle attached and an alcohol sponge.

For I.V. infusion administration, you will need prepared medication in I.V. solution, an administration set attached to the I.V. container with a 22G 1" needle attached and primed, an alcohol sponge, and tape.

For both methods, you will need two 3-ml syringes filled with saline solution, each with a 22G 1" needle attached, and dilute heparin solution (concentration determined by physician's order) in an appropriate syringe with needle attached, for flushing the heparin lock.

Steps
• Confirm the identity of the patient by checking the name, room number, and bed

number on his wristband. Explain the procedure.
- Check the venipuncture site for infiltration, phlebitis, or infection.
- Wipe the injection port of the heparin lock with an alcohol sponge, and insert the needle of a saline-filled syringe (see illustration below).
- Pull back on the plunger slightly and observe for blood return. If no blood is aspirated, begin to inject the saline solution slowly. Stop immediately if you feel any resistance; this indicates that the heparin lock is occluded and needs to be replaced.

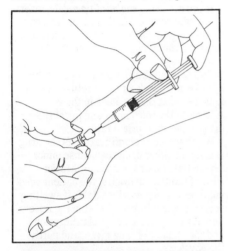

- If you feel no resistance, watch for signs of infiltration (puffiness or pain at the site) as you slowly inject the saline solution. If you note either of these signs, replace the heparin lock.
- If there are no signs of infiltration, administer the medication by the I.V. push or I.V. infusion method.
- After administering medication by I.V. push or I.V. infusion (see steps below), dispose of needles and syringes according to institutional policy.
- Document that the medication was given on the medication cardex.
- Record the amount of I.V. solution used (if any) on the intake and output sheet.
- Continue to assess the patient's response to drug therapy.

I.V. push
- Insert the needle of the syringe containing the medication into the injection port.
- Inject the medication at the suggested rate. Then remove the needle from the injection port.
- Insert the needle of the remaining saline-filled syringe into the injection port, and slowly inject the saline solution to flush all medication through the device. Withdraw the needle.
- Insert the needle of the heparin-filled syringe and inject the heparin flush solution to prevent clotting in the device.

I.V. infusion
- Insert the needle attached to the administration set into the injection port, and tape the connection securely.
- Open the flow clamp and adjust the flow rate.
- Infuse medication for the prescribed length of time; then flush the heparin lock with saline and heparin, as you would after an I.V. push injection.

Nursing considerations
- If you are giving an I.V. push injection of a drug that is incompatible with saline, flush the heparin lock with bacteriostatic water instead. In some institutions, the device is flushed with 2 to 3 ml of normal saline solution, instead of heparin flush solution, to prevent clotting in the cannula.
- Heparin locks should be changed regularly, according to institutional policy (usually every 48 to 72 hours).

Administering medication by I.V. push

I.V. push injection allows rapid I.V. administration of a bolus dose of a drug. The term *bolus* generally refers to a dose administered all at once. I.V. push may be used in an emergency to provide an immediate drug effect. It can also be used to achieve peak drug levels in the bloodstream, to deliver drugs that cannot be diluted (such as diazepam, digoxin, and phenytoin), or to administer drugs that cannot be given intramuscularly because they are toxic to muscle tissue or because the patient's ability to absorb them is impaired.

Bolus doses of medication may be injected directly into a vein, through an existing I.V. line, or through a heparin lock.

Because the medication administered takes effect rapidly, the patient must be monitored for adverse reactions such as cardiac arrhythmia. I.V. push injection is contraindicated when rapid administration of a drug could cause life-threatening complications or when the drug requires dilution. For certain drugs, the safe rate of injection specified by the manufacturer precludes administration by I.V. push.

Equipment and materials
For administration directly into the vein, you will need prepared medication in a syringe with a 20G 1" needle attached, a tourniquet, a povidone-iodine sponge, an alcohol sponge, a sterile 2" × 2" gauze pad, and an adhesive bandage. You may need a winged-tip needle with catheter and a 3-ml syringe filled with saline solution, with a 22G 1" needle attached.

A winged-tip needle is often used for an I.V. push largely because it can be quickly and easily inserted. This makes it ideal for the repeated administration of drugs, as in weekly or monthly chemotherapy.

For administration into an existing I.V. line, you will need prepared medication in a syringe with a 22G 1½" needle attached and an alcohol sponge.

For administration into a heparin lock, see "Infusing a drug through a heparin lock," pp. 110 and 111.

Steps
- Confirm the identity of the patient by checking his name, room number, and bed number on his wristband.
- Explain the procedure to him if this is the first time it is being performed.
- After administering medication directly into the vein or through an existing I.V. line or a heparin lock (see steps below), dispose of needles and syringes according to institutional policy.
- Document that the medication was given on the medication cardex.
- Continue to assess the patient's response to drug therapy.

I.V. push directly into the vein
- Select the largest vein suitable for an injection. The larger the vein, the more diluted the drug will become as it travels through it, minimizing vascular irritation. The antecubital or basilic veins are most commonly used, but, in an emergency, any accessible vein may be used.
- Apply a tourniquet above the injection site to distend the vein.
- Cleanse the injection site with the sterile povidone-iodine sponge. Then cleanse it with the sterile alcohol sponge, working outward from the puncture site in a circular motion to prevent recontamination with skin bacteria.
- If you are using the *syringe needle*, insert it into the vein at a 30° angle with the bevel up. The bevel should reach ¼" (0.6 cm) into the vein.
- If you are using a *winged-tip needle*, insert the needle with its bevel up, tape the butterfly wings in place when you see blood return in the tubing, and attach the drug-filled syringe.
- Pull back slightly on the plunger of the syringe and check for blood return, which indicates that the needle is in the vein.
- Remove the tourniquet and inject the drug at the appropriate rate.
- Watch for signs of infiltration as the drug is injected. Some drugs can cause minor-to-severe tissue damage upon infiltration. Also, if infiltration occurs, the patient does not receive the prescribed dose. If swelling occurs at the injection site, stop the injection. Estimate the amount of infiltration and the amount of drug given, and notify the physician.
- After the medication has been given, pull back slightly on the plunger of the syringe and check for blood return again. If blood appears, it indicates that the needle remained in place and all injected medication entered the vein.
- If you are using a *winged-tip needle*, flush the line with the normal saline solution from the second syringe to ensure delivery of all medication into the vein.
- Withdraw the needle and apply pressure to the injection site with the sterile gauze pad for 3 minutes to prevent hematoma formation.
- Apply the adhesive bandage to the site after bleeding has stopped.

I.V. push through an existing I.V. line
- Check the line for patency, and check the venipuncture site for infiltration, phlebitis, or infection.

- Check the compatibility of the medication with the existing I.V. solution. (If the drug is not compatible with the I.V. solution, close the flow clamp and flush the line with 3 to 5 ml of normal saline solution *before* and *after* the injection.)
- Close the flow clamp and wipe the injection port closest to the patient with a sterile alcohol sponge.

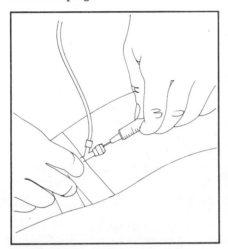

- Stabilize the injection port with one hand, and insert the needle (see illustration above).
- Inject the drug as you would for direct injection.
- After the injection, open the flow clamp and readjust the flow rate.

I.V. push through a heparin lock
- See "Infusing a drug through a heparin lock," pp. 110 and 111, in this chapter.

Nursing considerations
- Observe the patient for signs of respiratory or cardiac distress. Notify the physician immediately if any signs occur, and begin emergency procedures as necessary. Because drugs administered by I.V. push injection are delivered directly into the circulatory system and can produce an immediate effect, adverse reactions can develop rapidly.
- If you are giving a drug that is incompatible with saline, flush the infusion device with bacteriostatic water instead of saline to prevent drug precipitation due to incompatibility.

Managing a continuous narcotic infusion

Continuous narcotic infusion (CNI) is a safe, effective method of providing continuous parenteral (I.V.) analgesia when a patient's physical condition makes traditional administration routes ineffective (for example, when the oral route is ineffective because of an intestinal obstruction or when the I.M. or subcutaneous routes are ineffective because of bleeding problems, decreased muscle mass, or inadequate absorption). CNI is also effective when around-the-clock administration of oral, injected, or rectal narcotics no longer controls pain.

CNI is used in the treatment of cancer, severe burns, acute pancreatitis, fistulas, Crohn's disease, and acute postoperative pain. It does not produce addiction because patients receiving a continuous infusion do not develop a psychological need (as can patients who depend on p.r.n. narcotics). Furthermore, most patients taking narcotics for pain control will require decreased dosages as the pain subsides.

Narcotics commonly used for CNI are morphine, hydromorphone (Dilaudid), levorphanol (Levo-Dromoran), and methadone. Morphine is most often the drug of choice because it is less expensive than the other three. It is not recommended for the patient with biliary tract disease, however. Of all the narcotics, it produces the greatest constriction of the sphincter of Oddi, causing increased pressure within the biliary system and thereby increasing pain.

Equipment and materials
You will need prepared medication in a syringe with needle attached, an alcohol sponge, I.V. solution with administration set and volume-control set attached and primed, and an infusion pump with alarm. You may need venipuncture equipment.

Steps
- Confirm the identity of the patient by checking the name, room number, and bed number on his wristband.
- Explain the procedure to him to relieve anxiety.
- Wash your hands.

- If an I.V. line is not already in place, perform a venipuncture (see "Inserting a peripheral line," in Chapter 13, p. 195). If an existing line is in place, check it for patency, and check the site for infiltration, phlebitis, or infection.
- Administer a prescribed dose (usually a 1-hour dose) of the narcotic by I.V. push, as ordered. This provides quick, short-term relief until CNI takes effect.
- Before beginning CNI, check your institutional policy for specific guidelines. One way to begin is by putting 25 ml of I.V. fluid into the volume-control set and adding a 1-hour dose of the narcotic. Run this mixture through the infusion pump at 25 ml/hour.
- Repeat the procedure for the second hour. (Hourly doses allow easy adjustment of the dose according to the patient's response.)
- Continue hourly doses of the narcotic, adjusting the dose as ordered until the patient is comfortable.

PAIN MEDICATION FLOW SHEET

Date	Time	Medication	Pain Level (0 = no pain; 10 = worst pain imaginable) and Patient Comments	Respirations
10/1	12:30 p.m.	3/M	8 "Can't stand the pain"	22 (baseline)
	12:55 p.m.	Morphine, 5 mg, I.V. push	8	22
	1:00 p.m.	Morphine drip, 5 mg in 25 ml to run over 1 hour	7 "Beginning to ease somewhat"	18
	1:30 p.m.	3/M	7	18
	2:00 p.m.	Morphine drip, 5 mg in 25 ml to run over 1 hour	5 (Patient has slept some)	17
	2:30 p.m.	3/M	5	20
	3:00 p.m.	Morphine drip, 5 mg in 25 ml to run over 1 hour	5 "Feel sore"	17
	3:30 p.m.	3/M	6 "More cramping and aching"	22
	4:00 p.m.	Morphine drip, 7 mg in 25 ml to run over 1 hour	6	22
	4:30 p.m.	3/M	4 "Pain is easing"	18
	5:00 p.m.	Morphine drip, 28 mg in 100 ml to run over 4 hours	3 "Much more comfortable" (patient sleeping intermittently)	18
	9:00 p.m.	Morphine drip, 28 mg in 100 ml to run over 4 hours	3	18

- Once the patient is comfortable, begin infusion on a 4-hour schedule rather than a 1-hour schedule. Place 100 ml of I.V. fluid in the volume-control set and add a 4-hour dose of the narcotic (four times the hourly dose). Set the infusion pump at 25 ml per hour.
- Assess the patient's comfort level and respiratory rate at least every 30 minutes during the 1-hour infusions, then once every 4 hours during the 4-hour infusions. If necessary, the dose can be adjusted according to the patient's response.
- Document the date, time, dose, and medication on the medication record. Document the same information, along with the patient's pain level and respiratory rate, on a flow sheet to be kept at the patient's bedside. (See *Pain Medication Flow Sheet*.)

Nursing considerations
- Do not add the narcotic to the I.V. solution. An I.V. bottle or bag of 500 to 1,000 ml will hang for many hours; with prolonged exposure to light, morphine becomes discolored and should not be used.
- To assess patient response, develop a uniform system (a numerical scale or a set of

---

EQUIANALGESIA: SWITCHING TO ANOTHER ROUTE

Switching to another route of administration of narcotics may become necessary because of changes in the patient's condition, infiltration, patient comfort and convenience, or the need for better pain control. The physician will order the specific medication and route of administration, but you can suggest changes in the medication regimen based on observations of the patient, data in equianalgesic charts (which provide a general guide for converting from parenteral to oral drugs), and a few simple rules for switching from one route to another.

The equianalgesic chart and rules included below are only *guidelines* for determining the correct dose; dosage depends mostly on patient response.

Equianalgesic List: I.M. and P.O. Doses for Moderate-to-Severe Pain

Analgesic (narcotic)	I.M. (mg)	P.O. (mg)
Morphine*	10	30
Codeine	130	200
Hydromorphone (Dilaudid)	1.5	7.5
Levorphanol (Levo-Dromoran)	2	4
Meperidine (Demerol, Pethidine)	75	300
Methadone (Physeptone, Dolophine)	10	20
Oxycodone		30
Oxymorphone (Numorphan)	1	
Pentazocine (Fortral, Talwin)	60	180

*Morphine is the only drug for which the list's ratio of P.O. to I.M. is disputed; some experts maintain that while the 6:1 ratio applies to a one-dose administration, a 3:1 ratio is more accurate for prolonged administration.

This equianalgesic list is excerpted from the list distributed in 1980 by Analgesics Study Section, Sloan-Kettering Institute for Cancer Research, New York.

verbal descriptions, for example) for rating severity of pain.
- Make sure all staff members are aware of the rating system. This helps establish reliable guidelines for this subjective area of assessment and helps ensure the consistent monitoring necessary to adjust doses to patient need.
- If the I.V. infiltrates and CNI cannot be restarted right away, switch to another route immediately—preferably not the oral route. This will prevent withdrawal symptoms and keep the patient's pain from becoming unbearable before CNI can be restarted. As a precaution, calculate the dose for the alternative route beforehand. (See *Equianalgesia: Switching to Another Route*, p. 115.)
- Know the patient's baseline respiratory rate and his average rate during CNI to aid in accurate determination of the need to decrease or to stop CNI to prevent respiratory depression.
- If respiratory depression occurs, administer naloxone (Narcan) with caution. Narcan, as it is usually administered, reverses all analgesic effects and may cause withdrawal.
- If Narcan is needed, do not automatically use the whole vial in one dose. Small doses—0.2 to 0.8 mg—administered every 3 to 4 minutes can restore respiratory function without reversing all analgesic effects.
- If you see no improvement in the patient's breathing after administering a total of 10 mg of Narcan, respiratory depression may not be the result of the narcotic. Dying patients commonly experience periods of apnea or respiratory depression that stem entirely from their illness.
- If the patient experiences increased pain with certain activities (for example, whenever he is transported to or from treatments or during his bath), supplement CNI, as ordered, by giving an I.V. push dose of half the hourly dose p.r.n.
- Remember that the *patient* is the final authority on whether the pain exists and how severe it is. Even though the dose of narcotic may seem high, it is not excessive if his respiratory rate is stable and he has remained alert. If a patient's dose has been increased because he has developed a tolerance to the drug, he has also developed a respiratory tolerance, and administering a higher dose probably will not significantly depress respiration.

Switching from oral to I.V. administration
- Determine the total oral narcotic dose the patient receives in 24 hours.
- Convert the oral dose to an I.M. dose by using an equianalgesic list.
- Divide the 24-hour I.M. dose by 2 to derive the total I.V. dose. (In some patients it is appropriate to use the equivalent I.M. dose; others may require only half of the I.M. dose.)
- Divide the total I.V. dose by 24 to derive the hourly dose.

These steps are precise only to a point. The I.V. dose is the equivalent of the patient's oral dose. But if the oral dose was not adequate, the I.V. dose probably will not be adequate. The conversion gives the *equivalent* dose, not necessarily the effective dose. To determine the *effective* dose, the patient's overall condition, and especially the level of pain, must be considered.

Switching from parenteral to oral administration
- Although procedures vary, a common initial method is to administer half the parenteral dose, and then give the equivalent of the remaining half in oral form.
- After several such doses, the total dose is converted to an oral dose.
- Another approach is to administer a "loading dose" of the oral drug alone. This is an initial dose higher than the anticipated effective dose. It may initially produce some sedation but should convince the patient that the oral drug can relieve pain.
- This initial oral dose is then adjusted downward over several days, based on the patient's response, until the dosage provides satisfactory analgesia with minimal side effects and stable vital signs.
- The total oral dose is then reduced to the minimum dose necessary to achieve satisfactory analgesia.

Infusing a drug through an implantable infusion port

An implantable infusion port is a device that consists of catheter tubing attached to an injection port, which has a self-sealing entry septum. The device is implanted under the skin surgically, using local anesthesia. The catheter is then tunneled to various sites, such as a central vein leading into the right atrium, the peritoneal cavity, the epidural space, or the hepatic artery.

The port comes with catheters of varying lumen sizes, and its use determines the catheter size chosen. Currently available devices include Infuse-A-Port, Port-A-Cath, and MediPort (single and double lumen). They are used for patients who require long-term venous access for chemotherapy, other I.V. medications, fluids, or blood products. They can also be used for blood sampling.

Compared with right atrial catheters, such as the Hickman or Broviac catheter, the implantable infusion device needs no dressing changes, needs only monthly heparinization, and causes less restriction of everyday activity. (Catheters to the hepatic artery must be flushed weekly, however.) It also reduces the impact on body image and the risk of infection. For some patients, however, the right atrial catheter may be better because it is easier to manipulate and requires no needle insertion through the skin. Implantable infusion ports are contraindicated in those who have been unable to tolerate other implantable devices and in those who have or may develop peritonitis, an allergic reaction, or infections.

Equipment and materials
You will need a sterile towel to create a sterile field, a pair of sterile gloves, three povidone-iodine sponges, and sterile extension tubing with a stopcock (or other self-clamping mechanism) and a Luer-Lok.

For an I.V. bolus injection, gather these additional supplies:
- a sterile 22G 1½" straight Huber point needle (Note: Use only a Huber point needle to enter the port. The needle has an angled tip that slices the septum upon entry rather than coring it as a conventional needle will do. The septum then reseals upon withdrawal of the needle. Huber point needles come in various gauges and lengths; follow the manufacturer's recommendations in choosing the right one.)
- two sterile 6-ml syringes of saline solution
- two sterile 6-ml syringes of heparin solution (100 units/ml)
- a sterile syringe containing the prescribed drug
- alcohol sponges
- a small adhesive bandage.

For a continuous infusion, gather these additional supplies:
- a sterile 6-ml syringe of saline solution
- a sterile 6-ml syringe of heparin solution (100 units/ml)
- a sterile 22G 1" right-angled Huber point needle (Note: Choose the length of the needle so that when it is positioned in the port, the right angle is just above the surface of the skin so the patient can more easily cover the site with clothing and continue activities while receiving an infusion.)
- a sterile 3" × 3" gauze pad
- tincture of benzoin
- ½" Steri-Strips
- tape
- medium-sized transparent dressing such as Op-Site or Tegaderm
- prescribed I.V. solution or medication, and I.V. tubing connected to an infusion pump, if required. (An infusion pump is only necessary with arterial catheters.)

Steps
- Confirm the identity of the patient by checking the name, room number, and bed number on his wristband.
- Explain the procedure to him.
- Wash your hands.

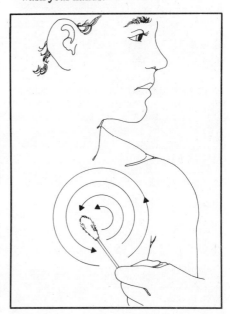

I.V. bolus injection
• Palpate the skin over the port to establish anatomical landmarks.
• Cleanse the injection site with a povidone-iodine swab. Start at the center of the septum and swab outward in a circular motion until you have cleaned an area at least 6" (15 cm) in diameter (see illustration on p. 117). Repeat this procedure twice, using a new swab each time.
• Allow the skin to air dry to activate the bactericidal, fungicidal, and sporicidal properties of povidone-iodine.
• Put on sterile gloves and attach a 6-ml syringe of heparin solution to the stopcock at the end of the extension tubing. Then connect the appropriate Huber point needle to the Luer-Lok at the other end and prime the tubing. Close the stopcock.
• Stabilize the port between the index finger and thumb of your nondominant hand and palpate the port entry system with your dominant hand to find the center of the septum.
• Holding the needle at a 90° angle to the skin surface like a dart, insert it into the center between the thumb and forefinger of the hand stabilizing the port, pushing until the needle stops. Then aspirate a small amount of blood to make sure the needle is properly positioned.
• Holding the needle firmly in place, open the stopcock. Using firm, steady pressure, flush the infusion port with 6 ml of heparin solution at a rate of less than 5 ml per minute. If swelling occurs or the patient complains of pain or a burning sensation as you are injecting the heparin solution, the needle is improperly positioned. Withdraw it from the injection port, re-prep the site, and insert another sterile needle.
• Close the stopcock, and disconnect the syringe and discard it.
• Attach a 6-ml syringe of saline solution to the stopcock, open it, and flush the injection port and catheter.
• Close the stopcock and disconnect the syringe and discard it.
• Attach the syringe containing the prescribed drug. Open the stopcock and slowly inject the drug.
• Close the stopcock and carefully disconnect the syringe to prevent any of the drug from dripping on the patient's skin.
• Attach the second 6-ml syringe of saline solution to the stopcock, open it, and inject the saline to clear the catheter of medication.
• Attach the second 6-ml syringe of heparin solution, open the stopcock, and inject all 6 ml to prevent occlusion at the catheter tip.
• Withdraw the needle, being careful not to twist or tilt it. (Twisting or tilting may cut the septum, causing extravasation.)
• Observe the injection site for signs of extravasation. Expect a small amount of serosanguinous drainage at the site upon needle withdrawal. If the patient complains of pain or an abnormal sensation at the site, notify the physician.
• Use alcohol sponges to remove the povidone-iodine from the area. Apply a small adhesive bandage if necessary.
• Document in the nurses' notes the medication, dose, time, patient tolerance of the procedure, appearance of the site, and any pertinent nursing interventions.
• Document on the medication cardex that the medication was given.

Continuous infusion
• Prepare the injection site, prime the extension tubing with heparin solution as for a bolus injection, close the stopcock, and insert the right-angled Huber point needle. Because this needle can rotate at the hub, use your finger to stabilize it at the angle during insertion. (See illustration below.)

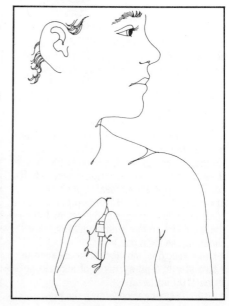

- Check for proper needle position by aspirating a small amount of blood.
- Holding the needle firmly in place, open the stopcock and flush the infusion port with 6 ml of heparin solution at a rate of less than 5 ml per minute. If swelling occurs or the patient complains of pain or a burning sensation, the needle is improperly positioned. Withdraw it from the injection port, re-prep the site, and insert another sterile needle.
- Close the stopcock, disconnect the syringe, and discard it.
- Attach a 6-ml syringe of saline solution to the stopcock, open it, and flush the port and catheter.
- Close the stopcock, disconnect the syringe, and discard it.
- Roll up the sterile 3" × 3" gauze pad and place it under the needle hub and Luer-Lok to support the needle.

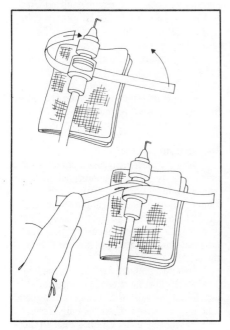

- Apply tincture of benzoin to the skin on both sides of the gauze pad to help the Steri-Strips adhere.
- Secure the needle and tubing by applying Steri-Strips across the needle hub, using chevron taping (see illustration above).
- Apply the transparent dressing to permit direct inspection of the insertion site.
- Attach the stopcock to the I.V. line from the infusion pump. Tape all connections to prevent accidental disconnections.
- Open the stopcock and begin continuous infusion at the prescribed rate.
- When infusion is completed, close the stopcock, disconnect the I.V. line, and attach a 6-ml syringe of saline to the stopcock.
- Inject the saline to clear the catheter of medication. Close the stopcock and discard the syringe.
- Attach a 6-ml syringe of heparin solution to the stopcock and flush the infusion port.
- Withdraw the needle without twisting or tilting it. Observe the site for signs of infection, infiltration, or bleeding. Remove the povidone-iodine and tincture of benzoin with alcohol, and apply a small adhesive bandage if necessary.
- Document in the nurses' notes the medication, dose, rate, time, patient tolerance of the procedure, appearance of the site, and pertinent nursing interventions.
- Document on the medication cardex that the medication was given.

Nursing considerations
- Make sure you know your facility's specific policies and procedures regarding use and care of implantable drug delivery systems, as well as the manufacturer's recommendations for the system in use.
- If the patient finds insertion of the needle painful, 0.1 to 0.15 cc of 2% lidocaine may be injected subcutaneously at the site before the Huber needle is inserted.
- Always flush the system with saline solution *after each drug* and *before heparinization* to prevent drug incompatibilities.
- Flush the port with heparin after each use to prevent occlusion.
- If the port is not used regularly, flush it with 5 ml of heparin solution (100 units/ml) every 4 weeks, or according to manufacturer's recommendations, to maintain patency. The frequency of flushing also depends on placement; for example, intraarterial placement requires weekly flushes.
- For patients requiring frequent blood sampling or intermittent I.V. drugs, the port may be used as a heparin lock by attaching a male adapter injection port to

the distal end of the extension tubing. Flush the system with 3 to 5 ml of heparin solution after each use.
- Inspect the area around the injection site daily for infection, hematoma, accumulation of serous fluid, and device rotation or extrusion.
- For a *continuous infusion*, change the I.V. line every 24 hours. The extension tubing and needle can remain in place 7 to 10 days unless a problem develops or unless institutional policy or manufacturer's recommendations differ. The dressing should be changed every 3 to 5 days, depending on the therapy and the condition of the site.
- If packed red blood cells are to be given through the port, "piggyback" the cells into normal saline and administer them at 15 to 20 cc per hour to reduce the risk of occlusion. Flush the system with a 15- to 20-ml bolus of normal saline between units.
- If you suspect the catheter is occluded, change the Huber point needle. Fibrin particles drawn into the catheter during blood sampling can occlude the needle.
- If changing the needle does not solve the problem, notify the physician. He may order alternation of gentle irrigation with aspiration using heparinized saline, or instillation of a fibrinolytic agent such as streptokinase or urokinase.
- Some patients may develop the nervous habit of "twiddling" the portals of their catheters (twiddler's syndrome), which may displace the catheter. Check the site regularly and note if the patient touches the site frequently. Patients must be instructed about the hazards of this behavior. Displacement is confirmed by X-ray.

INTRAARTERIAL
Managing an intraarterial infusion

Intraarterial infusion can deliver an antineoplastic drug through a catheter in a major artery directly to a localized, inoperable tumor. This procedure allows a high concentration of the drug to reach the tumor without metabolic breakdown by the liver or kidneys and with little dilution by the circulatory system. The intraarterial catheter is implanted surgically or threaded through a peripheral artery into branches of the celiac artery for liver tumors, into the external carotid artery for head and neck tumors, and into the internal carotid artery for brain tumors.

Intraarterial infusion can also deliver vasopressin to the site of gastrointestinal bleeding. Usually, the catheter is threaded from a peripheral site to the left gastric, celiac, or mesenteric artery, depending on the bleeding site.

To prevent blood backflow and clotting, infusion of heparinized saline begins in the operating room after implantation of the catheter, or in the X-ray department after insertion and confirmation of placement. Equipment for initial infusion must accompany the patient to either location. Because of arterial pressure, all fluids must be infused with either a pump or pressure cuff.

Equipment and materials
You will need a bag of heparinized saline solution for infusion, a bag of solution with medication for infusion, an I.V. pole, a volumetric infusion pump with tubing and cassette or a pressure cuff with pressure tubing and minidrip chamber, a stopcock, and sterile alcohol sponges. You may need a hemostat and a 4" × 4" gauze sponge.

The stopcock—placed between the catheter and the tubing—prevents blood leakage during bag and tubing changes.

Preparation
To prepare a volumetric infusion pump, wash your hands and hang the solution bag. Wipe the tubing insertion port with a sterile alcohol sponge, insert the tubing spike, and fill the drip chamber at least halfway. Then, according to the manufacturer's directions, open the flow clamp and prime the tubing and cassette.

To prepare a pressure cuff, insert the bag through the bottom of the pressure cuff, slip the tab through the hole in the bag, and hang the pressure cuff on the pole. Then wipe the tubing insertion port with an alcohol sponge, insert the tubing spike, and fill the drip chamber only one-quarter full, since the drip chamber will continue to fill when the cuff is being pressurized. Next, open the clamp, prime the tubing, and close the clamp. Inflate the pressure cuff.

Steps
Catheter insertion and monitoring
- Assess the patient's understanding of the procedure and correct any misconceptions. Make sure the patient knows the catheter insertion site. Tell him that insertion will take place in the operating room or X-ray department and that it will take 1 to 2 hours. If known, tell him how long the catheter will be in place and how it might restrict mobility or activity.
- If ordered, administer analgesics or sedatives before the procedure.
- After the procedure, take the patient's vital signs as ordered.
- Monitor the insertion site for bleeding, ecchymosis, hematoma, or catheter movement. Infection can follow catheter insertion but generally appears several days later.
- Watch for changes in catheter length, which indicate catheter displacement.
- If applicable, check the level of the pressure cuff. It should read at least 150 mm Hg and must be higher than the patient's systolic blood pressure (but not more than 300 mm Hg) to ensure an adequate drip rate for the infusion. After checking the pressure, close the inflation flow valve to prevent air leaks from the pressure cuff. If leaks occur, clamp the tubing between the pressure cuff and the bulb with a hemostat. To protect the rubber tubing from damage, wrap a 4" × 4" gauze sponge around the tubing before attaching the hemostat.
- Check the infusion tubing to detect kinks, external obstruction, or blood backflow. If backflow occurs, increase the pressure in the pressure cuff.

Changing a bag with an infusion pump
- Stop the infusion, turn the stopcock off, remove the tubing spike from the old bag, and insert it into the new one after cleansing the port with a sterile alcohol sponge.
- Hang the new bag, turn the stopcock on, and start the infusion pump.

Changing a bag with a pressure cuff
- Close the flow clamp, turn the stopcock off, and turn the pressure-release valve counterclockwise to deflate the pressure cuff.
- Remove the old bag from the pressure cuff and the tubing spike from the old bag. Put in the new bag and slip the tab through the hole on top of the bag.
- Wipe the port with an alcohol sponge. Insert the tubing spike, and hang the equipment on the I.V. pole.
- Turn the pressure-release valve clockwise to prevent air from escaping, and inflate the pressure cuff as necessary—to 150 to 300 mm Hg—to ensure an adequate drip rate.
- Open the stopcock and the flow clamp, and adjust to the desired drip rate.

Documentation
- Document that the medication was given on the medication cardex.
- Record the amount of solution infused on the intake and output sheet. To check the volume remaining in a bag using a pressure cuff, turn off the stopcock or clamp the line, deflate the pressure cuff, read the fluid level, and reinflate the pressure cuff.
- Record tubing and dressing changes, patient response to the infusion, assessment of catheter site, and signs of complications in the nurses' notes.

Nursing considerations
- Thrombus formation is the most common complication of intraarterial infusion; it usually requires removal of the catheter by the physician. Bleeding can occur at the catheter insertion site. Movement of the catheter can also occur, even when it is sutured in place. Fluoroscopic examination confirms catheter placement. Catheter-related sepsis may require administration of systemic antibiotics and catheter removal.
- Change the tubing every 24 hours with the solution. To do this, assemble new tubing and solution and a new pressure cuff or pump. Prime the new tubing. Then turn off the stopcock, switch the sets, and start the infusion.
- Change the dressing every 24 hours or when wet, following institutional procedures or using a subclavian dressing kit.
- The recent availability of mini-infusion pumps has made it possible for some patients to manage their intraarterial chemotherapy at home.

INTRATHECAL
Assisting with an intrathecal injection

An intrathecal injection allows direct administration of medication into the subarachnoid space of the spinal canal. Certain drugs—such as anti-infectives, or antineoplastics used to treat meningeal leukemia—are administered by this route because they cannot readily penetrate the subdural membrane through the bloodstream. Intrathecal injection may also be used to deliver anesthetics such as lidocaine hydrochloride to achieve regional anesthesia, as in spinal anesthesia or epidural block.

An invasive procedure performed by a physician under sterile conditions with a nurse assisting, intrathecal injection requires informed patient consent. The injection site is usually between the third and fourth (or fourth and fifth) lumbar vertebrae, well below the spinal cord, preventing the risk of paralysis. This procedure may be preceded by withdrawal of cerebrospinal fluid for laboratory analysis. Contraindications to intrathecal injection include inflammation or infection at the puncture site, septicemia, and spinal deformities (especially when the procedure is considered for anesthesia).

Equipment and materials
You will need a lumbar puncture tray, a fenestrated drape (if not on the lumbar puncture tray), antiseptic solution, povidone-iodine sponges (or cotton balls or gauze pads), sterile disposable gloves, local anesthetic, a package of sterile gauze pads, alcohol sponges, a 3- or 5-ml syringe, a 25G ⅝" needle, a syringe containing the prescribed drug, and an adhesive bandage.

You may need pillows, a shave preparation tray, and specimen containers with labels.

The lumbar puncture tray, drape, disposable gloves, and cotton balls and gauze pads should be sterile.

Steps
- Wash your hands.
- Make sure the patient or a responsible family member has signed the consent form.
- Reinforce the physician's explanation of the procedure to the patient. Tell him that he may experience a stinging sensation when the anesthetic is injected.
- Tell the patient to void just before the procedure, because he may have to stay in bed for several hours afterward.
- Provide privacy. If ordered, shave the injection site.
- Place the patient in the right or left lateral position, as directed by the physician. Use pillows, if permissible, to make the patient comfortable. Be sure the puncture site is well exposed and that lighting is adequate.
- Using sterile technique, open the lumbar puncture tray and the fenestrated drape. The tray serves as the sterile field.
- If povidone-iodine sponges are not available, pour the antiseptic solution over the cotton balls or gauze pads.
- The physician puts on the sterile gloves and cleanses the injection site with the povidone-iodine sponges or the saturated cotton balls or gauze pads.
- The patient is draped with the fenestrated drape so that the area surrounding the third and fourth lumbar vertebrae (or other appropriate site) is exposed.
- Wipe the diaphragm of the anesthetic bottle with the alcohol sponge. Leave the sponge on the bottle. Do not set the bottle on the sterile field.
- Using sterile technique, open the syringes and needle, and drop them onto the sterile field.
- Show the physician the label on the local anesthetic to verify its type and strength. Then turn the bottle upside down so he can fill the 3- or 5-ml syringe, using the 25G ⅝" needle, without contaminating the equipment.
- After the physician anesthetizes the skin and subcutaneous tissue, the lumbar puncture needle (from the tray) is inserted into the lumbar space. At this point, cerebrospinal fluid may be withdrawn for laboratory analysis. If so, label all specimen containers correctly and send them to the laboratory immediately after the procedure.
- Verify the type and amount of medication in the syringe with the physician.
- Using sterile technique, remove the needle from the syringe containing the prescribed medication, and hand the syringe to the physician.

- The physician attaches the syringe to the lumbar puncture needle and injects the medication into the subarachnoid space.
- Open a package of sterile gauze pads, using sterile technique.
- Put on sterile gloves and pick up a gauze pad.
- After the physician withdraws the needle, place a gauze pad over the injection site and apply gentle pressure to prevent medication seepage and bleeding.
- When there is no evidence of seepage or bleeding, apply an adhesive bandage to the site.
- Dispose of equipment according to institutional policy.
- Assist the patient to a position specified by the physician.
- Document the time and date of administration, the type and amount of medication given, the route of administration, and the name of the physician who administered the drug in the nurses' notes.
- Continue to assess the patient's response to drug therapy.

Nursing considerations
- If the patient cannot maintain the correct position, help him maintain back flexion by gently but firmly grasping him behind his neck and knees.
- Encourage the patient to drink fluids, as permitted, to help replace any cerebrospinal fluid loss.
- After injection of chemotherapeutic drugs, be especially alert for specific drug side effects.

INTRAARTICULAR

Assisting with an intraarticular injection

An intraarticular injection delivers drugs directly into a synovial cavity to relieve joint pain, to help preserve function and prevent contractures, and to delay muscle atrophy. It is most commonly used to administer a high concentration of steroid into an acutely inflamed joint (see *Common Intraarticular Injection Sites*, p. 124). Other drugs administered by this method are anesthetics and lubricants. Rarely, antiseptics, analgesics, and counterirritants may be injected by this route. Before intraarticular injection, synovial fluid may be withdrawn for relief of pressure or for laboratory analysis.

Usually performed by a physician with a nurse assisting, an intraarticular injection requires sterile technique to prevent introducing a pathogen into the joint and causing an infection. The procedure is painful, and the patient may require assistance in keeping the joint stable during injection. Intraarticular injection is contraindicated in patients with joint infection, joint instability or fracture, or systemic fungal infection.

Equipment and materials
You will need 3-ml and 5- or 10-ml syringes, prepared medication in a 5- or 10-ml syringe with an 18G 1½" needle attached, pillows, a sterile towel, sterile gloves, sterile cotton balls or gauze pads, a sterile emesis basin, antiseptic solution, a sterile fenestrated drape, local anesthetic, a 25G ⅝" needle, and an adhesive bandage.

You may need a 10- or 20-ml syringe for aspirating synovial fluid and sterile test tubes for synovial fluid aspirate, with appropriate additives and specimen labels.

Prepackaged sterile povidone-iodine sponges may be used. If they are used, you will not need the antiseptic solution, the sterile cotton balls or gauze pads, or the emesis basin.

Steps
- Confirm the identity of the patient by checking his name, room number, and bed number on his wristband.
- Explain the procedure to him, and provide privacy.
- Position the patient comfortably. The joint to be injected should be stabilized, supported (with pillows, if necessary), and fully exposed, with adequate lighting provided.
- Using sterile technique, open the sterile towel and place it on the bedside table, to create a sterile field.
- Using sterile technique, open the package containing the sterile emesis basin, and place it on the sterile field.
- Using sterile technique, open the syringes, needles, and cotton balls or gauze pads and drop them onto the sterile field.

124 Medication Administration and I.V. Therapy Manual

COMMON INTRAARTICULAR INJECTION SITES

- Acromioclavicular approach
- Anterior approach
- Humeroulnar approach
- Radiohumeral approach
- Anterior approach
- Lateral approach
- Anteromedial approach
- Dorsoradial approach
- Dorsolateral-ulnar approach
- Carpometacarpal injection
- Anteromedial approach
- Lateral approach
- Metatarsal approach

- After putting on the sterile gloves, the physician picks up the sterile cotton balls or gauze pads and holds them over the emesis basin.
- Pour the antiseptic solution over the cotton balls or gauze pads.
- Using sterile technique, open the package containing the sterile fenestrated drape, and hold it out so the physician can remove the drape.
- Hold up the local anesthetic bottle so the physician can read the label. Then turn the bottle upside down so he can insert the needle (25G ⅝") and fill the 3-ml syringe.
- The physician then anesthetizes the skin and subcutaneous tissue at the injection site.

Synovial fluid aspiration
- The physician withdraws synovial fluid with the 18G 1½" needle, using the 10-ml syringe. The needle is left in the joint for the subsequent injection of medication. The syringe with the specimen can be set aside until after the procedure.
- After completing the intraarticular injection, the physician will attach a needle to the specimen syringe and insert appropriate specimens into the test tubes. Label the test tubes appropriately and send them to the laboratory.

Intraarticular injection
- Verify the type and amount of medication in the prepared 5- or 10-ml syringe with the physician.
- Hand the syringe, with an 18G 1½" needle attached, to the physician. He then injects the medication into the synovial cavity. *If synovial fluid was aspirated,* hand the physician the medication syringe without a needle attached (remove it, using sterile technique). He attaches the syringe to the needle already in the joint and injects the medication.
- Using sterile technique, open a package of sterile gauze pads.
- Put on sterile gloves and pick up a gauze pad.
- After the physician withdraws the needle, place a gauze pad over the injection site and apply pressure to the site and (if appropriate) massage the area gently for 1 or 2 minutes, to aid absorption.
- Apply an adhesive bandage to the site.

- Dispose of needles and syringes according to institutional policy.
- In the nurses' notes document the time and date of administration, the type and amount of medication given, the route of administration, and the name of the physician who administered the drug. Also, note the amount of synovial fluid and any laboratory studies requested, if applicable.
- Continue to assess the patient's response to drug therapy.

Nursing considerations
- Advise the patient to avoid excessive use of the affected joint, because the injected medication may reduce pain while inflammation is still present.
- Because the medication may infiltrate and initially irritate surrounding tissue, local joint pain may increase for 24 to 48 hours after an intraarticular injection. This should subside within a couple of days. However, fever, persistent increased pain, redness, and swelling may indicate septic arthritis, a serious complication caused by contamination.

Review Questions

1. Why is it important to correctly identify an I.M. injection site?

2. Name the five I.M. injection sites.

3. In which injection site may no more than 2 ml of solution be injected?
   A. Deltoid
   B. Dorsogluteal
   C. Ventrogluteal
   D. Vastus lateralis
   E. Rectus femoris

4. Which is the most popular injection site in adults?
   A. Deltoid
   B. Dorsogluteal
   C. Ventrogluteal
   D. Vastus lateralis
   E. Rectus femoris

5. Name two methods of reducing the pain of an I.M. injection.

6. What is the purpose of the Z-track method of I.M. injection?
   A. To prevent injecting a blood vessel
   B. To prevent injecting a major nerve
   C. To seal off medication in the muscle
   D. To slow the absorption of the medication

7. Which injection site is safe to use in emaciated patients, infants, and children?
   A. Ventrogluteal
   B. Vastus lateralis
   C. Rectus femoris
   D. Dorsogluteal
   E. Deltoid

8. I.M. injections can traumatize local muscle cells. Which serum enzyme level may become elevated as a result of this trauma?
   A. CPK-MB/CPK$_2$
   B. LDH
   C. CPK
   D. SGOT

9. What three consequences may result from the failure to rotate injection sites?

10. If blood is aspirated into the syringe when giving an I.M. injection, what does this indicate, and what should you do next?
    A. The needle is in a blood vessel; inject the medication
    B. The needle is in the muscle; inject the medication
    C. The needle is in a blood vessel; withdraw the needle and prepare another injection
    D. The needle is in a joint; withdraw the needle and prepare another injection

11. Subcutaneous injections are contraindicated in:
    A. Patients with impaired coagulation mechanisms
    B. Areas of skin that are inflamed or edematous
    C. Sites within 2" of a scar, a bruise, or the umbilicus
    D. All of the above

12. Subcutaneous injections are performed using two different angles for the needle. State the two angles, and identify the necessary condition for the use of one of them.

13. An intradermal injection is used primarily for:
    A. Diagnostic purposes
    B. Producing a local effect
    C. Systemic absorption
    D. Answers A and B
    E. Answers A and C
    F. All of the above

14. When giving an intradermal injection, at what angle is the needle inserted? Is the bevel of the needle up or down? How far is the needle inserted?

15. If there is no wheal formation after you have given an intradermal injection, what does this indicate, and what should you do next?

16. A severe anaphylactic response, requiring immediate epinephrine injection and other emergency resuscitation procedures, can develop after an intradermal injection of an antigen. True or false?

17. To run a secondary line solely when using both a primary and a secondary I.V. line, the primary line is:
    A. Higher than the secondary line
    B. Lower than the secondary line
    C. At the same height as the secondary line

18. Which of the three types of volume-control sets can be damaged by squeezing the drip chamber with the lower clamp closed?

19. What are three reasons for maintaining a heparin lock in a patient?

20. What is a heparin flush, and why in some cases must it be preceded by sterile normal saline?

21. What are three indications of possible problems with a heparin lock?

22. What is the difference between I.V. push administration and I.V. bolus administration?

23. Name the two most common uses for intraarterial infusion.

24. Give five signs and symptoms of possible complications of an intraarterial infusion, and list their possible causes.

25. State the purposes of intrathecal and intraarticular injections.

26. When is continuous narcotic infusion (CNI) indicated?

27. Why is a 1-hour dose of narcotic given by I.V. push before CNI is started?

28. How should naloxone (Narcan) be administered if respiratory depression occurs in a patient on CNI? Why?

29. List three advantages of an implantable infusion device over the Hickman and Broviac catheters.

30. How (with what), when, and why should an implantable infusion device be flushed?

Speciale, J.L., and Kaalaas, J. "Infuse-a-Port—New Path for I.V. Chemotherapy," *Nursing 85* 5(10):40-43, October 1985.

Wilkes, G., et al. "Long-Term Venous Access...Subcutaneous Venous Access Device," *American Journal of Nursing* 85(7):793-96, July 1985.

Selected References

American Diabetes Association. "Continuous Subcutaneous Insulin Infusion," *Diabetes Care* 8(5):516, September/October 1985.

Childs, B.P. "Insulin Infusion Pumps—New Solution to an Old Problem," *Nursing 83* 13(11):54-57, November 1983.

Drugs, 2nd ed. Nurse's Reference Library. Springhouse, Pa.: Springhouse Corp., 1984.

Giving Medications. Nursing Photobook Series. Springhouse, Pa.: Springhouse Corp., 1982.

Holmes, W. "SQ Chemotherapy at Home," *American Journal of Nursing* 85(2):168-69, February 1985.

Managing I.V. Therapy. Nursing Photobook Series. Springhouse, Pa.: Springhouse Corp., 1983.

McGuire, L., and Wright, A. "Continuous Narcotic Infusion—It's Not Just for Cancer Patients," *Nursing 84* 14(12):50-55, December 1984.

Procedures. Nurse's Reference Library. Springhouse, Pa.: Springhouse Corp., 1983.

Application of Medication to the Eye, Ear, Nose, and Throat

Administering eye, ear, nose, or throat medications involves simple procedures. However, careful attention to the details of each procedure is necessary to ensure correct application of the medication for maximal therapeutic effect and to prevent unnecessary discomfort, local injury, infection, or other complications. This chapter discusses how to administer eye, ear, nose, and throat medications safely and effectively.

Administering eye medications

Eye medications—drops, ointments, and disks—serve both diagnostic and therapeutic purposes. During an eye examination, eye drops can be used to anesthetize the eye, dilate the pupil to facilitate refraction, and stain the cornea to identify corneal abrasions or scars. Eye medications can also be used to lubricate the eye, treat certain eye conditions (such as glaucoma and infections), protect the vision of neonates, and lubricate the eye socket for insertion of an artificial eye. Administration of eye medications requires sterile technique to avoid irritation or infection.

Equipment and materials
You will need prescribed eye medication at room temperature, cotton balls, warm water or normal saline solution, gauze pads, and tissues. You may need an eye dressing.
 All equipment and materials should be sterile.

Steps
• Confirm the identity of the patient by checking the name, room number, and bed number on his identification bracelet.
• Explain the procedure to him, and provide privacy.
• Make sure you know which eye to treat. Different medications or doses may be ordered for each eye.
• Wash your hands.
• If the patient is wearing an eye dressing, remove it by gently pulling it down and away from his forehead. Take care not to contaminate your hands.
• Remove any discharge by cleansing around the eye with cotton balls moistened with warm water or normal saline solution. With the patient's eye closed, cleanse from the inner canthus to the outer canthus, using a fresh cotton ball for each stroke.
• To remove crusted secretions around the eye, moisten a gauze pad with warm water or normal saline solution. Ask the patient to close the eye, then place the gauze pad over it for a minute or two. Remove the pad, then reapply moist sterile gauze pads, as necessary, until the secretions are soft enough to be removed without traumatizing the mucosa.
• Before instilling eye drops, applying ointment, or inserting an eye disk (see steps below), have the patient sit or lie in the supine position. If he is to be given eye drops or an ointment, instruct him to tilt his head back and toward the side of the eye to be treated, so excess medication flows away from the tear duct; this prevents systemic absorption through the nasal mucosa.
• After administration, remove any excess solution or ointment surrounding the eye

INSERTING AND REMOVING AN EYE MEDICATION DISK

A medication disk inserted into the eye can release medication for up to 1 week. Pilocarpine, for example, can be administered this way to treat glaucoma. The small, flexible oval disk consists of three layers: two soft outer layers and a middle layer containing the medication. Floating between the eyelids and the sclera, the disk stays in the eye while the patient sleeps and even during swimming and athletic activities. Once the disk is in place, the fluid in the eye moistens it, releasing the medication. Eye moisture or contact lenses do not adversely affect the disk. Eye medication disks offer the advantage of continuous release of medication. The patient never has to worry about forgetting to instill eye drops. Contraindications include conjunctivitis, keratitis, retinal detachment, and any condition where constriction of the pupil should be avoided.

To insert an eye medication disk
- Arrange to insert the disk before the patient goes to bed. This minimizes problems caused by the blurring that occurs immediately after the disk is inserted.
- Wash your hands.
- Press your fingertip against the oval disk so its length lies horizontally across your fingertip. It should stick to your finger. Lift it out of its packet.
- Evert the patient's lower eyelid and place the disk in the conjunctival sac. It should lie horizontally, not vertically. The disk will automatically stick to the eye.
- Pull the lower eyelid out, up, and over the disk. Tell the patient to blink several times. If the disk is still visible, lift the lower lid out and over the disk again. Tell the patient that once the disk is in place, he can adjust its position by gently pressing his finger against his closed lid. Caution him against rubbing his eye or moving the disk across the iris.
- If the disk falls out, wash your hands, rinse the disk in cool water, and reinsert it. If the disk bends out of shape, replace it. If both of the patient's eyes are being treated with medication disks, replace both disks at the same time, so both eyes receive medication at the same rate.
- If the disk continually slips out of position, reinsert the disk under the upper eyelid. To do this, gently lift and evert the upper eyelid and insert the disk in the conjunctival sac. Then, gently pull the lid back into position and tell the patient to blink several times. To adjust the disk to the most comfortable position, have the patient gently press on the closed lid. The longer the patient uses the disk, the easier it should be for him to retain it. If he cannot retain it, notify the physician.
- Before discharge, if the patient will continue therapy with an eye medication disk, teach him to insert and remove it himself. To check his mastery of these skills, have him insert and remove it for you.
- Also, teach the patient about possible side effects. Foreign-body sensation in the eye, mild tearing or redness, increased mucous discharge, eyelid redness, and itchiness can occur with the use of disks. Blurred vision, stinging, swelling, and headaches can occur with pilocarpine, specifically. Mild symptoms are common but should subside within the first 6 weeks of use. Tell the patient to report persistent or severe symptoms to his physician.

To remove an eye medication disk
- You can remove an eye medication disk with one or two fingers. To use *one finger*, evert the lower eyelid with one hand so you expose the disk. Then, use the forefinger of your other hand to slide the disk onto the lid and out of the patient's eye. To use *two fingers*, evert the lower lid with one hand to expose the disk. Then, pinch the disk with the thumb and forefinger of your other hand and remove it from the eye.
- If the disk is in the upper eyelid, apply long, circular strokes to the patient's closed eyelid with your finger until you can see the disk in the corner of the patient's eye. Once the disk is visible, place your finger directly on the disk and move it to the lower sclera. Then remove it as you would a disk in the lower lid.

HOW TO APPLY EYE MEDICATIONS

After you have checked the medication and positioned the patient correctly, you are ready to apply or instill the medication into the eye. The illustrations below summarize the essential steps necessary for safe and effective administration of eye drops or eye ointment.

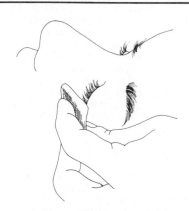

1. Moving from the inner to the outer canthus, cleanse the eye with a sterile gauze pad moistened with warm water or normal saline solution.

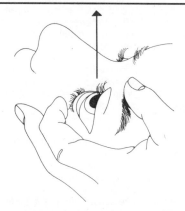

2. Ask the patient to tilt his head back and slightly toward the side to be treated, and have him look up and away. Place your index finger on the patient's cheekbone and gently pull down the skin, exposing the lower conjunctival sac.

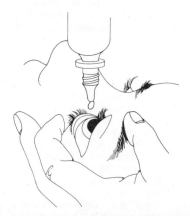

3. To instill eye drops, hold the squeeze bottle or the dropper in your other hand and squeeze the prescribed number of drops into the conjunctival sac. Release the patient's eye and let him blink to distribute medication over the eye. Blot away excess fluid with a clean cotton ball or tissue. Repeat the procedure in the other eye, as ordered.

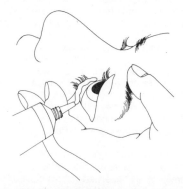

4. To apply eye ointment, squeeze a thin ribbon of ointment along the conjunctival sac starting at the inner canthus. As you approach the outer canthus, rotate the tube to detach the ointment. Release the patient's eye and ask him to close his eyes and roll them to distribute the medication. Wipe away excess ointment with a clean tissue. Repeat the procedure in the other eye, as ordered.

HOW TO APPLY AN EYE PATCH

An eye patch is used to prevent further injury after trauma or surgery by discouraging eye movement, to avoid damage to the eye after administration of a local anesthetic, to prevent contamination, or to promote healing. A surface bacterial infection contraindicates an eye patch because it enhances bacterial growth.

Although an eye patch must be ordered by the physician, it is a nursing responsibility to apply it. First, wash your hands. Then, ask the patient to close both eyes. Use as many sterile gauze pads as necessary to fill the orbital space so that the patch will be level with the edge of the frontal bone. Grasp the sterile eye patch in the center and place it over the gauze pads. Secure the patch with two parallel strips of nonallergenic tape, working from the patient's midforehead to the cheekbone, as shown. If added protection is needed, apply a plastic or metal shield over the patch, as ordered. The patch is easily removed by loosening the tape on the forehead and gently easing the patch down and off.

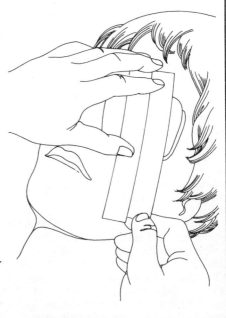

with a cotton ball or clean tissue. Use a separate cotton ball or tissue for each eye.
• Apply a new eye dressing if necessary. (See *How to Apply an Eye Patch*.)
• Document that the medication was given on the medication cardex.
• Return the medication to the storage area. Make sure you store it according to the label's instructions.
• Wash your hands.

Instilling eye drops
• Remove the dropper cap. Be careful to avoid contaminating the bottle top. Fill the dropper, as necessary.
• Before instilling drops, instruct the patient to look up and away. This moves the cornea away from the lower lid and minimizes the risk of touching the cornea with the dropper if the patient blinks.
• Steady the hand in which you are holding the dropper against the patient's forehead.
• With your other hand, gently pull down the lower lid of the affected eye, and instill drops in the conjunctival sac. (See *How to Apply Eye Medications*.)
• Tell the patient to close his eyes gently, without squeezing the lids shut, and to blink gently.

Applying eye ointment
• Remove the cap from the tube. Be careful to avoid contaminating the tip.
• Gently pull down the lower lid of the affected eye and squeeze a small ribbon of medication on the conjunctival sac from the inner to the outer canthus. Cut off the ribbon by turning the tube.
• If you wish, you can steady the hand holding the medication tube by bracing it against the patient's forehead or cheek. (See *How to Apply Eye Medications*.)
• Tell the patient to close his eyes gently and roll them to help distribute the medication over the surface of the eyeball.

Inserting an eye disk
See *Inserting and Removing an Eye Medication Disk*, p. 129.

Nursing considerations
- Administer eye drops that are at least at room temperature. Instilling cold drops is startling and uncomfortable.
- Never instill eye drops directly onto the eyeball. The cornea is sensitive and easily injured.
- After administering an eye medication that may be absorbed systemically (such as atropine), gently place your thumb over the inner canthus for 1 to 2 minutes while the patient closes his eyes. This helps prevent medication from flowing into the tear duct.
- Discard solution remaining in a dropper before returning it to the bottle.
- If the dropper has become contaminated, discard it and obtain another sterile dropper.
- To avoid cross-infection, never use a container of eye medication for more than one patient.
- When using an eyedropper, hold the bulb uppermost to prevent contaminating the medication with particles from inside the bulb.
- Instillation of some eye medications may cause transient burning, itching, and redness. Explain this to the patient beforehand, and document any reaction in your notes.
- Teach the patient not to rub his eyes after the instillation of drops or ointment to prevent irritating them.
- Work carefully and gently to prevent injury, especially when the lids are swollen, inflamed, and tender.

Instilling eardrops

Eardrops may be instilled to treat infection and inflammation, to soften cerumen for later removal, to produce a local anesthetic effect, or to facilitate removal of an insect trapped in the ear by immobilizing and smothering it. If the patient has a perforated eardrum, instillation of eardrops is usually contraindicated; however, certain medications may be instilled using sterile technique. Other conditions may also prohibit instillation of eardrops. For instance, instillation of drops containing hydrocortisone is contraindicated if the patient has herpes, another viral infection, or a fungal infection.

Equipment and materials
You will need prescribed eardrops, a bowl of warm water, a light source, and a tissue or a cotton-tipped applicator. You may need a cotton ball.

Preparation
To avoid side effects (such as vertigo, nausea, and pain) resulting from instillation of eardrops that are too cold, *warm the medication to body temperature* in the bowl of warm water or carry it in your pocket for 30 minutes before administration. If necessary, test the temperature of the medication by placing a drop on your wrist. If the medication is too hot, it may burn the patient's eardrum or, at the very least, be ineffective.

To avoid injury to the ear canal, inspect a glass dropper before using it to make sure it is not chipped.

Steps
- Confirm the identity of the patient by checking the name, room number, and bed number on his wristband.
- Explain the procedure to him, and provide privacy, if possible.
- Have him lie on the side opposite the affected ear.
- Wash your hands.
- Straighten the patient's ear canal. For an adult, pull the auricle of the ear up and back. For a child, pull the auricle of the ear down and back. (See "Instilling ear medications," p. 295.)
- Using the light source, examine the ear canal for drainage. If you find any drainage, remove it with the tissue or cotton-tipped applicator; drainage can interfere with the effectiveness of the medication.
- To avoid damaging the ear canal with the dropper, gently support the hand holding the dropper against the patient's head. Straighten the ear canal once again and instill the number of drops ordered. To avoid patient discomfort, direct the drops against the sides of the ear canal, not on the eardrum.
- Instruct the patient to remain on his side for 5 to 10 minutes to allow the medication to run down into the ear canal.
- *If ordered,* tuck a cotton ball *loosely* into the opening of the ear canal to prevent the medication from leaking out. Be careful not to insert it too deeply into the canal; this

would prevent drainage of secretions and increase pressure on the eardrum.
- Clean and dry the outer ear.
- If ordered, repeat the procedure in the other ear after 5 to 10 minutes.
- Assist the patient into a comfortable position.
- Wash your hands.
- Document that the medication was given on the medication cardex.

Nursing considerations
- Remember that some conditions make the normally tender ear canal even more sensitive, so be especially gentle when performing this procedure.
- *To prevent injury to the eardrum,* never insert a cotton-tipped applicator into the ear canal past the point where you can see the tip.
- Always wash your hands before and after instilling eardrops and between instilling them in both ears. Aseptic technique is especially vital if the patient's middle or inner ear has been opened by surgery or trauma.
- After applying eardrops to soften cerumen, irrigate the ear as ordered to facilitate cerumen removal.
- If the patient has vertigo, keep the side rails of his bed up and assist him during the procedure, as necessary. Also, move slowly and unhurriedly to avoid exacerbating his vertigo.
- Teach the patient to instill the eardrops correctly, so he can continue treatment at home, if necessary. Review the procedure and let him try it himself while you observe.
- Never place a cotton ball in the ear after administering eardrops unless specifically ordered to do so; it may interfere with outward movement of normal secretions and create undue pressure in the ear canal.

Instilling nasal medications

Nasal medications may be instilled by means of drops, a spray (atomizer), or an aerosol (nebulizer). Most drugs instilled by these methods produce local rather than systemic effects. Drops can be directed at a specific area; sprays and aerosols diffuse medication throughout the nose. Instilling nasal medications is a clean technique.

Most nasal medications, such as phenylephrine, are vasoconstrictors, which relieve nasal congestion by coating and shrinking swollen mucous membranes. Because vasoconstrictors may be absorbed systemically, they are usually contraindicated in hypertensive patients. Other classifications of nasal medications are antiseptics, anesthetics, and corticosteroids.

Nasal medications are usually aqueous, isotonic, slightly acidic, and nonirritating. Oily medications are never instilled into the nose because ciliary activity would be inhibited and the risk of respiratory infection increased. In addition, accidental inhalation of an oily medication may result in development of lipoid pneumonia.

Equipment and materials
You will need prescribed medication, an emesis basin (with nose drops only), and facial tissues. You may need a pillow, a small piece of soft rubber or plastic tubing, and a rubber nipple from a baby bottle.

Steps
- Confirm the identity of the patient by checking his name, room number, and bed number on his wristband.
- Explain the procedure to him, and provide privacy.
- Wash your hands.
- Follow the procedure for administering nose drops, a nasal spray, or a nasal aerosol (see steps below).
- Document that the medication was given on the medication cardex.

Instilling nose drops
- When possible, position the patient so the drops flow back into the nostrils, toward the affected area.
- *For drops to reach the eustachian tube opening,* position him in a supine position, with his head tilted slightly to the affected side.
- *For drops to reach the ethmoidal and the sphenoidal sinuses,* place him in the Proetz position. (See *Positioning the Patient for Instillation of Nose Drops,* p. 134.)
- *For drops to reach the maxillary and the frontal sinuses and the nasal passages,* place him in the Parkinson position. (See *Positioning the Patient for Instillation of Nose Drops,* p. 134.)

POSITIONING THE PATIENT FOR INSTILLATION OF NOSE DROPS

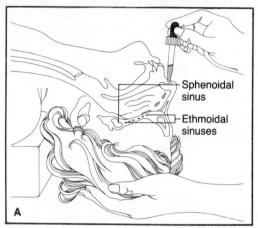

A. To reach the ethmoidal and sphenoidal sinuses, place the patient in the *Proetz position*. Place him on his back, with his shoulders elevated and his head tilted back over the edge of the bed; support the patient's head with one hand to prevent neck strain.

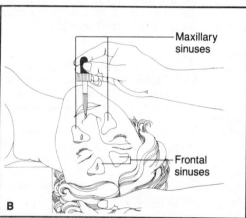

B. To reach the maxillary and frontal sinuses, place the patient in the *Parkinson position*. Place him on his back with his head toward the affected side and hanging slightly over the edge of the bed; support the patient's head with one hand to prevent neck strain.

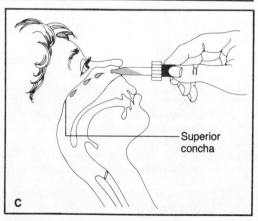

C. Place the patient *upright with his head tilted back* to instill nose drops for ordinary nasal congestion.

- To prevent undue strain on the patient's neck muscles, support his head with one hand, as necessary.
- If the patient suffers only from nasal congestion or if he cannot assume either the Proetz or the Parkinson position, place him in a supine position, and put a large pillow under his shoulders so his head tilts back over his shoulders. Tilt his head as far back as possible to prevent the drops from running into the throat.
- If the patient suffers only from ordinary nasal congestion and is able to sit up, position him upright with his head tilted back.
- Draw up some medication in the dropper.
- Push up the tip of the patient's nose slightly. Position the dropper just above or in front of the nostril, and direct its tip toward the midline of the nose (superior concha), so the drops flow toward the back of the nasal cavity rather than toward its base, where they would flow down the throat.
- Insert the dropper about ⅜" (1 cm) into the nostril. Make sure the dropper does not touch the sides of the nostril; this would contaminate the dropper and could cause the patient to sneeze. (Besides, you have to see the dropper tip to count the drops.)
- Instill the prescribed number of drops, observing the patient carefully for any signs of discomfort.
- To prevent the drops from leaking out of the nostrils, ask him to keep his head tilted back for at least 5 minutes and to breathe through his mouth. This also allows sufficient time for the medication to work.
- Keep an emesis basin handy, so the patient can expectorate any medication that flows into the oropharynx and mouth. Use a facial tissue to wipe any excess medication from his nostrils and face.
- Clean the dropper by separating the plunger and pipette and flushing them with warm water. Allow to air dry.

Administering a nasal spray
- Have the patient sit upright, with his head tilted back slightly.
- Remove the protective cap from the atomizer.
- To prevent air from entering the nasal cavity and to allow the medication to flow in properly, occlude one nostril with your finger. Insert the atomizer tip into the open nostril.
- Instruct the patient to inhale, and as he does so, squeeze the atomizer once, quickly and firmly. Use just enough force to coat the inside of the nose with medication. Too much force may drive the solution and contamination into the sinuses and eustachian tubes.
- If ordered, spray the nostril again. Then, repeat the procedure in the other nostril.
- Instruct the patient to keep his head tilted back for several minutes and to breathe slowly through his nose so the medication has time to work. Tell him not to blow his nose.
- Rinse the atomizer tip with warm water to prevent contamination of the medication with nasal secretions.

Administering a nasal aerosol
- Instruct the patient to clear his nostrils by gently blowing his nose.
- Insert the medication cartridge according to the manufacturer's directions. With some models, you will fit the medication cartridge over a small hole in the adapter. (When inserting a refill cartridge, first remove the protective cap from the stem.)
- Shake the aerosol well immediately before each use, and remove the protective cap from the adapter tip.
- Hold the aerosol between your thumb and index finger, with your index finger on top of the medication cartridge.
- Tilt the patient's head back, and carefully insert the adapter tip in one nostril, while occluding the other nostril with your finger.
- Press the adapter and cartridge together firmly to release one measured dose of medication.
- Shake the aerosol, and repeat the procedure to instill medication into the other nostril.
- Remove the medication cartridge and wash the nasal adapter in lukewarm water according to manufacturer's instructions. Allow the adapter to dry thoroughly before reinserting the cartridge.

Nursing considerations
- Before instilling nose drops in a young child or an uncooperative patient, attach a small piece of tubing to the end of the dropper to prevent damage to mucous membranes.
- When using an aerosol, be careful not to puncture or incinerate the pressurized car-

tridge. Store it at temperatures below 120° F. (48.9° C.).
- To prevent the spread of infection, label the medication bottle, and use it again only for that patient.
- Ideally, nasal medications should be self-administered by the patient. Teach him how to instill them correctly so he can continue treatment after discharge, if necessary. Caution him against using nasal medications longer than prescribed; they may cause a rebound effect that worsens the condition. During rebound, the medication loses its effectiveness and relaxes the vessels in the nasal turbinates, producing a stuffiness that can be relieved only by discontinuing the medication.
- Inform the patient of possible side effects. For example, explain that some nasal medications may cause restlessness, palpitations, nervousness, and other systemic effects. Instruct the patient to report these to his physician.

Applying throat medications

Throat medications are usually applied by means of a pharyngeal spray (atomizer or spray pump), a mouthwash, or a lozenge (troche). Drugs applied by these methods produce local rather than systemic effects and are classified as antibiotics, antiseptics, or anesthetics.

Equipment and materials
For a spray, you will need prescribed throat medication, an atomizer or spray pump, a tongue blade or a spoon, and tissues.
For a mouthwash, you will need prescribed solution, the patient's medication record and chart, a drinking cup, an emesis basin, and tissues.
For a lozenge, you will need a prescribed lozenge and the patient's medication record and chart.

Steps
- Confirm the identity of the patient by checking the name, room number, and bed number on his identification bracelet.
- Explain the procedure to him.
- Wash your hands.
- Follow the procedure for administering a pharyngeal spray, a mouthwash, or a lozenge (see steps below).

- Document that the medication was given on the medication cardex.

Applying a pharyngeal spray
- Assist the patient to an upright position. If he cannot sit up, ask the physician if another form of medication can be substituted. Spraying the throat of a supine patient increases the risk of aspiration.
- Ask the patient to open his mouth. If you are administering an anesthetic, such as Chloraseptic, invert the bowl of a teaspoon or place the tongue blade over the patient's tongue *before* you spray. Ask him to hold the spoon or tongue blade. This will keep his tongue from getting numb. It will also help you see the irritated area of his throat.
- Instruct the patient to avoid inhaling as the medication is being administered.
- To use a *spray pump,* hold the nozzle just *outside* his mouth, and direct the medication toward his throat.
- To use an *atomizer,* insert its tip just *inside* his mouth, and direct the medication toward the back of his throat.
- Squeeze the container quickly and firmly, using enough force to propel the spray to the inflamed throat tissues.
- Caution the patient not to swallow immediately, so the medication can run down his throat and coat the mucous membranes. Observe for aspiration.

Administering a mouthwash
- Assist the patient to an upright position.
- For a *mouthwash,* give him ⅛ to ½ cup (30 to 120 ml) of the solution and instruct him to swish it around in his mouth, especially over his teeth and gums. Warn him not to swallow it but to spit it into the emesis basin. Hand him a tissue so he can wipe his mouth.
- For a *gargle,* instruct the patient to tilt his head back slightly and take a deep breath. Give him ⅛ cup of the solution, and tell him to hold it in his mouth. Then, instruct him to exhale slowly to create the gargling action. Warn him not to aspirate the solution. Tell him to spit it into the emesis basin. Then give him a tissue to wipe his mouth.
- If the physician has ordered a medication such as lidocaine hydrochloride (Xylocaine Viscous), instruct the patient to *swallow*

the solution, so it coats and soothes irritated throat tissue. Tell him not to eat or drink for a half hour afterward.

Administering a lozenge
• Assist the patient to an upright position.
• Give him the lozenge or place it in his mouth, and tell him to keep it in his mouth until it dissolves. Instruct him not to chew it or swallow it; this renders it largely ineffective.

Nursing considerations
• Instruct the patient to eat or drink nothing for at least 30 minutes after receiving throat medications to avoid decreasing the effectiveness of the drug.
• If you have administered an anesthetic spray, warn the patient to eat or drink nothing for at least 1 hour afterward. The anesthetic will inhibit his gag reflex and increase the risk of aspiration.
• Some lozenges contain sugar. If the patient is on a sugar-restricted diet, consult the physician for a substitute medication.
• Applying throat medications is best done by the patient himself. Teach him to apply throat medications correctly, so he can continue treatment at home if necessary. Review the procedure and let the patient try it himself while you observe.

Review Questions

1. In instilling eye drops, which one of the following techniques is in *error*?
   A. The nurse has the patient look up and away
   B. The nurse holds the bulb of the eyedropper uppermost
   C. The nurse carefully drops solution onto the white surface of the eye
   D. The nurse exposes the conjunctival sac by placing an index finger on the patient's cheekbone and gently pulling down on the skin under the lower lid

2. In administering an eye ointment, where and how is the medication applied?

3. In instilling eardrops in an adult, which one of the following techniques is in *error*?
   A. The nurse uses clean technique for the procedure
   B. The nurse warms the solution before instilling it
   C. The nurse straightens the ear canal by pulling the auricle upward and backward
   D. The nurse allows the drops to fall gently onto the eardrum

4. Why should a cotton ball *not* be placed in the ear canal after instilling eardrops?

5. Nasal medications are usually aqueous solutions. Cite three reasons why oily medications are not used for nasal instillation.

6. How should the patient be positioned when receiving nose drops for nasal congestion?

7. Describe two ways to position the patient for instillation of nose drops to treat a sinus condition.

8. How are nose drops instilled so that they do not flow down the throat?

9. What is the correct patient position for applying throat medications? Why?

10. How long should the patient refrain from eating or drinking after receiving throat medications?

Selected References

Emergencies. Nurse's Reference Library. Springhouse, Pa.: Springhouse Corp., 1985.
Giving Medications. Nursing Photobook Series. Springhouse, Pa.: Springhouse Corp., 1982.
Procedures. Nurse's Reference Library. Springhouse, Pa.: Springhouse Corp., 1983.

Topical Application of Medication

Topical application refers to giving a drug by placing it on the *skin* or *mucous membranes*. This includes transdermal, vaginal, rectal, sublingual, and buccal administration, as well as instillation, irrigation, and inunction (rubbing the medication into the skin). Except for nitroglycerin and certain drugs given rectally, topical medications are usually used for their local rather than systemic effects. (See *Topical Medications: Pros and Cons* for a discussion of the benefits and drawbacks of topical administration.) This chapter discusses how to administer topical medications effectively.

SKIN APPLICATION
Applying medication to the skin

Medications that are applied to the skin come in several dosage forms: powders, lotions, creams, and pastes. Each dosage form is ordered for its particular benefits. (See *Guide to Topical Dosage Forms.*) Application is a simple nursing procedure that is often easily taught to the patient himself.

Equipment and materials
You will need a container of prescribed medication, tongue depressors, 4"x 4" gauze sponges, tape, and gloves.
   The tongue depressors and gauze sponges should be sterile.

Steps
• Confirm the identity of the patient by checking the name, room number, and bed number on his wristband.
• Explain the procedure thoroughly to him, and provide privacy.
• Wash your hands.
• Expose the area to be treated. Make sure the skin is intact, unless the medication has been ordered to treat a skin lesion such as an ulcer. Application of ointment to broken or abraded skin may cause systemic absorption.
• Help the patient assume a comfortable position that provides access to the area to be treated.
• Open the container of medication. Place the lid upside down to prevent contamination of the inside.
• Wear gloves to prevent the absorption of medication by your own skin and to protect yourself.
• After applying a powder, lotion, ointment, or paste (see steps below), document that the medication was given on the medication cardex.

Applying a powder
• Apply to clean, dry skin.
• To prevent inhalation of powder particles, instruct the patient to turn his head to one side during application.
• If you are applying powder to the patient's face or neck, give him a cloth or gauze to cover his mouth. Then, ask him to exhale as you apply the powder.

Applying a lotion
• Remove residue from previous applications with soap and water.
• To increase absorption in certain skin conditions, warm the patient's skin with heat packs or a bath.

TOPICAL MEDICATIONS: PROS AND CONS

Benefits
- Faster relief from surface pain and itching than with systemic drugs
- Less severe allergic reactions than with systemic drugs
- Fewer side effects than with systemic drugs
- Comforting for the patient, since he can witness the care
- Increased protection against infection for skin that has lost its natural protective capabilities

Drawbacks
- Difficult to deliver in precise doses
- May stain skin, clothing, furniture, or bed linen
- Application procedure may be time-consuming
- May be embarrassing to patient, depending on the site
- May be difficult for the patient to apply, depending on the site

GUIDE TO TOPICAL DOSAGE FORMS

As noted in the chart below, the different dosage forms of medications applied to the skin have varied uses. The physician will order the appropriate one based on the desired therapeutic effect.

Type	Use
Powder (an inert chemical that may contain medication)	• Promotes skin drying • Reduces moisture, maceration, friction
Lotion (a suspension of insoluble powder in water or an emulsion without powder)	• Creates sensation of dryness • Leaves uniform surface film of powder • Soothes, cools, protects the skin
Cream (an oil-in-water emulsion in semisolid form)	• Lubricates as a barrier
Ointment (a suspension of oil and water in semisolid form)	• Retains body heat • Provides prolonged medication contact • Lubricates, softens, and protects skin and mucous membranes
Paste (a stiff mixture of powder and ointment)	• Provides a uniform coat • Reduces and repels moisture

- Shake the container well.
- Using gloves, apply medication and thoroughly massage it into the skin.
- Dry the skin.

Applying an ointment
- Remove residue from previous applications. (See *How to Remove an Ointment*, p. 140.)
- Remove a tongue depressor from its sterile wrapper and cover one end with ointment from the tube, or lift out a dollop from the jar. Then, transfer the ointment from the tongue depressor to your gloved hand.
- Apply the ointment to the affected area with long, smooth strokes that follow the direction of hair growth. This avoids forcing medication into hair follicles, which can cause irritation and lead to folliculitis. Avoid excessive pressure, which could abrade the skin.
- To prevent contamination of the ointment, use a new tongue depressor each time you remove ointment from the container.
- To protect the applied ointment and keep it from soiling the patient's clothes and bedding, tape an appropriate amount of sterile gauze over the treated area. If you are applying ointment to the patient's hands or feet, cover the site with white cotton gloves or terrycloth scuffs. If you are applying ointment to his entire body, have him wear a loose cotton gown or pajamas.
- To apply nitroglycerin ointment transdermally, see *Applying Transdermal Drugs*, p. 141.

HOW TO REMOVE AN OINTMENT

The first step in *reapplying* an ointment is to *remove* any previously applied ointment from the skin. To do so, follow these steps:
• Wash your hands.
• Rub a solvent such as cottonseed oil on your hands and apply it liberally to the treated area in the direction of hair growth, or saturate a sterile gauze sponge with the solvent and use this to gently remove the ointment. Repeat this procedure until you have removed all the ointment.
• Remove excess oil by gently wiping the area with the sterile gauze sponge. Do not rub too hard; *this could irritate the skin.*
• Assess the patient's skin condition for signs of irritation, allergic reaction, or skin breakdown.
• Reapply the prescribed ointment, as ordered. Complete removal of previously applied ointment will prevent skin irritation from an accumulation of ointment and will maximize the therapeutic effect of any freshly applied ointment.

Applying a paste
• Remove residue from previous applications.
• Apply medication to clean, dry skin.
• Cover medication to increase absorption and to protect the patient's clothing and bed linen.

Nursing considerations
• Never apply medication without first removing previously applied medication, to prevent skin irritation from an accumulation of medication.
• Do not apply too much ointment to any skin area. It may cause irritation and discomfort, stain clothing and bedding, and make removal difficult.
• Never apply medications formulated for the skin to the mucous membranes. Drug absorption through mucous membranes is rapid, and overmedication may result. The membrane surfaces are moist and easily penetrated and lack the skin's tough outer layer of dead cells.
• Do not apply ointment to moist, creased, or folded skin because it can cause irritation in such circumstances.
• Never apply ointment to the eyelids or ear canal unless ordered. It may congeal and occlude the tear duct or ear canal.
• Inspect the treated area frequently for signs of an adverse reaction, such as irritation, rash, or allergic reaction.
• Notify the physician of any of the following: a change in the amount, color, consistency, or odor of any drainage; or increased redness or swelling.

Giving a medicated shampoo

Medicated shampoos include keratolytic and cytostatic agents, coal tar preparations, and lindane (gamma benzene hexachloride) solutions. Keratolytic and cytostatic shampoos are commonly used to treat dandruff. Concentrated formulas, and frequent or extended use, increase their effectiveness. Coal tar shampoos are generally used for their antipruritic effects in the treatment of psoriasis. However, they are recommended only in refractory cases because they may cause photosensitivity and retard wound healing. Lindane solutions are used most often to treat head lice.

Equipment and materials
You will need a prescribed medicated shampoo, two bath towels, and a comb. You may need a gown, gloves, a surgical cap (if desired), and tweezers or a fine-tooth comb (for head lice).

Steps
• Confirm the identity of the patient by checking the name, room number, and bed number on his wristband.
• Explain the procedure to him, and provide privacy.
• Wash your hands, and follow the procedure for using a keratolytic or cytostatic, coal tar, or lindane shampoo (see steps below).
• Document that the medicated shampoo was given on the medication cardex

Using a keratolytic or cytostatic shampoo
• Shake the bottle of shampoo well to mix the solution evenly.
• Wet the patient's hair thoroughly.

APPLYING TRANSDERMAL DRUGS

Through an adhesive disk or measured dose of ointment applied to the skin, transdermal drugs supply constant, controlled medication directly into the bloodstream for prolonged systemic effect. Nitroglycerin is often applied transdermally. Most drugs have molecules too large for absorption through the skin. Transdermal drugs should not be applied to broken or irritated skin because they would increase irritation; or to scarred or calloused skin, because they may not be readily absorbed.

To apply transdermal ointments
- Place the prescribed amount of ointment on the application strip or measuring paper, taking care not to get any on your skin.
- Apply the strip to any dry, hairless area of the body. Do not rub the ointment into the skin. (If necessary, carefully shave an area for application of the medication.)
- Tape the application strip and ointment to the skin.
- If desired, cover the application strip with plastic wrap, and tape the wrap in place.
- Instruct the patient to keep the area around the ointment as dry as possible.
- Wash your hands immediately after applying the ointment to avoid absorbing any of the drug yourself.

To apply transdermal disks
- Open the package and remove the disk.
- Without touching the adhesive surface, remove the clear-plastic backing.
- Apply the disk to a dry, hairless area (scopolamine is usually applied behind the ear). If necessary, carefully shave an area for application of the disk.
- Instruct the patient to keep the area around the disk as dry as possible.
- Wash your hands immediately after applying the disk to avoid absorbing the drug yourself.
- Record the type of medication, the date and time of application, and the dose on the patient's medication record and chart. Also note any side effects and the patient's response.
- When applying transdermal medications, reapply them at the same time every day to ensure a continuous effect, but alternate the application sites to avoid skin irritation.
- Before reapplying nitroglycerin ointment, remove the plastic wrap, application strip, and any remaining ointment from the patient's skin.
- Teach the patient how to apply his transdermal medication so he can continue treatment at home. Have him demonstrate the procedure for you.
- Explain to the patient that skin irritation, such as pruritus or a rash, may occur; he should report this to his physician.
- Explain to the patient that he may experience side effects of the drug administered. For example, transdermal nitroglycerin medications may cause headaches and, in the elderly, postural hypotension.

- Apply the proper amount of shampoo, as directed on the label.
- Work the shampoo into a lather, adding water as necessary.
- If the shampoo is a *cytostatic* agent, rinse the hair immediately. If it is a *keratolytic* agent, leave it on the scalp and hair for as long as instructed (usually 5 to 10 minutes) to soften and loosen scales. Then rinse the hair thoroughly.
- Apply the same amount of shampoo again, and lather and rinse.
- Towel-dry the patient's hair and comb out any tangles.

Using a coal tar shampoo
- Wet the patient's hair thoroughly.
- Massage the shampoo into the scalp.
- Rinse completely.
- Massage the shampoo into the scalp again, but this time leave it on for 5 to 10 minutes, as directed on the label.
- Rinse completely.
- Towel-dry the patient's hair and comb out any tangles.

Using a lindane solution
- Put on the gown and gloves before entering the patient's room. If desired, protect your own hair with a surgical cap.

- Apply the correct amount of shampoo to dry hair, starting at the scalp and working through to the ends. Pay special attention to obviously infested areas.
- After the shampoo has thoroughly coated the scalp and hair, add small amounts of water and work the shampoo into a lather.
- Lather the scalp and hair for 4 to 6 minutes.
- Rinse completely. Do not repeat the procedure.
- Towel-dry the patient's hair.
- After the hair is dry, comb the hair with a fine-tooth comb to remove nits or nit shells. If necessary, remove dead lice or nits with tweezers.
- Remove your gown and gloves (and cap, if worn), and dispose of them and the towels according to institutional policy, to prevent the spread of lice.

Nursing considerations
- Check the label on the shampoo before starting the procedure to ensure use of the correct amount; instructions may vary among brands.
- Keep the shampoo away from the patient's eyes. If any shampoo should accidentally get in his eyes, irrigate them promptly with water.
- Repeated shampooing with lindane may cause skin irritation and possibly systemic toxicity, especially in children. Warn patients not to use it repeatedly or excessively.
- Medicated shampoos are contraindicated in patients with broken or abraded skin.

Giving a therapeutic bath

Therapeutic baths combine water with oatmeal, starch, oil, alkaline salts, or tar preparations. They are used primarily to relieve pruritus and inflammation. They are also used to soften and remove crusts, scales, and old medications, and to soothe and relax the patient. Baths relieve pruritus by coating irritated skin with a soothing, protective film; they reduce inflammation by producing vasoconstriction in surface blood vessels.

The colloid bath—using instant oatmeal or oatmeal powder, cornstarch, or laundry starch—has a drying effect on eczematous lesions. The oil bath—using mineral or cottonseed oil or commercial bath oils—has an antipruritic and emollient effect that helps treat acute and subacute eczematous lesions and also soothes dry skin. The alkaline bath—using alkaline salts, such as sodium bicarbonate—has a cooling effect that helps relieve pruritus. The medicated tar bath leaves a film of tar on the skin that works with ultraviolet light to inhibit the rapid cell turnover characteristic of psoriasis.

Equipment and materials
You will need a bathtub, a cloth bathmat, a rubber mat, a bath (utility) thermometer, a therapeutic additive, a measuring device, a colander or sieve for oatmeal powder, two washcloths, two towels, a hospital gown or loose-fitting cotton pajamas, and lubricating cream or ointment, if ordered.

Preparation
Assemble supplies and draw the bath before bringing the patient to the bath area, to prevent chilling him. Begin by cleaning and disinfecting the tub, because the patient with skin breakdown is particularly vulnerable to infection. Place the cloth bathmat next to the tub. Place the rubber mat in the tub to prevent falls; the therapeutic additive may make the tub slippery. Fill the tub with 6″ to 8″ (15.2 to 20.3 cm) of water no hotter than 95° to 100° F. (35° to 37.8° C.) to prevent vasodilation, which could aggravate pruritus.

Measure the correct amount of therapeutic additive, according to the physician's order or package instructions. As the tub is filling, thoroughly mix the additive into the water. Add most substances directly to the water, but place oatmeal powder in a sieve or colander under the tub faucet to help it dissolve. Regulate the thickness of the oatmeal bath by adding more water or more oatmeal or oatmeal powder as needed. When giving a tar bath, wear a plastic apron or protective gown, because tar preparations stain clothing.

Steps
- Confirm the identity of the patient by checking the name, room number, and bed number on his wristband.

- Explain the procedure to him, and have him void.
- Escort him to the bath area, and close the door to provide privacy and eliminate drafts.
- Wash your hands.
- Assist the patient to undress, and help him into the tub, if necessary. Advise him to use the safety rails to prevent falls.
- Tell him the bath may feel unpleasant at first, because his skin is irritated, but assure him that the medication will soon coat and soothe his skin.
- Ask the patient to stretch out in the tub and submerge his body up to the chin. Give him a washcloth to apply the bath solution gently to his face and other body areas not immersed, if he is capable. (Note: If the patient is taking a tar bath, tell him not to get the bath solution in his eyes, because tar is an eye irritant.)
- Warn the patient against scrubbing his skin, to prevent further irritation.
- Add warm water to the bath as needed to maintain a comfortable temperature.
- Allow the patient to soak for 15 to 30 minutes. If you must stay with him, pull the bath curtain to give him privacy and protect him from drafts. If you must leave the room, show him how to use the call button, and ensure his privacy.
- After the bath, help him from the tub. Have him use the safety rails to prevent falls.
- Help the patient pat his skin dry with towels. Do not rub the skin because friction increases pruritus.
- Apply lubricating cream or ointment, if ordered, while the skin is moist and most permeable.
- Provide a fresh hospital gown or loose-fitting pajamas.
- Escort the patient to his room, and make sure he is comfortable.
- Drain the bath water, clean and disinfect the tub, and dispose of soiled materials properly. If you have given an oatmeal powder bath, rinse the tub immediately after draining it or the powder will cake, making later removal difficult.
- Document that the therapeutic bath was given on the medication cardex and/or nurses' notes. In the nurses' notes state the duration of the bath, water temperature, type and amount of additive, skin appearance before and after the bath, patient's tolerance for treatment, and any patient comments regarding effectiveness of the bath.

Nursing considerations
- Because pruritus seems worse at night, give a therapeutic bath before bedtime, unless otherwise ordered, to promote restful sleep.
- Because the patient with a skin disorder may be self-conscious, maintain eye contact during conversation and avoid staring at his skin. Also, avoid nonverbal expressions and gestures that show revulsion. If the patient wishes, allow him to talk about his condition and how it affects his self-esteem.
- Refrain from using soap during a therapeutic bath, because its drying effect counteracts the bath emollient.
- Because the patient with skin breakdown chills easily, protect him from drafts.
- After the bath, avoid covering or dressing him too warmly, because perspiration aggravates pruritus.
- To prevent excoriation and infection, instruct the patient not to scratch his skin.
- Advise the patient to wear loose-fitting cotton pajamas, underwear, and other clothing. Tight clothing and scratchy or synthetic materials can aggravate skin conditions by causing friction and increasing perspiration.
- If the patient is confined to bed, place the therapeutic additive in a basin of water (95° to 100° F., 35° to 37.8° C.) and apply it with a washcloth, using light, gentle strokes.
- Teach the patient how to give himself a medicated bath so therapy can be continued at home if needed.

Applying a medicated soak

A soak is the immersion of a body part in warm water or a medicated solution. This treatment helps soften exudates, facilitate debridement, enhance suppuration, cleanse wounds or burns, apply medication to infected areas, and increase local blood supply and circulation. Typical medications used in soaks include hydrogen peroxide, povidone-iodine, magnesium sulfate (Epsom salts), and magnesium permanganate.

WET DRESSINGS

Wet dressings, or continuous soaks, are used in wound management and in the treatment of inflammatory skin conditions when the patient is unable to tolerate a medicated bath, when the area to be treated cannot be immersed, when the condition needs long-term treatment and protection, or when a wound needs mild debridement.

The same technique is used for application of a wet dressing as for a dry dressing, with one exception—the gauze pad is soaked in a wetting solution or medication for a few moments before being placed on the wound or affected area. The area is then wrapped in an insulating covering, such as Kerlix, a towel, or linen-saver pad, for a prescribed length of time. The most commonly used wetting solutions and medications include:

- **isotonic solutions,** such as sterile normal saline or lactated Ringer's solution, which aid mechanical debridement.
- **hydrogen peroxide** (commonly used half-strength), which irrigates the wound and aids mechanical debridement. Its foaming action also warms the wound, promoting vasodilation and reducing inflammation.
- **acetic acid,** which treats *Pseudomonas* infection.
- **sodium hypochlorite** (Dakin's solution), is an antiseptic that also slightly dissolves necrotic tissue. This solution is unstable and must be freshly prepared every 24 hours.
- **povidone-iodine,** a broad-spectrum, fast-acting antimicrobial. Watch for patient sensitivity to it. Also, protect the surrounding skin from contact, because this solution can dry and stain the skin.
- **antibiotic solutions** containing neomycin, chloramphenicol, gentamicin, and carbenicillin. Their use is controversial, because some physicians believe they cause overgrowth of resistant organisms.
- **enzymatic agents** (collagenase, sutilains, and fibrinolysin and desoxyribonuclease), which digest and liquefy necrotic debris. Their use is controversial, because some physicians consider their effectiveness unproven.
- **aluminum acetate** (Burow's solution), which is used to treat mild skin irritation and inflammation from insect bites, poison ivy, and exposure to soaps, detergents, and chemicals.
- **aluminum sulfate** (Domeboro powder), which is used to relieve inflammation from insect bites, poison ivy, and other contact dermatoses. When this solution is prepared, the clear portion is decanted and used for the soak. The precipitate is discarded.

Most soaks are applied with clean tap water using clean technique, but sterile solution and sterile equipment are required for treating wounds, burns, or other breaks in the skin.

A medicated wet dressing or compress may also be known as a soak. This type of soak is used when the affected area cannot be immersed. (See *Wet Dressings*.)

Equipment and materials
You will need a basin or an arm or foot tub, a bath (utility) thermometer, hot tap water or prescribed medicated solution, a cup and a pitcher, a linen-saver pad, an overbed table, a footstool, pillows, and towels. You may need gauze sponges and other dressing materials.

Preparation
Clean and disinfect the basin or tub. Run hot tap water into a pitcher, or heat the prescribed solution, as applicable. Measure the temperature of the water or solution with a bath thermometer. If it is not within the prescribed range (usually 105° to 110° F., or 40.6° to 43.3° C.), add hot or cold water or reheat or cool the solution, as applicable. If you are preparing the soak away from the patient's room, heat the liquid slightly above the correct temperature to allow for cooling during transport. If the solution for a medicated soak is not premixed, prepare the dilution and heat it.

Steps

- Confirm the identity of the patient by checking the name, room number, and bed number on his wristband.
- Explain the procedure to him, and provide privacy.
- Wash your hands.
- If the soak basin or tub will be placed in bed, make sure the bed is flat beneath it to prevent spills.
- For an arm soak, have the patient sit erect. For a leg or foot soak, have him lie down and bend the appropriate knee. For a foot soak in the sitting position, have him sit on the edge of the bed or transfer him to a chair.
- Place a linen-saver pad under the treatment area, and if necessary, cover the pad with a towel to absorb spillage.
- Expose the treatment area. Remove any dressing and dispose of it properly. If the dressing is encrusted and stuck to the wound, leave it in place, proceed with the soak, and remove the dressing after a few minutes. Or, soak the dressing with sterile water or saline, and then remove it.
- Position the soak basin under the treatment area on the bed, overbed table, footstool, or floor, as appropriate. Pour the heated, medicated liquid into the soak basin or tub. Then *gradually* lower the arm or leg into the basin to allow adjustment to the temperature change. Make sure the soak solution covers the treatment area.
- Support other body parts with pillows or towels as needed to prevent undue pressure and muscle strain. Make the patient comfortable, and ensure good body alignment.
- Check the temperature of the soak solution with the bath thermometer every 5 minutes. If the temperature drops below the prescribed range, remove some of the cooled solution with a cup. Then, lift the patient's arm or leg from the basin to avoid burns, and add hot water or solution to the basin. Mix the liquid thoroughly, and then check its temperature. If the temperature is within the prescribed range, lower the patient's arm or leg into the basin again.
- After 15 to 20 minutes, or as ordered, lift the patient's arm or leg from the basin and remove the basin.
- Dry the arm or leg thoroughly with a clean towel. If the patient has a wound, dry the skin around it without touching the wound.
- While the skin is hydrated from the soak, use gauze sponges to remove any loose scales or crusts.
- Observe the treatment area for general appearance, degree of swelling, debridement, suppuration, and healing.
- Redress the wound, if appropriate.
- Remove the towel and linen-saver pad, and make the patient comfortable in bed.
- Discard the soak solution, dispose of soiled materials properly, and clean and disinfect the basin. If the treatment is to be repeated, store the equipment in the patient's room.
- Record in the nurses' notes the date, time, and duration of the soak; area treated; solution and its temperature; skin and wound appearance before, during, and after treatment; and the patient's tolerance.
- If a medicated soak was given, document this on the medication cardex.

Nursing considerations

- To treat large areas, particularly burns, a soak may be administered in a whirlpool or Hubbard tank, using sterile technique.
- Observe the patient for signs of tissue intolerance: extreme redness at the treatment site, excessive drainage, bleeding, or maceration. If such signs develop or the patient complains of pain, discontinue the treatment and notify the physician.
- Teach the patient how to apply a medicated soak so that therapy can be continued at home, if necessary. Have him demonstrate the procedure for you.

MUCOUS MEMBRANE APPLICATION

Administering buccal and sublingual medications

Buccal and sublingual administration of certain drugs prevents their destruction or transformation in the stomach or small intestine. These drugs take effect quickly because the thin epithelium and abundant vasculature of the oral mucosa allow direct absorption into the bloodstream. Only a few drugs are given this way (see *Most Commonly Used Buccal and Sublingual Drugs, p. 146*). The patient must be observed carefully so he does not swallow the drug or suffer localized mucosal irritation.

MOST COMMONLY USED BUCCAL AND SUBLINGUAL DRUGS

Buccal
erythrityl tetranitrate (Cardilate)
methyltestosterone (Oreton Methyl)

Sublingual
ergotamine tartrate (Ergomar)
erythrityl tetranitrate (Cardilate)
isoproterenol hydrochloride (Isuprel Glossets)
isosorbide dinitrate (Sorbitrate)
nitroglycerin (Nitrostat)

Equipment and materials
You will need prescribed medication and a medication cup.

Steps
- Confirm the identity of the patient by checking the name, room number, and bed number on his wristband.
- Explain the procedure to him if he has never taken a drug buccally or sublingually before.
- Wash your hands.
- *For buccal administration,* place the tablet in the upper or lower buccal pouch, between the cheek and gum.
- *For sublingual administration,* place the tablet under the tongue.
- Instruct the patient to keep buccal or sublingual medication in place until it dissolves completely, to ensure absorption.
- Document that the medication was given on the medication cardex.

Nursing considerations
- Caution the patient against chewing the tablet, and tell him not to touch it with his tongue because he may swallow it accidentally.
- Tell him not to smoke before it has dissolved because nicotine's vasoconstrictive effects slow absorption.
- Do not give liquids with either form of medication, and tell the patient not to drink anything until the medication has completely dissolved.
- Teach the patient to take sublingual nitroglycerin at the *first* sign of angina. The tablet should be wetted with saliva and placed under the tongue until completely absorbed.
- Some buccal medications may cause mucosal irritation. Alternate sides of the mouth for repeat doses to prevent continuous irritation of the same site.
- Some sublingual medications—erythrityl tetranitrate, for example—may cause a tingling sensation under the tongue. Explain that this is normal. If the patient finds it annoying, erythrityl tetranitrate can be placed in the buccal pouch instead, another acceptable route for administering this drug.

Inserting vaginal medications

Vaginal medications include suppositories, creams, gels, and ointments. These medications can be inserted as topical treatments for infection (particularly *Trichomonas* vaginitis and monilial vaginitis) or inflammation. They can also be used as contraceptives. Suppositories have a cocoa butter base; they melt when they contact the vaginal mucosa and then diffuse topically, as effectively as creams, gels, and ointments.

Vaginal medications usually come with disposable applicators that enable placement in the anterior and posterior fornices. Vaginal administration is most effective when the patient can remain lying down to retain the medication.

Equipment and materials
You will need clean gloves; prescribed medication and an applicator, if necessary; water-soluble lubricant; and a small sanitary pad.

Steps
- Confirm the identity of the patient by checking the name, room number, and bed number on her wristband.
- Explain the procedure to her, and provide privacy.
- Wash your hands.
- Ask the patient to void.
- Ask her if she would rather insert the medication herself. If so, provide appropriate instructions. If not, proceed with the following steps.
- Help her into the lithotomy position.

- Expose only the perineum, and follow the procedure for inserting a suppository or an ointment, cream, or gel (see steps below).
- When finished, remove and discard the gloves.
- Wash the applicator with soap and warm water and store it, unless it is disposable. If the applicator can be used again, label it so it will be used only for the same patient.
- To prevent medication from soiling the patient's clothing and bedding, provide a sanitary pad.
- Help her return to a comfortable position.
- Wash your hands thoroughly.
- Document that the medication was given on the medication cardex.

Inserting a suppository
- Remove the suppository from the wrapper, and lubricate it with water-soluble lubricant.
- Put on gloves and expose the vagina.
- With the forefinger of your free hand, insert the suppository about 2″ (5 cm) into the vagina. To ensure patient comfort, direct your finger *down* initially (toward the spine), and then *up* and *back* (toward the cervix).
- If the suppository is small, insert it in the tip of an applicator. Then, lubricate the applicator, hold it by the cylinder, and insert it into the vagina. When the suppository reaches the distal end of the vagina, depress the plunger. Remove the applicator while the plunger is still depressed.

Inserting ointments, creams, or gels
- Insert the plunger into the applicator. Then, fit the applicator to the tube of medication.
- Gently squeeze the tube to fill the applicator with the prescribed amount of medication. Lubricate the applicator.
- Put on gloves and expose the vagina.
- Insert the applicator as you would a small suppository, and administer the medication.

Nursing considerations
- Refrigerate vaginal suppositories that melt at room temperature.
- If possible, teach the patient how to insert vaginal medication. She may have to administer it herself after she is discharged. Give her a patient instruction chart if one is available.
- Instruct the patient not to wear a tampon after inserting vaginal medication, because it would absorb the medication and decrease its effectiveness.
- Explain to the patient that vaginal medications may cause transient local irritation.

Administering medication by vaginal irrigation

A vaginal irrigation, or douche, is the instillation of fluid into the vaginal cavity to remove odor or foul discharge, to preoperatively disinfect the vagina, or to administer antiseptic drugs. It may also be performed to stop bleeding (using a cold solution) or to relieve pain and inflammation (using a warm solution). When performed after delivery or gynecologic surgery, vaginal irrigation requires sterile technique. Patient teaching is necessary, since the patient may have to repeat the procedure herself. Vaginal irrigation is usually contraindicated during pregnancy; for 4 to 6 weeks after miscarriage or postpartum; or in untreated venereal disease.

Equipment and materials
You will need a plastic irrigation container or bag; tubing, a clamp, and a curved plastic vaginal tip; prescribed solution; a bath (utility) thermometer; a straight-back chair or short I.V. pole; pillows; a linen-saver pad; bedpan with cover; clean gloves; water-soluble lubricant; toilet tissue; and a perineal pad. You may need a container to mix the douche solution. Vaginal irrigation sets are also available.

Preparation
Prepare the prescribed irrigating solution, as ordered. Heat the solution to a temperature between 105° to 110° F. (40.6° to 43.3° C.), as ordered. Avoid overheating to prevent injury to vaginal mucous membranes and the skin of the meatus. Hang the irrigation bag, with its tubing clamp closed, on the I.V. pole or straight-back chair.

Steps
- Confirm the identity of the patient by checking the name, room number, and bed number on her wristband.

- Explain the procedure to her, and provide privacy.
- Wash your hands.
- Have her urinate to prevent discomfort from a distended bladder and to allow full distention of the vagina with the solution.
- If the patient's condition permits, ask her if she would rather perform the irrigation herself. If so, provide appropriate instructions. If not, proceed with the following steps.
- Lower the head of the bed, and help the patient into the dorsal recumbent position. Place a pillow under her head and a linen-saver pad beneath her buttocks.
- Position her on the bedpan and drape her as you would for a pelvic examination. Place a pillow under her back to provide comfort.
- Adjust the height of the irrigation bag to no more than 2' (0.6 m) above the level of the vagina to ensure a slow, steady flow of solution.
- Put on clean gloves.
- Lubricate the end of the plastic vaginal tip with water-soluble lubricant to facilitate insertion.
- Separate the labia and open the tubing clamp to allow a small amount of solution to flow over the meatus. This reduces the risk of introducing external organisms into the vagina. Then reclamp the tubing.
- Gently insert the vaginal tip 2" to 2½" (5.1 to 6.4 cm) into the vagina at approximately a 45-degree angle, following the vaginal curvature to prevent patient discomfort.
- Open the clamp to allow solution to flow into the vagina. Then gently rotate the vaginal tip to make sure that fluid reaches all areas of the vagina. (If retention of the solution is ordered, clamp the tube and use your free hand to close the labia around the tip for 30 to 60 seconds.)
- When the irrigating container is empty, close the clamp and remove the tip from the vagina.
- Help the patient into a sitting position on the bedpan to allow the solution to drain from the vagina.
- Remove the bedpan and inspect the return flow.
- Offer the patient toilet tissue to dry the perineum. Instruct her to wipe from front to back to avoid fecal contamination of the urethra and vagina. Then provide her with a perineal pad to keep the bed dry and to promote her comfort.
- Rinse and dry the equipment, and set it aside for subsequent use. After final use of the equipment, discard the disposable irrigation set or send the nondisposable set to the institution's central supply department for sterilization.
- Wash your hands.
- Document that the medication was given on the medication cardex.

Nursing considerations
- Teach the patient how to perform vaginal irrigation so she may continue therapy at home if needed.
- Supervise her the first time she performs vaginal irrigation.
- Instruct her not to attempt irrigation while sitting on the toilet or standing in the shower, *because only the supine position ensures thorough vaginal irrigation.*
- Emphasize to her that irrigation is necessary only in the presence of inflammation, hyperacidity, odorous discharge, pain, or bleeding.

Administering rectal medications

The rectal route is often used if the patient is unconscious or otherwise unable to swallow. Also, drugs are administered rectally because they would be destroyed by digestive enzymes in the stomach and small intestine, or because they taste too offensive for oral use. Dosage forms include suppositories, ointments, and enemas. (See "Giving a Retention or Irrigating Enema," p. 150.)

A rectal suppository is a small, solid, medicated mass—usually cone-shaped—with a cocoa butter or glycerin base. It melts at body temperature, and the medication is absorbed slowly. Rectal suppositories commonly contain drugs that stimulate peristalsis and defecation; relieve pain, vomiting, and local irritation; reduce fever; or induce relaxation. Because insertion may stimulate the vagus nerve, this procedure is contraindicated in patients with potential cardiac dysrhythmias. It may have to be avoided in patients with recent rectal or prostate surgery because of the risk of local trauma or discomfort during insertion.

Topical Application of Medication

An ointment is a semisolid medication that is used for local effects only and may be applied externally to the anus or internally to the rectum. Rectal ointments commonly contain drugs that reduce inflammation, or relieve pain and itching.

Equipment and materials
You will need a clean finger cot (or glove), water-soluble lubricant, an applicator (for ointment), several 4"x 4" gauze pads (for ointment), and a linen-saver pad. You may need a bedpan.

Steps
- Confirm the identity of the patient by checking the name, room number, and bed number on his wristband.
- Explain the procedure and the purpose of the medication to him, and provide privacy.
- Wash your hands.
- Place the patient on his left side in the Sims' position. Drape him with the bedcovers to expose only the rectal area. Protect the bedding with a linen-saver pad.
- Follow the procedure for inserting a suppository or applying ointment (see steps below).
- Document that the medication was given on the medication cardex.

Inserting a suppository
- Put the finger cot on the index finger of your dominant hand. (If a finger cot is not readily available, use a glove.)
- Remove the suppository from its wrapper, and lubricate it with water-soluble lubricant.
- Lift the upper buttock with your nondominant hand to expose the anus.
- Instruct the patient to take several deep breaths through his mouth to help relax the anal sphincters and reduce anxiety or discomfort during insertion.
- Using the index finger of your dominant hand, insert the suppository—tapered end first—about 1" to 1½" (2.5 to 3.8 cm), until you feel it pass the internal anal sphincter. Try to direct the tapered end toward the side of the rectum, so it contacts the membranes.
- Encourage the patient to lie quietly and, if applicable, to retain the suppository for the appropriate length of time. A suppository administered to relieve constipation should be retained as long as possible (at least 20 minutes) to be effective.
- Ensure the patient's comfort. Offer the bedpan, if appropriate.
- Discard the used equipment.

Applying an ointment
- *To apply externally,* wear gloves or use a gauze pad to spread medication over the anal area.
- *To apply internally,* attach the applicator to the tube of ointment and coat the applicator with water-soluble lubricant.
- Lift the upper buttock with your nondominant hand to expose the anus.
- Instruct the patient to take several deep breaths through his mouth to relax the anal sphincters and reduce anxiety or discomfort during insertion.
- Gently insert the applicator, directing it toward the umbilicus.
- Slowly squeeze the tube to eject the medication. Follow the physician's orders and instructions on the drug label to determine how much to administer.
- Remove the applicator and place a folded 4"x 4" gauze pad between the patient's buttocks to absorb excess ointment.
- Disassemble the tube and applicator. Recap the tube, and clean the applicator thoroughly with warm soap and water.

Nursing considerations
- Provide continuous reassurance and support throughout any rectal procedure; a tactful and compassionate approach is just as important as your skill in giving the medication.
- To preserve the patient's dignity, *ensure privacy* and *avoid exposing him unnecessarily.*
- Keep rectal suppositories in the refrigerator until needed to prevent softening and, possibly, decreased effectiveness. A softened suppository is difficult to handle and insert. To harden it again, hold the suppository (in its wrapper) under cold running water.
- Because intake of food and fluid stimulates peristalsis, insert a suppository for relieving constipation about 30 minutes before mealtime to help soften the feces in the rectum and facilitate defecation.

- Insert a medicated retention suppository between meals. Tell the patient to avoid expelling it, but if he has difficulty retaining it, place him on a bedpan immediately after the procedure.
- Make sure his call button is handy and watch for his signal, because he may be unable to suppress the urge to defecate long enough to wait for the bedpan.
- Advise him that the suppository may discolor his next bowel movement. Anusol suppositories, for example, give feces a silver-gray, pasty appearance.

Giving a retention or irrigating enema

Enemas involve the instillation of solution into the rectum and usually into the colon. The retention enema, as its name implies, is held within the rectum or colon longer than the irrigating enema, which is almost completely expelled within 15 minutes. Both types of enemas stimulate peristalsis through mechanical distention of the colon and stimulation of the nerves in the rectal wall.

Enemas serve to cleanse the lower bowel in preparation for diagnostic or surgical procedures. This cleansing permits direct visualization of the intestinal mucosa in such procedures as sigmoidoscopy and colonoscopy, and it also allows instillation of a contrast medium, such as barium, for radiographic examination. It also reduces contamination of the operative site during certain surgical procedures.

Enemas also relieve constipation and are often administered after a barium enema to prevent impaction of retained barium. Certain enemas, such as the Harris flush, relieve gas or distention from paralytic ileus.

The retention enema has additional uses that include acting as an emollient—soothing irritated tissues of the colon—and administering medication. In hepatic coma, a drug-solution enema, such as neomycin sulfate (Mycifradin), reduces blood ammonia levels by decreasing intestinal flora; lactulose (Cephulac), a drug-solution enema, acidifies colon contents and lowers blood ammonia levels. A sodium polystyrene sulfonate (Kayexalate) enema releases sodium ions for exchange by potassium ions in hyperkalemia.

Enemas are contraindicated after recent colon or rectal surgery or myocardial infarction, and in acute abdominal conditions of unknown etiology, such as suspected appendicitis. They should be administered cautiously to patients with dysrhythmias.

Equipment and materials

You will need prescribed solution; a bath (utility) thermometer; an enema administration bag with attached rectal tube and clamp; an I.V. pole; clean examination gloves, if desired; linen-saver pads; a bath blanket; two bedpans with covers, or a bedside commode; toilet tissue; and water-soluble lubricant. For the patient who may have difficulty retaining the solution, you may need a Foley catheter or Verden rectal catheter with 30-ml balloon and syringe, or a plastic rectal tube guard.

Commercially packaged disposable enema administration sets are readily available, as are commercially prepared, small-volume enema solutions in both irrigating and retention types.

Preparation

Prepare the prescribed type and amount of solution, as indicated (see *Types of Irrigating and Retention Enemas*). The volume for an irrigating enema is usually 750 to 1,000 ml for an adult, and less for a retention enema. Because the ingredients may be mucosal irritants, make sure the proportions are correct and the agents are thoroughly mixed to avoid localized irritation. Note that some solutions, such as the Mayo enema, require full or partial preparation at bedside immediately before administration.

Warm the solution to reduce patient discomfort. Note that some enemas, such as milk-and-molasses and starch, must be heated to high temperatures for proper mixing, and then cooled to 100° to 105° F. (37.8° to 40.6° C.). Test the solution's temperature with the bath thermometer. In the absence of a specific order, administer an enema to an adult at 100° to 105° F. to avoid burning rectal tissues.

Clamp the tubing and fill the solution bag with the prescribed solution. Unclamp the tubing and allow a small amount of solution to run through the tubing and out the cath-

TYPES OF IRRIGATING AND RETENTION ENEMAS

SOLUTION	PREPARATION	PURPOSE
Irrigating enemas		
Harris flush	1,000 ml of tap water	Cleansing
Magnesium sulfate	Add 3 tbsp of magnesium sulfate to 3 tbsp of salt in 1,500 ml of tap water.	Carminative
Saline	If a commercially prepared solution is not available, add 2 tsp of salt to 1,000 ml of tap water.	Cleansing
Soap and water	Add 1 packet of mild soap to 1,000 ml of tap water and remove all bubbles before administering.	Cleansing
Retention enemas		
Mayo	Dissolve 60 ml of white sugar in 240 ml of warmed tap water. Add 30 ml of sodium bicarbonate to mixture immediately before administering.	Carminative
Milk and molasses	Add 175 to 200 ml of hot milk to 175 to 200 ml of molasses. Heat mixture to 160° F. (71.1° C.) and then cool to 105° F. (40.5° C.).	Carminative
Oil	150 ml of mineral, olive, or cottonseed oil	Cleansing, emollient
Olive oil and glycerin	Add 60 ml of olive oil to 60 ml of glycerin.	Cleansing, emollient
1-2-3	Add 30 ml of magnesium sulfate 50% to 60 ml of glycerin. Add mixture to 90 ml of warm tap water.	Cleansing
Starch	Add 1 tsp of powdered starch to 60 ml of cold tap water and add to 160 ml of boiling tap water, or add 30 ml of liquid starch mix to the boiling water. Boil the mixture for 2 minutes and then cool to 105° F. (40.5° C.).	Emollient

eter. Then, reclamp the tubing to detect leaks and remove air that could cause discomfort if introduced into the colon. Hang the solution container on the I.V. pole and take all supplies to the patient's room. If you are using a Foley or Verden rectal catheter, fill the syringe for the balloon with 30 ml of water.

Steps
- Confirm the identity of the patient by checking the name, room number, and bed number on his wristband.
- Provide privacy, and explain the procedure to him.
- To determine the need for the rectal tube guard or the Verden rectal or Foley cathe-

ter, ask him if he has had previous difficulty retaining an enema.
• Wash your hands thoroughly. Put on clean examination gloves, if desired.
• Assist the patient, as necessary, in putting on a hospital gown. The gown makes enema administration easier and reduces the patient's worries about soiled clothing.
• If not contraindicated, place the patient in the left lateral Sims' position. This will facilitate the solution's flow by gravity into the descending colon. If this position is contraindicated or the patient finds it uncomfortable, position him on his back or right side. (Note: Instructions on some commercially prepared small-volume enemas recommend the knee-chest position, if it is not contraindicated, because it helps the solution flow farther into the colon and distributes it over as much of the lower colon's surface as possible.) Follow package instructions when administering these enemas.
• Place linen-saver pads under the patient's buttocks to prevent soiling the linens. Replace the top bed linens with a bath blanket to provide privacy and warmth.
• If necessary, finish preparing the enema solution. (See *Types of Irrigating and Retention Enemas*, p. 151.)
• Lubricate the distal tip of the rectal catheter with water-soluble lubricant to facilitate rectal insertion and reduce irritation.
• Separate the patient's buttocks and touch the anal sphincter with the rectal tube to stimulate contraction. Then, as the sphincter relaxes, tell the patient to breathe deeply through his mouth as you gently advance the tube toward the umbilicus. Insert the tube about 4" (10 cm) for an adult. Avoid forcing the catheter to prevent rectal wall trauma.
• If the tube does not advance easily, allow a little solution to flow in to relax the inner sphincter enough to ease passage.
• If the patient feels pain or the tube meets continued resistance, notify the physician. This may signal an unknown stricture or abscess.
• If the patient has poor sphincter control, use a rectal tube guard, or slip the tube through the cut end of a baby bottle nipple. You can also use a Verden rectal catheter or Foley catheter as a rectal tube, if institutional policy permits. Insert the lubricated catheter as you would a rectal tube. Then, gently inflate the balloon with 20 to 30 ml of water. Gently pull the catheter back against the patient's internal anal sphincter to seal off the rectum. If leakage still occurs with the balloon in place, add more water to the balloon in small amounts. Avoid inflating the balloon above 45 ml, since overinflation can cause compromised blood flow to rectal tissue.
• Hold the solution container slightly above bed level and release the tubing clamp. Then raise the container gradually to start the flow—usually at a rate of 75 to 100 ml/minute for an *irrigating* enema, but at the slowest possible rate for a *retention* enema to avoid stimulating peristalsis and to promote retention.
• Adjust the flow rate of an irrigating enema by raising or lowering the solution container according to the patient's retention and comfort. However, do not raise it higher than 24" (70 cm) for an adult, because excessive pressure can force colonic bacteria into the small intestine or rupture the colon.
• When performing a *Harris flush*, stop the flow by lowering the solution container below bed level and allowing gravity to siphon the enema out of the colon. Continue to raise and lower the container until gas bubbles cease or the patient feels more comfortable and abdominal distention subsides. Do not allow the solution container to empty completely before lowering it, because this may introduce air into the bowel.
• Hold the rectal tube in place throughout the procedure since bowel contractions and the pressure of the tube against the anal sphincter can promote tube displacement.
• Assess the patient's tolerance frequently.
• If the patient complains of discomfort, cramps, or the need to defecate, stop the flow by pinching or clamping the tubing. Then, hold the patient's buttocks together or firmly press toilet tissue against the anus. Instruct him to gently massage his abdomen and breathe slowly and deeply through his mouth to help relax abdominal muscles and promote retention. Resume administration of the enema at a slower rate of flow after a few minutes have passed, but interrupt the flow any time the patient feels uncomfortable.

- If the flow slows or stops, the catheter tip may be clogged with feces or pressed against the rectal wall. Gently turn the catheter slightly to free it without stimulating defecation. If the catheter tip remains clogged, withdraw the catheter, flush with solution, and reinsert.
- After administering most of the prescribed amount of solution, clamp the tubing. Stop the flow before the container empties completely, to avoid introducing air into the bowel.
- If you are using a Foley or Verden rectal catheter, leave the catheter in place to promote retention. Or, gently remove the catheter and apply firm pressure with toilet tissue or a rolled washcloth against the anus to stimulate sphincter contraction and enema retention.
- For an *irrigating* enema, instruct the patient to retain the solution for 15 minutes, if possible. For a *retention* enema, instruct him to avoid defecation for the prescribed length of time or as follows: 30 minutes or longer for oil retention, milk-and-molasses, and Mayo enemas; and 15 to 30 minutes for anthelmintic and emollient enemas. (If the patient is apprehensive, position him on a bedpan and allow him to hold the tissue or washcloth against his anus.)
- Have a bedpan or commode nearby so it is available when the patient needs it. If he is allowed to use the bathroom, make sure it will be available. Place toilet tissue within reach of the bed and the toilet or commode.
- Place the call signal within his reach. If he will be using the bathroom or the commode, instruct him to call for help before attempting to get out of bed, because the procedure may make him feel weak or faint—particularly if he is elderly. Also instruct him to call you if he experiences weakness at any time.
- When the solution has remained in the colon for the recommended time or for as long as the patient can tolerate it, assist him onto a bedpan or to the commode or bathroom, as required. (First, deflate the balloon and remove the catheter, if applicable). Provide privacy while he is expelling the enema. Instruct him not to flush the toilet.
- Assist with cleansing, if necessary, and return the patient to bed. Make sure he is clean, comfortable, and can easily reach the call signal. Place a clean linen-saver pad under him to absorb rectal drainage, and tell him he may need to expel additional stool or flatus later.
- Observe the contents of the bedpan, commode, or toilet. Carefully note fecal color, consistency, approximate amount (small, medium, or large), and the presence of blood, rectal tissue, worms, pus, mucus, or other unusual matter.
- Properly clean and/or dispose of the enema equipment. If additional enemas are scheduled, store clean, reusable equipment in a closed plastic bag in the patient's bathroom.
- Discard your gloves and wash your hands.
- Record in the nurses' notes the date and time of enema administration; special equipment used; type and amount of solution; retention time; approximate amount returned; color, consistency, and amount of feces; abnormalities in the return; any complications that occurred; and the patient's tolerance for the treatment.
- Document the administration of drug-solution enemas on the medication cardex.

Nursing considerations
- Since patients with salt-retention disorders, such as congestive heart failure, may absorb sodium from a saline enema solution, administer these to such patients with caution and monitor electrolyte status.
- Schedule a retention enema before meals, since a full stomach may stimulate peristalsis and make retention difficult.
- An oil-retention enema is frequently followed 1 hour later by a soap-and-water enema to help expel softened feces completely.
- Administer less solution when giving a hypertonic enema, since osmotic pull moves fluid into the colon from body tissues, increasing the volume of the colon's contents.
- Alternative means of instilling the solution include using a bulb syringe or a funnel with the rectal tube.
- For a patient who cannot tolerate a flat position—because of dyspnea, for example— administer the enema with the head of the bed in the lowest position he can safely and comfortably maintain.

- For a bedridden patient using a bedpan to expel the enema, raise the head of the bed so his position approximates sitting or squatting.
- Unless absolutely necessary, do not give an enema to a patient who is in a sitting position, because the solution will not flow high enough into the colon and will only distend the rectum and trigger rapid expulsion. In addition, attempting to insert the rectal catheter into a seated patient may injure the rectal wall.
- If the patient has hemorrhoids, instruct him to bear down gently during tube insertion. This causes the anus to open and facilitates insertion.
- If the physician orders enemas until clear, give no more than three to avoid excessive irritation of the rectal mucosa. Advise the physician if the return is not clear after three administrations.
- In patients with fluid and electrolyte disturbances, measure the amount of expelled solution to assess for retention of enema fluid.
- Enemas may produce dizziness or faintness; excessive irritation of the colonic mucosa, from repeated administration or from patient sensitivity to enema ingredients; hyponatremia or hypokalemia, from repeated administration of hypotonic solutions; colonic water absorption, from prolonged retention of hypotonic solutions (which may in turn cause hypervolemia, or water intoxication); and cardiac dysrhythmias, from vasovagal reflex stimulation after insertion of the rectal catheter.
- Sodium polystyrene sulfonate enemas should be given cautiously to a patient with low sodium tolerance.

Instilling medication into the bladder

Bladder instillation of medication is an uncommon procedure, but it may be used to treat bladder infections by introducing medicated irrigating solution into the patient's bladder for a prescribed time. More often, it is used for instillation of a radiopaque substance in diagnostic testing. A catheter must be in place before medication can be instilled.

Equipment and materials
You will need prescribed medicated irrigating solution, a sterile irrigating syringe, a sterile solution bowl, alcohol sponges, a Kelly clamp, sterile gloves, and a linen-saver pad.
Commercially prepared sterile irrigation sets are available and include an irrigating solution container, a graduated receptacle, and a bulb or 50-ml catheter-tipped syringe. If the patient does not have a catheter in place, gather the appropriate equipment.

Preparation
Warm the medicated solution to room temperature to prevent vesical spasms during instillation.

Steps
- Confirm the identity of the patient by checking the name, room number, and bed number on his wristband.
- Explain the procedure to him, and provide privacy.
- Wash your hands.
- If a catheter is not already in place, catheterize the patient, draining the bladder completely. If one is already in place, proceed with the following steps.
- Position the patient and place a linen-saver pad under the buttocks.
- Pour the ordered amount of medicated solution into the sterile container or bowl.
- Put on the gloves, and disconnect the end of the catheter from the drainage bag.
- Clean the end of the catheter and the end of the drainage tube with an alcohol sponge; place the sponge over the end of the drainage tube.
- Fill the irrigating syringe with the prescribed medication.
- Drain any excess urine from the bladder.
- Then, *slowly* instill the prescribed volume of medication (via gravity or gentle syringe pressure) into the catheter, and clamp it below the arm of the catheter balloon with the Kelly clamp.
- If the catheter has been placed for this procedure only, remove it, and instruct the patient to retain the medicated solution for the prescribed amount of time—usually 15 to 30 minutes—before voiding. A sterile gauze sponge can be pressed against the external urinary meatus to minimize the sensation of having to void.
- If an indwelling catheter is in place, reopen the catheter after the prescribed amount of time.

- Clean the ends of the catheter and drainage tube with an alcohol sponge before reconnecting them.
- Record in the nurses' notes the type and amount of medicated solution used; the amount, color, and consistency of return flow; and the patient's tolerance of the procedure. Also, note any resistance encountered during instillation of the solution. If the return flow volume is less than the prescribed amount of instilled solution, note this on the intake and output sheets and in the nurses' notes.
- Document that the medication was given on the medication cardex.

Nursing considerations
- If you encounter any resistance during instillation of the medicated solution, do not use excessive pressure to force the solution into the bladder. Stop the procedure and notify the physician.
- If frequent instillations become necessary, the physician may order a closed (or continuous) irrigation system. This decreases the risk of further infection by eliminating the need to disconnect the catheter and drainage tube repeatedly. (See "Administering medication by continuous bladder irrigation" below.)
- Explain to the patient who does not have an indwelling catheter in place that a urinal or bedpan must be used each time he voids and that he may experience a burning sensation the first few voidings.
- If the patient has not voided 6 to 8 hours after removal of the catheter, notify the physician.

Administering medication by continuous bladder irrigation

Continuous, or closed, bladder irrigation delivers a continuous flow of medicated irrigating solution through a triple-lumen catheter. (See *Set-up for Continuous Bladder Irrigation*, p. 156.) It is used in the treatment of an irritated, inflamed, or infected bladder. Maintaining a closed urinary drainage system reduces the risk of further infection. Continuous bladder irrigation also helps prevent urinary tract obstruction by flushing out small blood clots that form after prostate or bladder surgery. The continuous flow of irrigating solution also creates a mild tamponade that may help prevent venous hemorrhaging.

Equipment and materials
You will need two containers of prescribed medicated irrigating solution, Y-type I.V. tubing, and a sterile alcohol or povidone-iodine sponge.

(Note: Continous bladder irrigation requires that a triple-lumen catheter be in place. The irrigation tubing is connected to the third port (or lumen) of the catheter.)

Normal saline solution at room temperature is usually prescribed for bladder irrigation after prostate or bladder surgery. An antibiotic solution may also be ordered postoperatively but is most often used to treat infections. Large volumes of irrigating solution are usually required for continuous bladder irrigation during the first 24 to 48 hours after surgery. This explains the advantage of the Y-type I.V. tubing, which allows immediate irrigation with reserve solution.

Steps
- Confirm the identity of the patient by checking the name, room number, and bed number on his wristband.
- Explain the procedure to him, and provide privacy.
- Wash your hands.
- Insert one spike of the Y-type tubing into each container.
- Squeeze the drip chamber on each spike of the tubing.
- Open the flow clamps to remove air from the tubing that could cause bladder distention. Then close them.

Beginning irrigation
- Hang the two containers of irrigating solution on the I.V. pole.
- Clean the opening of the inflow lumen of the catheter with the sterile alcohol or povidone-iodine sponge.
- Insert the distal end of the I.V. tubing securely into the inflow lumen of the catheter. (The outflow lumen should already be attached to tubing leading to the drainage collection bag.)
- Open the flow clamp under one of the containers of irrigating solution, and set the drip rate, as ordered.

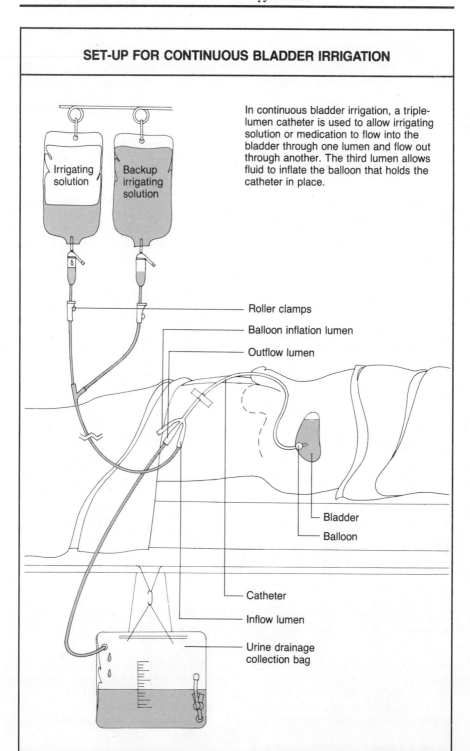

Using the reserve container

- To prevent air from entering the system, do not allow the primary container to empty completely. Close the flow clamp under the *near-empty* container and simultaneously open the flow clamp under the reserve container. This prevents a reflux of irrigation solution from the reserve container into the near-empty one.
- Adjust the drip rate, as ordered.
- Disconnect the tubing from the near-empty container with a twisting motion. Be careful not to contaminate the tip of the tube.
- Hang a new reserve container on the I.V. pole and insert the tubing, maintaining asepsis.
- Discard the empty container appropriately.
- When the first reserve container is nearly empty, repeat the procedure.
- After replacing a container of solution, record the time and the amount of fluid given on the intake and output record. Also record the time and amount of fluid drained each time you empty the collection bag.
- Record in the nurses' notes the time, date, appearance of drainage, and any complaints the patient may have.
- Document the administration of medicated solutions on the medication cardex.

Nursing considerations

- Always have a second container of irrigating solution available to replace the one that is nearly empty.
- Check inflow and outflow lines periodically for kinks to make sure the solution is running freely. If the flow rate is rapid, check the lines frequently.
- Measure outflow volume accurately. It should equal or, allowing for urine production, slightly surpass inflow volume. If inflow volume exceeds outflow volume in a patient who has had surgery, suspect bladder rupture at the suture lines or renal damage. Notify the physician immediately.
- Empty drainage collection bags frequently—as often as every 4 hours, or as needed.
- When the irrigating solution contains a medication, label the container with the drug name, dose, rate, and time added.

Review Questions

1. Define topical application, and list the routes of administration included under this method.

2. What is the first step in applying medication to the skin? Why?

3. What are the purposes of giving therapeutic baths?

4. When is the best time to give a therapeutic bath?

5. True or false:
   A. Creams and some lotions should be rubbed in by hand.
   B. If there is any ointment left on the tongue blade after application, you may scrape it off into the container.
   C. When removing the cap of a medication jar or bottle, the cap should be placed upside down on the tray or cart.
   D. A wet dressing is applied when the area to be treated cannot be immersed, when a wound needs mild debridement, or when the condition needs long-term treatment.

6. Is it all right to use skin medication on mucous membranes? Why or why not?

7. Nitroglycerin is commonly administered by what routes?

8. What is the benefit of applying nitroglycerin transdermally?

9. What effects do the following therapeutic baths produce?
   A. Colloid bath
   B. Oil bath
   C. Alkaline bath
   D. Tar bath

10. When you are applying a medicated soak, how should dressings be removed if they are encrusted and stuck to the wound?

11. Why are some drugs administered sublingually and buccally?

12. What can you do to prevent mucosal irritation when administering a buccal medication?

13. In what direction is a vaginal suppository inserted into the vagina?

14. What is the purpose of warming the solution for a vaginal irrigation?

15. In what instances should rectal administration of medication be avoided? Why?

16. How should the patient be positioned for insertion of rectal medication?

17. Why is the left lateral Sims' position chosen for enema administration? What is an alternative position?

18. If the patient complains of discomfort, cramps, or the need to defecate during instillation of an enema, what nursing action should you take?

19. Why should you warm medicated irrigating solution before instillation into the bladder?

20. What is the benefit of continuous bladder irrigation over frequent intermittent bladder irrigation?

Selected References

Brunner, L., and Suddarth, D. *The Lippincott Manual of Nursing Practice*, 3rd ed. Philadelphia: J.B. Lippincott Co., 1982.

Giving Medications. Nursing Photobook Series. Springhouse, Pa.: Springhouse Corp., 1982.

Procedures. Nurse's Reference Library. Springhouse, Pa.: Springhouse Corp., 1983.

Inhalation Administration of Medication

Administration of medications directly to the respiratory tract is accomplished via *inhalation*. For a medication to be inhaled, machines or devices must be used to produce a mist containing tiny droplets of the medication. Drugs inhaled in this form can travel deep into the lungs. They are absorbed directly through the linings of the respiratory tract or through the alveoli, depending on droplet size. This chapter details proper use of the equipment necessary to ensure safe, effective administration of medication via inhalation.

Using a hand-held inhaler

Hand-held inhalers include the metered-dose nebulizer, the turbo-inhaler, and the nasal inhaler (see *Types of Inhalers*, p. 160). These devices deliver topical medications to the respiratory tract, producing both local and systemic effects. The mucosal lining of the respiratory tract absorbs the inhalant almost immediately. Examples of common inhalants are bronchodilators, used to facilitate mucous drainage, and mucolytics, which attain a high local concentration to liquefy tenacious bronchial secretions.

Use of a hand-held inhaler may be contraindicated in patients who cannot form an airtight seal around the device, and in patients who lack the coordination or clear vision necessary to assemble a turbo-inhaler. There are also specific contraindications for inhalant drugs. For example, tachycardia or a history of cardiac dysrhythmias associated with tachycardia contraindicates the use of bronchodilators.

Equipment and materials

You will need an inhaler, prescribed medication, and normal saline solution (or another appropriate solution) for gargling. You may need an emesis basin.

Steps

• Confirm the identity of the patient by checking his name, room number, and bed number on his wristband.
• Explain the procedure to him.
• Wash your hands.
• Administer the medication, using a metered-dose nebulizer, a turbo-inhaler, or a nasal inhaler (see steps below).
• On the patient's medication record, note the inhalant administered, the dose, and the time. Note any significant change in the heart rate after bronchodilation, and any other side effects.

Using a metered-dose nebulizer
• Remove the mouthpiece and cap from the bottle.
• Insert the metal stem on the bottle into the small hole on the flattened portion of the mouthpiece. Then, turn the bottle upside down.
• Have the patient exhale, and then place the mouthpiece in his mouth and tell him to close his lips around it.
• Instruct him to inhale slowly as you firmly push the bottle down against the mouthpiece once, and to continue inhaling until his lungs feel full.
• Remove the mouthpiece from the patient's mouth, and tell him to hold his breath for several seconds, to allow the medication to reach the alveoli. Then, instruct him to exhale slowly through pursed lips to keep the distal bronchioles open and to allow increased absorption and diffusion of the drug and better gas exchange.

TYPES OF INHALERS

Nasal inhaler

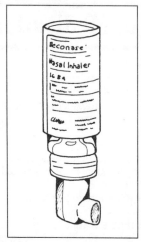

Metered-dose nebulizer

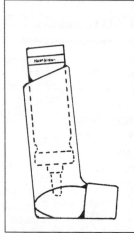

Turbo-inhaler

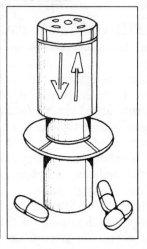

• Have the patient gargle with normal saline solution, if desired, to remove medication from the mouth and back of the throat. (The lungs retain only about 10% of the inhalant; most of the remainder is exhaled, but substantial amounts may remain in the oropharynx.)
• Rinse the mouthpiece thoroughly with warm water to prevent accumulation of residue.

Using a turbo-inhaler
• Hold the mouthpiece in one hand. With the other hand, slide the gray sleeve away from the mouthpiece as far as it will go.
• Unscrew the tip of the mouthpiece by turning it counterclockwise.
• Firmly press the colored portion of the medication capsule into the propeller stem of the mouthpiece.
• Screw the inhaler together again securely.
• Holding the inhaler with the mouthpiece at the bottom, slide the gray sleeve all the way down and then up again to puncture the capsule and release the medication. Do this only once.
• Have the patient exhale completely and tilt his head back. Then, instruct him to place the mouthpiece in his mouth, close his lips around it, and inhale once, quickly and deeply, through the mouthpiece.
• Tell the patient to hold his breath for several seconds to allow the medication to reach the alveoli. (Instruct him not to exhale through the mouthpiece.)
• Remove the inhaler from the patient's mouth, and tell him to exhale as much air as possible.
• Repeat the procedure until all the medication in the device is inhaled.
• Have the patient gargle with normal saline solution, if desired, to remove medication from the mouth and back of the throat. Be sure to provide an emesis basin if needed.
• Discard the empty medication capsule, put the inhaler in its can, and secure the lid. Rinse the inhaler with warm water at least once a week.

Using a nasal inhaler
• Have the patient blow his nose to clear his nostrils.
• Insert the medication cartridge in the adapter. (When inserting a refill cartridge, first remove the protective cap from the stem.)

Inhalation Administration of Medication

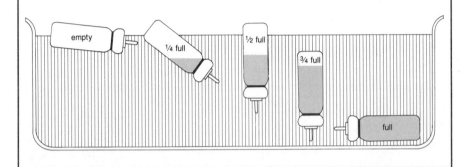

DETERMINING HOW MUCH INHALANT IS LEFT

To find out how much inhalant is left in the canister, drop it into a pan of water. Its position in the water tells you how much inhalant remains.

- Shake the inhaler well, and remove the protective cap.
- Hold the inhaler with your index finger on top of the cartridge and your thumb under the nasal adapter. The adapter tip should be pointing toward the patient.
- Have the patient tilt his head back. Then, tell him to place the adapter tip in one nostril while occluding the other nostril with his finger.
- Instruct him to inhale gently as he presses the adapter and the cartridge together firmly to release a measured dose of medication. (Note: Follow manufacturer's instructions. Some medications should not be inhaled during administration; Turbinaire is an example.)
- Tell the patient to remove the inhaler from his nostril and to exhale through his mouth.
- Shake the inhaler, and have him repeat the procedure in the other nostril.
- Have him gargle with normal saline solution to remove medication from the mouth and throat.
- Remove the medication cartridge from the nasal inhaler, and wash the nasal adapter in lukewarm water. Let the adapter dry thoroughly before reinserting the cartridge.

Nursing considerations

- When using a turbo-inhaler or a nasal inhaler, make sure the pressurized cartridge is not punctured or incinerated. Store the medication cartridge below 120° F. (48.9° C.).
- If you are using a turbo-inhaler, keep the medication capsules wrapped until needed so they do not deteriorate.
- Teach the patient how to use the inhaler so he can continue treatments himself after discharge, if necessary.
- Explain that most canisters contain 200 puffs and he need not spray a dose of medication into the air to see how much is left. Show him how to estimate the amount of medication left. (See *Determining How Much Inhalant Is Left.*)
- Explain that overdosage—which is common—can make the drug ineffective for him. Tell him to record the date and time of each inhalation and his response, to prevent overdosage and to help the physician determine the drug's effectiveness.
- Also, note if the patient uses an unusual amount of medication—more than one metered cartridge every 3 weeks, for example, with the metered-dose nebulizer.
- Caution the patient not to use over-the-counter drugs in addition to his prescribed drug because they may be incompatible.
- Inform him of possible side effects, such as palpitations, tremors, dizziness, and headaches. Instruct him to notify the physician if these occur.

Administering medication through a nebulizer

Used to deliver moisture or medication, nebulizers produce 100% humidity in a fine aerosol mist of fluid droplets that, ideally, slowly settle deep into the lungs. Drugs commonly administered via nebulizer include bronchodilators, mucolytics, immunosuppressants, corticosteroids, and antibiotics.

The large-volume nebulizer and the ultrasonic nebulizer usually deliver moisture rather than medication. The side-stream nebulizer and the mini-nebulizer deliver aerosolized medication. The side-stream nebulizer attaches to a ventilator or to an intermittent positive-pressure breathing (IPPB) machine. The mini-nebulizer is hand-held. (See *Nebulizers Used to Deliver Medication*.)

Nebulization should be used cautiously in patients with delicate fluid balance and in asthmatic patients with active or potential bronchospasm.

Equipment and materials

For using the side-stream nebulizer, you will need a pressurized gas source; prescribed medication; diluent, usually sterile normal saline solution or sterile distilled water; and an appropriate syringe and needle. You may need suction equipment.

The nebulizer and tubing may be connected to a ventilator or an IPPB machine. Use of an IPPB machine also requires a mouthpiece or mask.

For using the mini-nebulizer, you will need a nebulizer cup with lid; a pressurized gas source; a flow meter, as necessary; oxygen tubing; a T-piece; a mouthpiece or mask, or other appropriate gas-delivery device; pre-

NEBULIZERS USED TO DELIVER MEDICATION

Type	Advantages	Disadvantages
Mini-nebulizer or Maxi-mist 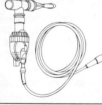	• Conforms to patient's physiology, allowing him to inhale and exhale on his own power. • Can cause less air trapping than medication administered by intermittent positive-pressure breathing (IPPB). • May be used with compressed air, oxygen, or compressor pump. • Compact and disposable.	• Procedure takes a long time if patient needs nurse's assistance. • Medication distributed unevenly if patient does not breathe properly.
Side-stream nebulizer 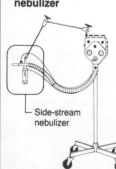 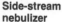	• Delivers medication to patient on ventilator or during IPPB therapy.	• Those disadvantages associated with ventilators or IPPB therapy. • Adverse reaction to medication.

scribed medication; diluent, usually sterile normal saline solution or sterile distilled water; and a 5-ml syringe and needle. You may need suction equipment.

Disposable units are commercially available.

Preparation

To prepare a side-stream nebulizer, draw up the medication and diluent, if required, into the syringe. Or, draw the medication into the syringe and use a premeasured container of sterile saline solution or water.

To prepare a mini-nebulizer, draw up the medication into the syringe, and inject it into the medication cup. Add the prescribed amount of sterile saline solution or water. Keep the cup upright to prevent spillage. Attach the T-piece and the mouthpiece, mask, or other gas-delivery device. Attach one end of the oxygen tubing to the nebulizer.

Steps

- Confirm the identity of the patient by checking the name, room number, and bed number on his wristband.
- Explain the procedure to him.
- Wash your hands.

Using a side-stream nebulizer

- Take vital signs and auscultate lungs to establish a baseline.
- Remove the nebulizer cup, inject the medication, and replace the cup. If using an IPPB machine, attach the mouthpiece or mask to the machine.
- If possible, place the patient in a sitting or high Fowler's position to facilitate maximal lung expansion and promote aerosol dispersion. Encourage him to take slow, deep, even breaths. Turn on the machine and check for an ample quantity of mist, indicating proper operation.
- Remain with the patient during treatment (usually 15 to 20 minutes), and take vital signs to detect adverse reactions to the medication. If the patient must rest, turn off the nebulizer to avoid wasting medication.
- Encourage and assist the patient to cough and expectorate, or perform suction as necessary. Auscultate the lungs again to evaluate the effectiveness of therapy.

Using a mini-nebulizer

- Take the patient's vital signs to establish a baseline.
- If possible, place the patient in a sitting or high Fowler's position to facilitate lung expansion and aerosol dispersion.
- Attach the free end of the oxygen tubing to the pressurized gas source. Turn on the gas source and check the outflow port for proper misting. If you are administering oxygen, adjust the flow meter to provide proper misting. Usually a setting of 5 to 6 liters/minute is adequate.
- Instruct the patient to breathe slowly, deeply, and evenly through his mouth, and to hold his breath for 2 to 3 seconds on full inspiration to receive the full benefit of the medication.
- If possible, remain with the patient during treatment (usually 15 to 20 minutes). Take vital signs to detect adverse reactions to the medication.
- Encourage and assist the patient to cough and expectorate, or perform suction as necessary. Briefly stop the treatment if he needs to rest.

Concluding nebulizer procedures

- Make sure the patient is comfortable and breathing easily before you leave.
- Clean all equipment, as appropriate, and return it to the proper area.
- Record the date, time, and duration of therapy; type and amount of medication added to the nebulizer; fraction of inspired oxygen (FIO_2), if analyzed; baseline and subsequent vital signs and breath sounds; result of the therapy, such as loosened secretions; any complications and the nursing actions taken; and the patient's tolerance of the treatment.

Nursing considerations

- Instruct the patient to rinse out his mouth after inhaling the mist of medication to avoid swallowing it.
- A nebulizer is inadequate for humidification. For this purpose, a large-volume humidifier must be incorporated into the flow line.
- If the nebulizer is used to deliver an antibiotic meant to remain in the lungs, caution the patient to avoid coughing. (This is not always possible because the moistened air may cause tracheal irritation and a cough reflex.)

- Provide emotional support during treatment; many patients find nebulizer treatments uncomfortable because they are frightened or feel they are drowning.

Administering medication using IPPB

Intermittent positive-pressure breathing (IPPB) delivers room air or oxygen into the lungs at a pressure higher than atmospheric pressure. Delivery ceases when pressure in the mouth or in the breathing circuit tube rises to a predetermined positive pressure. Although IPPB was once the mainstay of pulmonary therapy, its *routine* use is currently controversial.

Critics contend that it is costly, complicated, and easily replaced by properly performed deep-breathing exercises and incentive spirometry. Despite these claims, IPPB is performed in many institutions by both specially trained nurses and respiratory therapists.

Proponents believe that IPPB treatments expand lung volumes more fully, promote an effective cough, deliver aerosolized medications deeper into the air passages, decrease the work of breathing, and help mobilize secretions.

IPPB is contraindicated in uncompensated pneumothorax and tracheoesophageal fistula. Active hemoptysis or recent gastric surgery may also contraindicate this therapy.

Equipment and materials

You will need the IPPB machine, breathing circuit tubing, other necessary tubing (usually one or two sections), a mouthpiece or mask, prescribed medication, a 3-ml syringe with needle, a sphygmomanometer, a stethoscope, tissues, and a waste bag or specimen cup. You may need noseclips, a source of pressurized gas at 50 pounds/square inch (psi), oxygen, and suction equipment.

Some IPPB machines have internal compression units; others require a source of pressurized air or oxygen.

Individual plastic ampules with premeasured doses of routine IPPB medications are commercially available.

Preparation

Attach the breathing circuit tube to the appropriate opening(s), and any other tubes as required, according to the manufacturer's instructions. Draw up the ordered medication in the syringe and inject it into the nebulizer cup, making sure the cup remains upright. Or, snap off the top of the plastic ampule and squeeze its contents into the nebulizer cup.

Steps

- Confirm the identity of the patient by checking his name, room number, and bed number on his wristband.
- Explain the procedure to him to ensure his cooperation.
- Wash your hands.
- Take baseline blood pressure and heart rate, especially if a bronchodilator is to be administered. Listen to breath sounds for comparison with later auscultations.
- If the machine is not already set up, attach the appropriate tubing to the pressure source. Refrain from using a flow meter, because the IPPB machine requires a pressure higher than a flow meter can provide.
- Check the system for proper operation and leaks. Adjust the pressure as ordered, or to 15 centimeters of water pressure (cm H_2O). Remove the mouthpiece or mask and occlude the end of the tubing. Then, manually cycle the machine on and check that it cycles off at the desired pressure. If the machine fails to reach pressure, check for a leak in the system—a small hole in the tubing or a disconnection in the circuit or nebulizer.
- Set the nebulizer control, if necessary.
- If you are administering oxygen, set the dilution as ordered. If the patient has chronic obstructive pulmonary disease and cannot tolerate increased FIO_2, compressed air may be used to power the machine.
- Instruct the patient to sit erect in a chair, if possible, to allow for optimal lung expansion. Otherwise, place him in a high Fowler's position.
- Replace the mouthpiece or mask on the tubing. Place it on the patient, or show him how to position it to achieve a tight seal.
- Tell the patient to breathe deeply and slowly through his mouth, allowing the machine to do the work during the treatment.

This will cycle the machine and deliver a breath to the patient. When the preset pressure is met, the machine will cycle off, ending inspiration.
- Instruct him to hold his breath for a few seconds after full inspiration to allow greater distribution of gas and dispersion of nebulized particles. Then instruct him to inhale normally.
- While the patient is breathing, adjust the machine settings, as necessary, to match his inspiratory flow pattern. This may require changing the pressure setting or the inspiratory flow, sensitivity, or terminal flow setting, if present.
- If the patient is unable to maintain a tight seal with the mouthpiece, decrease the pressure until he appears comfortable and then gradually increase the pressure. Apply a noseclip when using a mouthpiece, or use a mask instead.
- During treatment, take the patient's blood pressure and heart rate. *IPPB increases intrathoracic pressure and may temporarily decrease cardiac output and venous return, resulting in tachycardia, hypotension, or headache.* Monitoring also detects reactions to bronchodilators. If you find a sudden change in blood pressure or an elevation in heart rate by 20 or more beats, stop the treatment and notify the physician.
- If the patient is tolerating the treatment, continue until the medication in the nebulizer is exhausted, usually after 15 to 20 minutes.
- After treatment, or as needed, have the patient expectorate into tissues or a specimen cup, or perform suction as necessary. Listen to his breath sounds and compare them with pretreatment sounds.
- Wash the mouthpiece or mask, the nebulizer, and all other accessories with a warm detergent solution. Rinse and dry them thoroughly to prevent bacterial growth. Store the tubing pieces in a clear plastic bag and replace them according to institutional policy, usually every day. Discard soiled tissues in a waste bag and dispose of it properly.
- Record the date, time, and duration of treatment; medication administered; pressure used; vital signs; breath sounds before and after treatment; amount of sputum produced; any complications and nursing actions taken; and the patient's tolerance of the procedure.

Nursing considerations
- To assess IPPB appropriately, measure the volume delivered to the patient to make sure breathing is deep.
- Be sure to explain the machinery carefully and provide emotional support during therapy; the work of breathing can be increased if the patient is uncomfortable or anxious.
- If possible, avoid administering IPPB immediately before or after meals because it may induce nausea, and because a full stomach reduces lung expansion.
- Never administer IPPB without medication in the nebulizer because it could dry the patient's airways and make secretions more difficult to mobilize.
- In treatment to mobilize secretions, use a specimen cup to measure secretions obtained.
- If the patient wears dentures, leave them in place to ensure a proper seal with the mouthpiece, but remove them if they slide out of position.
- If the patient has an artificial airway, use a special adapter, such as mechanical ventilation tubing, during IPPB.
- When using a mask to administer treatments, allow the patient frequent rest periods and observe for gastric distention. Gastric insufflation occurs more commonly with a mask than with a mouthpiece.
- If blood pressure is stable during the initial treatment, you may not need to check it during subsequent treatments unless the patient has a history of cardiovascular disease, hypotension, or sensitivity to the drug delivered in IPPB.
- Dizziness can result from hyperventilation.
- Decreased blood pressure can result from decreased venous return, especially in a patient with hypovolemia or cardiovascular disease.
- Spontaneous pneumothorax may result from increased intrathoracic pressure; it is rare but most likely to occur in patients with emphysematous blebs.

Review Questions

1. How are drugs absorbed in the respiratory tract?

2. The use of a hand-held inhaler requires what abilities?

3. For a drug to be inhaled, how does its form need to be changed?

4. Name four devices or machines used to deliver medications for inhalation.

5. Why should the patient using a nebulizer be in a sitting position or high Fowler's position if at all possible?

6. Define IPPB.

7. What is the supposed benefit of delivering medications via IPPB?

8. When administering medications via inhalation, what nursing action can be taken to allow greater dispersion of aerosolized droplets of medications?

9. Why should IPPB not be administered immediately before or after a meal?

10. During IPPB, why is it important to take vital signs?

Selected References

Dunlap, C., and Marchionno, P. "Help Your COPD Patient Take a Better Breath with Inhalers," *Nursing83*:42-43, May 1983.
Procedures. Nurse's Reference Library. Springhouse, Pa.: Springhouse Corp., 1983.

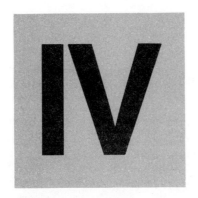

Principles and Procedures in I.V. Therapy

12 Preparing for I.V. Therapy 168

13 Performing I.V. Therapy Procedures 195

14 Maintaining I.V. Therapy 210

15 Parenteral Nutrition 232

16 Blood and Blood Component Therapy 256

Preparing for I.V. Therapy

Today, more than 25% of all patients receive some form of I.V. therapy during hospitalization, and more than 200 commercially prepared I.V. fluids are available. The purposes of I.V. therapy are to restore or maintain fluids and electrolytes, administer medications (see Chapter 8, Parenteral Administration of Medication), provide nutrition (see Chapter 15, Parenteral Nutrition), facilitate transfusion therapy (see Chapter 16, Blood and Blood Component Transfusion), and serve as a route for blood sampling.

The decision to implement I.V. therapy is a medical one. However, nursing assessment of the patient may help the physician decide whether or not to start I.V. therapy. Once this is decided, a nursing-care plan must focus first on properly preparing the patient, then on maintaining aseptic technique and preventing potential complications through meticulous maintenance of the I.V. line and insertion site.

This chapter covers key points of preparing for I.V. therapy and provides the basic information necessary to make educated decisions in the choice of sites and equipment for I.V. therapy. Patient preparation, peripheral and central venipuncture devices, infusion equipment, and documentation are highlighted.

Components of an I.V. order

A complete order for I.V. therapy should specify the following:
- type of solution (see *Abbreviations for I.V. Solutions*)
- any additives and their concentration (such as 10 mEq KCl in 50 ml D_5W)
- rate or volume of infusion (see *Calculating Flow Rates*, p. 182)
- duration of infusion.

A sample order may read as follows:
Date: (specify)
Time: (specify)
Give $D_5$0.2NaCl with 20 mEq KCl per 500 ml at 60 ml/hr x 48 hr.
Signature, MD

Fluids and solutions for I.V. therapy are ordered by the physician. Orders may be standardized for different illnesses and therapies (such as burn treatment) or individualized. Some institutional policies dictate an automatic stoporder for I.V. fluids (for example, I.V. orders are good for 24 hours from the time of writing, unless otherwise specified). If an order is not complete, however, consult with the physician.

Types of solutions

A *solution* is a liquid containing one or more dissolved substances called *solutes*. Most solutes are dissolved in water, and 1 ml of water weighs 1 g. Grams and milliliters, therefore, are used synonymously in reference to solutions. For example, a 5% dextrose solution contains 5 ml or 5 g of dextrose (solute) in 100 ml of water (solvent).

ABBREVIATIONS FOR I.V. SOLUTIONS

AA: .... Amino acids
D: .... Dextrose solution (percentage unspecified)
D₅LR: .... Dextrose 5% in Ringer's injection, lactated
D₅R: .... Dextrose 5% in Ringer's injection
D-S: .... Dextrose-saline combinations
D₂.₅½NS or D₂.₅½NaCl: .... Dextrose 2.5% in sodium chloride 0.45%
D₂.₅NS or D₂.₅NaCl: .... Dextrose 2.5% in sodium chloride 0.9%
D₅¼NS or D₅0.2 NaCl: ..... Dextrose 5% in sodium chloride 0.225%
D₅½NS or D₅0.45 NaCl: ...... Dextrose 5% in sodium chloride 0.45%
D₅NS or D₅/0.9 NaCl: .... Dextrose 5% in sodium chloride 0.9%
D₁₀NS or D₁₀/0.9 NaCl: .... Dextrose 10% in sodium chloride 0.9%
D₅W: .... Dextrose 5% in water
D₁₀W: .... Dextrose 10% in water
DXN-NS: .... Dextran 6% in sodium chloride 0.9%
IS: .... Invert sugar
LR or RL: .... Ringer's injection, lactated
NS or NSS: .... Sodium chloride 0.9%
R: .... Ringer's injection
TPN: .... Total parenteral nutrition
W: .... Sterile water for injection

The *tonicity* of an I.V. fluid, or how the fluid compares with normal blood plasma, is an important characteristic. (Normal plasma tonicity is 290 milliosmoles per liter, or 290 mOsm/L.) I.V. fluids that have higher osmolality are considered *hypertonic;* they draw fluid from the cells and are irritating when infused. I.V. fluids that have lower osmolality are considered *hypotonic;* they draw fluids into the cells. Fluids that approximate the osmolality of blood plasma are called *isotonic;* they are usually chosen for peripheral administration.

Commonly used solutions, their contents, tonicity, and indications are listed in *Types of I.V. Solutions,* pp. 170-171.

Administration equipment

Fluid containers
Sterile, evacuated glass containers for fluid and blood became available in 1929. Since then, glass containers have largely been replaced by plastic bags for parenteral fluids. However, glass I.V. containers are still used regularly in some hospitals and occasionally they must be used to deliver specific medications that are adsorbed by plastic (for example, diazepam and insulin).

Glass I.V. bottles are evacuated, or have a vacuum inside, so any additives that are injected into the stopper of a glass I.V. bottle are "pulled in" quickly. To balance the outflow of fluid from a glass bottle, air intake is essential for the solution to flow correctly, and a vented I.V. administration set must be used. (Vented administration sets have an extra filtered port near the spike, to allow air entry.) Because glass bottles are more difficult to store and more likely to break, extra care must be taken in their use.

Plastic fluid containers are more widely used for routine administration of I.V. fluids. They may be soft, flexible bags or semi-rigid rectangular containers, allowing easy storage, transport, and disposal. Because plastic I.V. containers are flexible, they collapse as fluid flows out, and they are not evacuated. Consequently, air venting is not required, and the chance of air embolism or airborne contamination is reduced.

Administration sets
I.V. administration sets differ mainly in the drop factor (the rate of flow they can produce), the number of Y-site ports, and the

TYPES OF I.V. SOLUTIONS

Description	Dextrose (g/100 ml)	Calories/ 100 ml	Electrolytes (mEq/100 ml)			
			Na^+	K^+	Ca^{++}	Mg^{++}
Carbohydrates in water						
D_5W	5	17	0	0	0	0
$D_{10}W$	10	34	0	0	0	0
Carbohydrates in sodium chloride solution						
$D_5$0.2 NaCl	5	17	3.4	0	0	0
$D_5$0.45 NaCl	5	17	7.7	0	0	0
$D_5$0.9 NaCl	5	17	15.4	0	0	0
Sodium chloride solution						
0.45 NaCl	0	0	7.7	0	0	0
0.9 NaCl or NSS (normal saline)	0	0	15.4	0	0	0
3% NaCl	0	0	51.3	0	0	0
Electrolyte solutions						
D_5 lactated Ringer's (D5LR)	5	17	13.0	0.4	0.3	0
Lactated Ringer's (LR, Hartmann's)	0	0	13.0	0.4	0.3	0
D_5 Ringer's (D5R)	5	17	14.7	0.4	0.4	0
Ringer's	0	0	14.7	0.4	0.4	0

Preparing for I.V. Therapy

Electrolytes (mEq/100ml)				Tonicity	Benefits from administration
Cl⁻	HPO₄⁻⁻	Acetate	Lactate		
0	0	0	0	Isotonic	• Prevents dehydration
0	0	0	0	Hypertonic	• Prevents and treats ketosis
					• Promotes sodium diuresis (particularly following excessive administration of electrolyte solution)
					• Supplies calories (for energy)
					• Supplies water (for body needs)
					• Vehicle for I.V. medication
3.4	0	0	0	Isotonic	• Promotes diuresis
7.7	0	0	0	Hypertonic	• Corrects moderate fluid loss
15.4	0	0	0	Hypertonic	• Prevents alkalosis
					• Provides calories and sodium chloride
					• Treats sickle-cell crisis
7.7	0	0	0	Hypotonic	• Treats alkalosis
15.4	0	0	0	Isotonic	• Corrects excessive fluid loss
					• Treats diabetic ketoacidosis
51.3	0	0	0	Hypertonic	• Treats adrenocortical insufficiency
					• Treats vomiting from pyloric stenosis
					• Used before or during blood administration
10.9	0	0	2.8	Hypertonic	• Treats dehydration
					• Treats electrolyte imbalance
10.9	0	0	2.8	Isotonic	• Restores normal fluid balance after extracellular fluid shift (lactated Ringer's)
15.5	0	0	0	Hypertonic	
					• Replaces fluid lost through vomiting or G.I. suction
15.5	0	0	0	Isotonic	

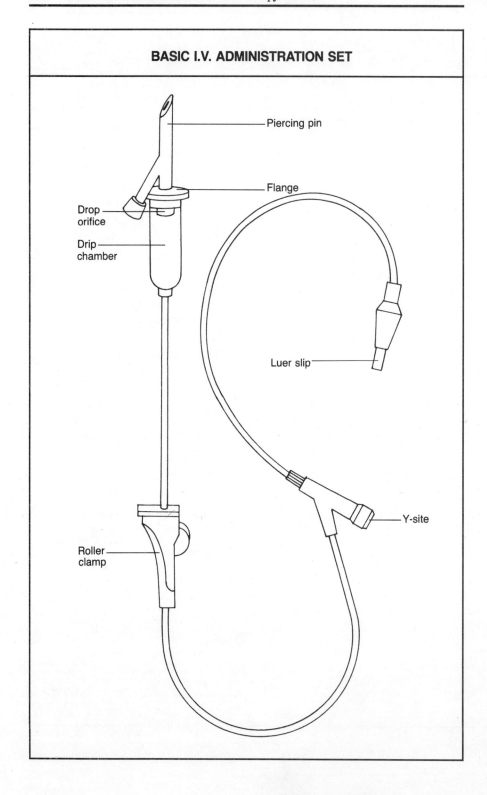

presence or absence of an in-line filter. (See *Basic I.V. Administration Set.*) Selection of a particular set reflects the rate and type of infusion and the type of fluid container.

Two types of drip systems are available: macrodrip and microdrip. A macrodrip set can deliver a solution in large quantities and at rapid rates; it delivers a larger

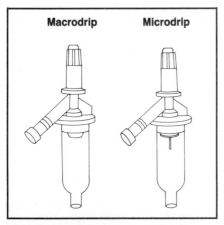

amount of solution with each drop than does the microdrip set. (See illustration above.) The microdrip set, used for pediatric and certain adult patients requiring small or closely regulated amounts of I.V. solution, delivers a smaller quantity of solution with each drop.

Administration tubing with a secondary injection port permits separate or simultaneous infusion of two solutions. (See illustration at bottom left.) Tubing with a

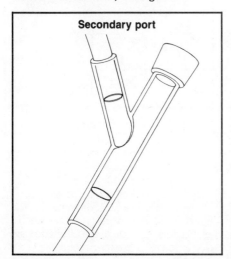

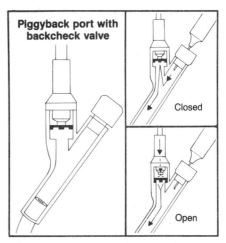

piggyback port and a backcheck valve permits intermittent infusion of a secondary solution and, on its completion, automatic return to infusion of the primary solution. (See illustration above.)

Vented I.V. tubing is used for a solution contained in a nonvented bottle; nonvented tubing, for a solution contained in a bag or vented bottle. (See illustration below.)

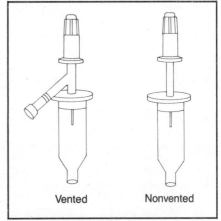

For a typical I.V. set-up for fluid and intermittent medication administration, see *Piggyback Set*, p. 106, in Chapter 8.)

Volume control sets with fluid chambers calibrated in milliliters (also called buretrols, solusets, or metrisets) are used to administer small, precise amounts of fluid or medications, as with pediatric patients, or to deliver potent intermittent or continuous medications (see *Volume Control Set*, p. 174). Macrodrip and microdrip sets are available.

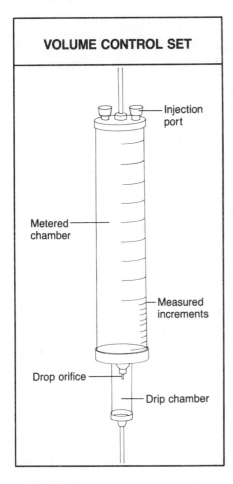

VOLUME CONTROL SET
- Injection port
- Metered chamber
- Measured increments
- Drop orifice
- Drip chamber

In-line filters
An in-line I.V. filter is a device placed in the fluid pathway between the I.V. tubing and the venipuncture device to remove pathogens and particles from I.V. solutions. Some filters are already built into the line; others need to be added, always using aseptic technique. In-line filters help reduce the risk of infusion phlebitis. (See illustration at right.) Ideally, filters used for routine in-line filtration are also able to prevent air from entering a patient's circulation by venting it through the filter housing.

Filters range in size from 0.22 microns (smallest) to 170 microns (largest) and are chosen according to the type of fluid infused and the desired effect. The 0.22-micron filter is the most commonly used filter in I.V. setups. National Intravenous Therapy Association standards recommend routine usage of 0.22-micron final in-line filters, although this usually depends on institutional policy.

Filters used with infusion pumps must be able to withstand the pressure generated by the pump. Some filters are made only for use with gravity flow; when pressure exceeds a certain level, the filter cases may crack.

In-line filters must be primed when you set up the fluid system. Follow the manufacturer's directions for the filter you are using.

Guidelines for using in-line filters
In general, use an in-line filter:
- with any infusion for an immunodeficient patient
- for hyperalimentation
- when using additives comprising many separate particles, such as antibiotics requiring reconstitution, or when administering several additives
- when phlebitis is likely to occur.

Avoid using an in-line filter:
- when administering solutions with large particles that will clog the filter and stop I.V. flow—for example, suspensions (such as amphotericin B), emulsions (such as Liposyn), and high-molecular-volume plasma expanders (such as dextran)
- when administering a small dose of a drug (5 mg or less), because the filter may absorb it.

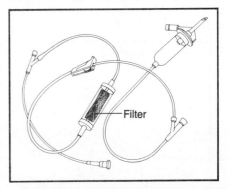

Filter

Be sure to change an in-line I.V. filter according to the schedule specified in the manufacturer's directions. Changes are necessary because bacteria trapped in the filter release endotoxins, pyrogens small enough to pass through the filter into the bloodstream.

I.V. controllers and pumps

Various types of controllers and pumps electronically regulate the flow of I.V. solutions or drugs when extreme accuracy is required (for example, during infusion of hyperalimentation solutions and of chemotherapeutic and cardiovascular agents).

Controllers regulate gravity flow by counting drops. They are less expensive to use, work well with uncomplicated adult infusions, and are less likely to cause I.V. complications. However, because controllers simply count drops, which are not always of equal size, these devices fail to achieve the accuracy of pumps, which measure flow rate in milliliters per hour. Controller alarms also may be triggered frequently by changes in patient position.

Pumps have mechanisms to propel the solution at the desired rate under pressure. They are more accurate and come in many sizes and types. However, pumps are more expensive to use and may increase the chances of infiltration or phlebitis because of the pressure used to infuse the fluid.

The peristaltic action pump applies pressure to the I.V. tubing to force the solution through it. This pump is easy to prime but is not recommended for use with "delicate" infusions such as blood cells, which might be broken down under pressure. The piston-cylinder pump acts much like a syringe; a specific volume of fluid is infused via a small plunger. Two types are syringe pumps and volumetric pumps.

In a syringe pump, a prefilled syringe is placed in a chamber, the rate is set, and the infusion is delivered when the syringe plunger is pushed forward by the pump. Syringe pumps are used for small doses and are portable, making them ideal for home care. They are also used for administering fluids to infants and for delivering intraarterial drugs. Volumetric pumps run on a system in which fluid is pulled from a container by a special disposable cassette and delivered at a certain rate over a specific period. Most volumetric pumps operate at high pressures (up to 45 psi) and can deliver 1 to 999 ml/hour with 97% to 98% accuracy.

Specialized pumps and infusers include implantable pumps that are surgically inserted under the patient's skin, prefilled with medication, and programmed to deliver very small amounts of potent medications. These may be periodically refilled with medication by the insertion of a needle through the skin; otherwise, minimal care is required.

Both controllers and pumps have detectors and alarms that automatically signal or respond to the completion of an infusion, the presence of air in line, low battery power, and occlusion or inability to deliver at the set rate. Depending on the problem, these devices may shut off, sound or flash an alarm, or switch to a keep-vein-open rate. For more information on selecting an infusion device appropriate for specific solutions, see *Selecting the Right Infusion Device*, p. 176.

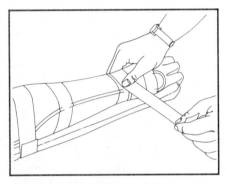

Armboards and restraints

Armboards are used to support areas of joint flexion, or to restrain I.V. sites in extremely active patients and in children. Armboards should be padded to maintain comfort and prevent nerve damage. Normal joint configuration should be maintained by supplemental padding, with gauze under areas such as the wrist in adult patients, and the sole of the foot in pediatric patients. Tape should not be wrapped completely around the patient's arm, nor should it be applied too tightly because it will act as a tourniquet, decreasing peripheral circulation distal to the I.V. site. (See illustration above.) The circulatory and neurologic status of the extremity distal to the I.V. site should be assessed at least once a shift in adults and hourly in children to make sure that capillary refill is present (for example, fingernails should blanch when squeezed,

SELECTING THE RIGHT INFUSION DEVICE

Infusion	Device	Administration set	Points to remember
TPN (in-hospital and home use)	• Volumetric pump	• Set specific to pump • Vented set for fat emulsion	• Use 0.22-micron filter for hyperalimentation solution. • Fat emulsion often piggybacked and run by gravity.
Blood and blood products	• Gravity controller • Nonperistaltic volumetric pump	• Set specific to pump or controller • Y-type set with in-line filter • Add microaggregate blood filter to line.	• Peristaltic pump may cause hemolysis.
Nitroglycerin	• Volumetric pump	• Use special non-PVC tubing.	• PVC sets adsorb nitroglycerin, reducing dose.
Drugs with high therapeutic/ toxic ratio (e.g., streptokinase, nitroprusside, dopamine, aminocaproic acid, oxytocin)	• Volumetric pump • Computer-interfaced pump	• Set specific to pump • Burette set may be used for secondary line measurement or add-on medications.	• Use 0.22-micron filter for immune-compromised patients and those at risk for air embolism. • Use 5-micron filter for highly particulated solutions.
Chemotherapy drugs	• Gravity controller • Volumetric pump • Syringe pump • Implantable pump	• Set specific to pump or controller • Syringe and extension set for syringe pump • Implantable pump with a Huber-tip needle and syringe	• Use 0.22-micron filter for immune-compromised patients. • Small volumes for syringe or implantable pump should be drawn up using filter needle or filter straw.
Vesicant drugs	• Syringe pump • Implantable pump • Gravity controller	• Set specific to pump or controller	• Pump should be used only on central lines, such as Hickman or Broviac catheters. • Use of pumps is not recommended on peripheral lines because skin sloughing and necrosis can occur with infiltration.
Long-term drug infusions (such as insulin, heparin, and chemotherapy)	• Syringe pump • Implantable pump	• Set specific to pump	• Patient must be taught how to use and maintain pump.
Limited volumes, pain control	• Volumetric micropump • Syringe pump	• Set specific to pump • Burette set may be used for secondary line measurement or add-on medications.	• Flow rate: 0.1 ml/hr to 99 ml/hr. • Microsets have low priming volume. • Use minimum diluent in mixing drugs.
Arterial infusions	• Volumetric pump • Computer-interfaced pump • Volumetric micropump	• Set specific to pump	• Use air-trapping or air-eliminating filter. • Pumps with variable-output pressure allow pressure to be adjusted to the patient's intraarterial pressure.

then return to pink when released) and that the patient has no complaints of numbness, tingling, or paresthesias.

Restraints are not normally used unless the patient is extremely combative or extremely active, or is not in control of limb movement. Some armboards come with straps that may be secured to the bed (not the siderail) to immobilize the I.V. site. A physician's order is required for restraints and judgment should be used in requesting them.

Temporary restraints may be used for starting an I.V. in a child (such as mummy restraints, or the assistance of a coworker). Restraints should not be placed proximal to or above the I.V. site because they may impede the flow of solution. They should be loosened hourly, and color and circulatory status of the involved extremity should be assessed.

Setting up a fluid system

Proper selection, assembly, and preparation of equipment is necessary to ensure accurate delivery of an I.V. solution. Assembly requires aseptic technique to prevent pathogenic contamination, which can cause local or systemic infection. You should first gather the necessary equipment and materials, then wash your hands thoroughly before setting up the I.V. system. You will need:
- solution, as ordered
- infusion tubing
- filter, if ordered
- 20g or 22g needle for piggybacking the tubing into the injection cap or side port.

Inspecting the container and solution
- Check the label, noting the correct infusate, size of container, and expiration date. Discard an outdated solution.
- Look for cracks or chips in glass bottles, or tears in plastic bags. Squeeze the bag to detect leaks. Plastic bags often come with an outer wrapper, which must be removed to inspect the solution container. Small cracks or leaks may admit microorganisms; discard the container if they are detected, even if the solution looks clear.
- Assess the clarity of the solution. If it is not clear, discard it and notify the pharmacy or dispensing department. Solutions may vary in color, but should be clear—not cloudy, turbid (thick), or separated (for example, lipid emulsions may separate, appearing in layers like salad dressing).
- Look at the cap to make sure it is intact. If the pharmacy has instilled additives into the I.V. container, the cap may have been resealed.

Preparing the solution
- Open the container, using sterile technique to remove the metal or pharmacy additive cap from a bottle, or the plastic pull-tab that is usually on a plastic container. Be careful not to contaminate the port.
- If the physician has ordered medications added to the I.V. container, swab the bottle top or side port of the bag with a disinfectant solution such as 70% alcohol, and inject the medication. A glass bottle with a vacuum will "pull" the medication into the bottle. Medications must be pushed into a plastic bag, with the bag hanging or lying on a table. Take care not to pierce the back wall of the bag. Gently rotate the container to disperse the additive equally in the solution.
- Label the container with the time, date, type, and amount of any additive; the patient's name; the bottle number; and your name.

Attaching and priming the tubing
- Choose the correct administration set for the type of I.V. container, the type of solution, and the patient. Examine the set for cracks, holes, and missing clamps.

Preparing a nonvented bottle
- Remove the bottle's metal cap and inner disk, if present.
- Place the bottle on a stable surface, and wipe the rubber stopper with an alcohol sponge.
- Remove the protective cap from the administration set spike, and push the spike through the center of the bottle's rubber stopper. Avoid twisting or angling the spike, to prevent pieces of the stopper from breaking off and falling into the solution.
- Invert the bottle. If its vacuum is intact, you will hear a hissing sound and see air bubbles rising (this may not occur if you have already added medication). If it is not intact, discard the bottle.

- Hang the bottle on the I.V. pole, and squeeze the drip chamber until it is half full.

Preparing a vented bottle
- Remove the bottle's metal cap and latex diaphragm to release the vacuum. If the vacuum is not intact (except after medication has been added), discard the bottle.
- Place the bottle on a stable surface, and wipe the rubber stopper with an alcohol sponge. Close the flow clamp on the infusion set.
- Remove the protective cap from the administration set spike, and push the spike through the insertion port next to the air vent tube opening.
- Hang the bottle on the I.V. pole, and squeeze the drip chamber until it is half full.

Preparing a bag
- Place the bag on a flat, stable surface or hang it on an I.V. pole. Then, remove the protective cap or tear the tab from the tubing insertion port, and wipe the port with an alcohol sponge. Close the flow clamp on the infusion set.
- Remove the protective cap from the administration set spike.
- Holding the port carefully and firmly with one hand, quickly insert the spike with your other hand.
- Hang the bag, if not already done, and squeeze the drip chamber until it is half full.

Priming the I.V. tubing
- If ordered, attach a filter to the opposite end of the I.V. tubing, and follow the manufacturer's instructions for filling and priming. Most filters are held with the air vent facing upward, so the filter membrane may be completely wet with solution, and all air bubbles eliminated from the line.
- If you are not using a filter, remove the protective cap on the tubing. Then, while maintaining the sterility of the end of the tubing, hold it over a wastebasket or sink, and open the flow clamp.
- Leave the clamp open until I.V. solution flows through the entire length of tubing, forcing out all air. Invert all Y-sites and backcheck valves, and tap them, if necessary, to fill them with solution.
- After priming the tubing, close the clamp and replace the protective cover. Then, loop the tubing over the I.V. pole.

Labeling and marking the container
The container should be labeled and marked with a time strip. (Note: In children, the volume-control set may be labeled, instead of the container.)
The label should include the following:
- Patient's name, identification number, and/or room number
- Date and time the container was hung
- Your name
- Any additives
- Container number.

The National Coordinating Committee of Large-Volume Parenterals recommends numbering each container sequentially over the course of I.V. therapy. For example, if 3,000 ml of solution are ordered on May 10, the day's 1,000-ml bottles are numbered 1, 2, 3. If 3,000 more ml are ordered on May 11, these bottles are numbered 4, 5, 6. This system minimizes administration errors. If a different solution is ordered, bottle numbers start again at 1.

A time strip attached to the container, using a piece of tape or a preprinted strip,

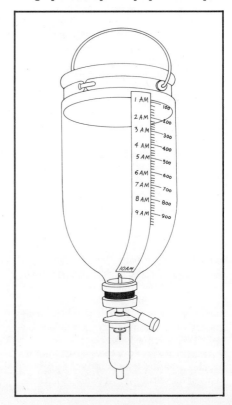

allows you to quickly determine if the infusion rate is correct by glancing at the bottle. It should be used even if an infusion control device is used. The tape length should coincide with the volume of solution. Mark hourly increments on the tape at levels indicating the volume of solution that should be infused. For example, for an infusion of 1,000 ml in 10 hours, there should be 10 marks on the tape, with each mark approximately 100 ml apart on the bag or bottle. Put the time strip in place with the container hanging, so that the top mark will align with the level of solution when the infusion starts, and the bottom mark will show when the solution should finish running. (See illustration on p. 178.)

Setting up a controller or pump

To set up a *controller*, first attach the controller to the I.V. pole. Then, swab the port on the I.V. container with alcohol, insert the administration set spike, and fill the drip chamber no more than halfway to avoid miscounting the drops. Rotate the chamber so the fluid touches all sides to remove any vapor that could interfere with correct drop counting. Now, prime the tubing and clamp it closed. Position the drop sensor above the fluid level in the drip chamber and below the drop port to ensure correct drop counting. Insert the tubing into the controller, close the door, and completely open the flow clamp.

To set up a *pump*, first attach the pump to the I.V. pole. Then, swab the port on the I.V. container with alcohol, insert the administration set spike, and completely fill the drip chamber to prevent air bubbles from entering the tubing. Next, prime the tubing and clamp it closed. Now, follow the manufacturer's instructions for placement of tubing. If you are using a peristaltic-action pump, you will usually place the tubing behind the door. (See the illustrations below.) If you are using a piston-cylinder pump, attach the tubing to the cassette.

PERISTALTIC PUMP AND PISTON-CYLINDER PUMP—ATTACHING THE TUBING

Tubing on linear peristaltic pumps and some controllers fits into slots or guides behind a door. On some models, it goes around a rotor over peristaltic fingers.

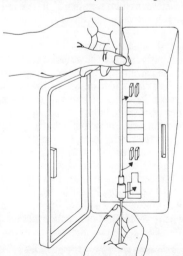

The cassette slides into a nest and is locked in. Cassettes may also be mounted outside the machine.

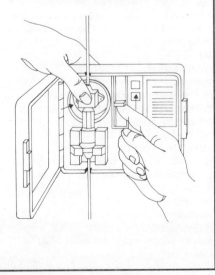

INFUSION PUMPS: HOW TO PREVENT PROBLEMS

An infusion pump is only as effective as the nurse operating it. Do not expect the pump to be a substitute for your own nursing skills. You still must check the patient regularly for complications, such as infiltration or infection. And the machine may not work properly all the time. Make sure you have easy access to the manufacturer's instructions and recommendations. But you can avoid several common infusion pump problems by using this checklist:
- Follow the manufacturer's instructions precisely when you insert the tubing. Remember, each model is a little different, and it is easy to make a mistake. Note: To avoid overloading the patient with fluid, be sure to clamp off the tubing when the pump door is open.)
- Take care to flush *all* air out of the tubing before connecting it to the patient. The danger of air embolism increases when the fluid is under pressure.
- Double-check the flow rate. Do not assume you will get an accurate rate just by setting the control. Monitor the flow rate yourself over a specific time span; once you determine how inaccurate the delivery rate is, you can adjust the flow accordingly.
- If your machine has a photoelectric drop sensor, position it properly. Align the top edge with the drip opening, and make sure the drip chamber is one-half to one-third full. Otherwise, the drop count will not be accurate.
- Do not let droplets cling to the sides of the drip chamber, or the drop count will be unreliable. Correct this problem by removing the drop sensor, clamping off the tubing below the chamber, and inverting the solution container and drip chamber. Repeat, if necessary. Then, replace the drop sensor, unclamp the tubing, and adjust the flow rate.
- Avoid turning the pump on and off excessively. This can clog the catheter.
- Before you attach an I.V. filter or infuse blood, check the manufacturer's recommendations. Not all pumps are designed for these purposes.

Steps
- Position the controller or pump on the same side of the bed as the I.V. or anticipated venipuncture site to avoid crisscrossing I.V. lines over the patient.
- Plug in the machine and attach its tubing to the needle or catheter hub. If you are using a controller, position the drip chamber 30" (76.2 cm) above the infusion site to ensure accurate gravity flow.
- Depending on the machine, set the appropriate dials on the front panel to the desired infusion rate and volume. Always set the volume dial 50 ml less than the prescribed volume or 50 ml less than the volume in the container, so you can hang a new container before the old one empties completely. Then, turn on the machine and press the start button.
- Check the patency of the I.V. line and watch for infiltration. If you are using a controller, monitor the accuracy of the infusion rate.
- Tape all connections and, if necessary, dress the I.V. site. Check the drip rate again because taping may alter it.
- Turn on the alarm switches. Then, explain the alarm system to the patient to prevent apprehension when a change in the infusion activates the alarm.

Special considerations
Frequently monitor the pump or controller and the patient to ensure correct operation and flow rate and to detect infiltration and complications such as infection or air embolism. If electrical failure occurs, a pump will automatically switch to battery power.

Move the tubing in controllers and peristaltic pumps every few hours to prevent permanent compression or tubing damage. For further information see *Infusion Pumps: How to Prevent Problems*. Change the tubing and cassette every 48 hours, or as the manufacturer or institutional policy dictates.

Complications with the use of I.V. controllers and pumps are the same as those associated with peripheral lines. Keep in mind that infiltration can develop rapidly with infusion by a volumetric pump.

Flow rate calculation

Maintaining proper flow rates for prescribed I.V. solutions is essential to prevent complications. Calculated from a physician's orders, flow rate is usually expressed as the total volume of solution infused over a prescribed interval or as the total volume given in milliliters per hour.

Two types of flow-regulating clamps are available. The screw clamp provides greater accuracy, but the roller clamp, used for standard fluid therapy, is faster and easier to use. (See illustration below.) A third type

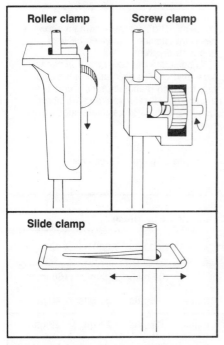

Roller clamp

Screw clamp

Slide clamp

of clamp, the slide clamp, can stop or start the flow, but cannot regulate the rate. (See illustration above.)

When regulated by a clamp, flow rate requires close monitoring and correction because such factors as venous spasm, venous pressure changes, patient movement or manipulations of the clamp, and bent or kinked tubing can cause the rate to vary markedly.

For steps you can take to solve problems with flow rate, see Chapter 14, Maintaining I.V. Therapy.

When regulated by a clamp or controller, flow rate is usually measured in drops per minute. When regulated by a volumetric pump, it is measured in milliliters per hour. With any device, flow rate can be easily monitored by using a time tape, which marks the prescribed solution level at hourly intervals. (See p. 178.) Usually, flow rate is recorded at the time a peripheral line is set up. However, if you adjust the rate, record the change, the date and time, and your initials.

I.V. administration sets are constructed to deliver a specific number of drops per milliliter. This drop factor can be found on the set's package label. Standard macrodrip sets deliver 10 to 20 drops/ml, depending on the manufacturer; microdrip sets, 60 drops/ml; and blood transfusion sets, 10 drop/ml. A commercially available adapter can convert a macrodrip set to a microdrip system.

To calculate and set the drip rate:
- Use the formula in *Calculating Flow Rates*, p. 182.
- After calculating the desired drip rate, remove your watch and hold it next to the drip chamber or position your wrist accordingly, to allow simultaneous observation of the watch and the drops. (See illustration below.)

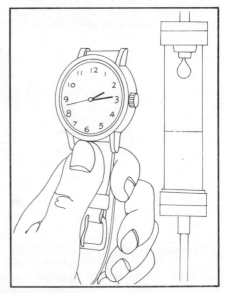

CALCULATING FLOW RATES

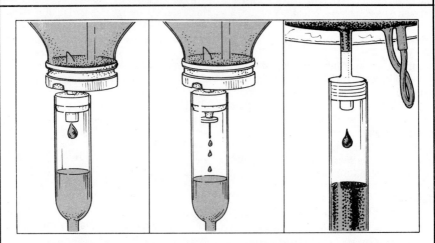

When calculating the flow rate of I.V. solutions, remember that the number of drops required to deliver 1 ml varies with the type of administration set used and the manufacturer. The illustration at left shows a standard (macrodrip) set, which delivers from 10 to 20 drops/ml. The illustration in the center shows a pediatric (microdrip) set, which delivers about 60 drops/ml. The illustration at right shows a blood transfusion set, which delivers about 10 drops/ml.

To calculate the flow rate, it is necessary to know the calibration of the drip rate for each manufacturer's product. As a quick guide, refer to the chart below. Use this formula to calculate specific drip rates.

$$\frac{\text{Volume of infusion (in ml)}}{\text{time of infusion (in minutes)}} \times \text{drop factor in drops/ml} = \text{drops/min}$$

Company name	Drop/ml	Drops/minute to infuse					
		500 ml/ 24 hr	1,000 ml/ 24 hr	1,000 ml/ 20 hr	1,000 ml/ 10 hr	1,000 ml/ 8 hr	1,000 ml/ 6 hr
		21 ml/hr	42 ml/hr	50 ml/hr	100 ml/hr	125 ml/hr	166 ml/hr
Abbott	15	5 gtts	10 gtts	12 gtts	25 gtts	31 gtts	42 gtts
Travenol	10	3 gtts	7 gtts	8 gtts	17 gtts	21 gtts	28 gtts
Cutter	20	7 gtts	14 gtts	17 gtts	34 gtts	42 gtts	56 gtts
IVAC	20	7 gtts	14 gtts	17 gtts	34 gtts	42 gtts	56 gtts
McGaw	13	4 gtts	9 gtts	11 gtts	22 gtts	27 gtts	36 gtts
Microdrip	60	21 gtts	42 gtts	50 gtts	100 gtts	125 gtts	166 gtts

(no matter which manufacturer)

- Release the clamp to the approximate drip rate. Then count drops for 1 minute to account for flow irregularities.
- Adjust the clamp, as necessary, and count drops for 1 minute. Continue to adjust the clamp and count drops until the rate is correct.
- If the infusion rate slows significantly, avoid increasing the rate to catch up; simply adjust the infusion to the ordered rate.

When infusing drugs, use an I.V. pump or controller, if possible, to avoid flow rate inaccuracies. An excessively slow flow rate may cause insufficient intake of fluids, drugs, and nutrients. An excessively rapid rate of fluid or drug infusion may cause circulatory overload, possibly leading to congestive heart failure and pulmonary edema, and drug side effects.

Preparing for venipuncture

Steps in preparing for venipuncture include selecting the appropriate I.V. device (needle, catheter, or infusion port) and choosing the best site. Device and site selection de-

COMMONLY USED PERIPHERAL I.V. DEVICES

GAUGE	AGE OF PATIENT	USAGE OF DEVICE
Teflon catheter-over-needle		
26	Neonates, infants	• Nonviscous medications, fluids
24	Neonates, infants, toddlers, school age	• All neonatal infusions • Fluids, nonviscous intermittent medications • Temporary repair of pediatric silastic catheter • Transfusions via I.V. pump
22	Infants, toddlers, school age, adolescents, adults	• O.R. use (anesthesia), transfusions • TPN, fluids, medications • Most routinely used device
20	Toddlers, school age, adolescents, adults	• O.R. use (anesthesia) • TPN, transfusion • Silastic catheter repair (Broviac)
18	School age, adolescents, adults	• O.R. use (anesthesia), transfusions (occasionally jugular in smaller child) • Silastic catheter repair
16	Adolescents, adults	• Possibly O.R. use, plasma pheresis, rarely used in children (occasionally for peritoneal tap) • Repair of larger silastic catheter (1.6 mm lumen size, e.g., Hickman)
Butterfly winged steel needle		
25	Neonates (½" or ⅝" needles), infants, toddlers	• Scalp vein and peripheral use • Fluids, nonviscous medications
23	Infants, toddlers, neonates, school age, adolescents, adults	• TPN, neonatal and infant transfusions, chemotherapy • Blood drawing, fluids
21	School age, adolescents, adults	• Possibly toddler transfusion, chemotherapy bolus • TPN, viscous medications, O.R. use (anesthesia), plasma pheresis
19	Adolescents, adults	• Transfusions, O.R. use (anesthesia) • Plasma pheresis, TPN

pend on the type of solution; the frequency and duration of infusion; the patient's age, size, and condition; and the patency and location of available veins.

Selecting an I.V. device

Because of the many sizes and shapes of devices available, choosing the best one can be difficult. As a general rule, select the smallest-gauge needle or catheter for the infusion (considering the size of the vein and the viscosity of the solution) unless subsequent therapy will require a larger device. (Note: The higher the number, the smaller the gauge.) Smaller gauges cause less trauma to veins and allow greater blood flow around their tips, thereby reducing the risk of clotting. For information on how to choose the appropriate gauge, see *Commonly Used Peripheral I.V. Devices*, p. 183.

Peripheral I.V. devices

Three types of needles and catheters are commonly used for peripheral lines:

• A *winged-tip or scalp-vein needle* (such as an E-Z Set or Butterfly) is ½" to 1¼" (1.3 to 3.1 cm) long and made of metal. It has tubing that is 3" to 12" (7.5 to 30 cm) long. Use this needle when a patient is in stable condition, has adequate veins, or needs I.V. fluids or medications for just a short time. You can also use it when a patient is receiving intermittent I.V. push injections over an indefinite period of time. (Straight metal needles, once commonly used in I.V. therapy, are difficult to secure and are now used mainly for blood withdrawal in adults and for temporary access to administer bolus medications.)

• An *over-the-needle catheter* (such as an Abbocath, Jelco, or Angiocath) is a radiopaque catheter and needle. This catheter is available in lengths ranging from 1¼" to 5½" (3.1 to 13.8 cm). Use one that is 1¼" to 2" (3.1 to 5 cm) long when a patient's condition is unstable (for instance, when he needs a large volume of fluids or blood); when only poor vein sites are available (such as the wrists or hands); or when caustic I.V. medications are to be administered. The longer catheters are used only in the operating room. An over-the-needle catheter with a resealable cap may be used for intermittent administration of I.V. medication.

• A *through-the-needle catheter* (such as Intracath) combines a 1½- to 2-inch-long (3.8- to 5-cm) needle with an 8- to 36-inch-long (20- to 90-cm) catheter. Use this catheter when venous access is poor, when I.V. therapy will be long term, or when extremely caustic medications (such as total parenteral nutrition or continuous chemotherapy) are ordered. It is easily inserted via a peripheral vein, although it may also be inserted into the jugular, subclavian, or femoral sites for central venous access. The needle must be sutured to the skin to stabilize it.

For more information on the advantages and disadvantages of each type, see *Needles and Catheters for Peripheral Lines*.

Another device used for peripheral lines is an *in-lying catheter*. This is used when a venesection is indicated but a vein cannot be entered percutaneously as a result of obesity, venous collapse or sclerosis, or peripheral vasoconstriction from massive, rapid blood loss. Performed by a physician with a nurse assisting, venesection is the sterile insertion of the catheter into the basilic or cephalic veins of the antecubital fossa—or less frequently, into the femoral and saphenous veins because of the risk of phlebitis and emboli—after surgical exposure and incision. After insertion, a sterile dressing is applied, and the catheter is used for the same purposes as a peripheral I.V. line.

Central I.V. devices

Central venous access may be accomplished using a through-the-needle catheter (as described above) or a silastic catheter such as the Hickman, Broviac, Hickman/Broviac, and Groshong catheters. The through-the-needle catheter is often used in the hospital for fluid replacement, total parenteral nutrition (TPN), and medication administration. Silastic catheters are usually chosen when long-term TPN and chemotherapy, either in the hospital or at home, are required.

The silastic catheter floats in the bloodstream, reducing the risk of intravascular trauma. The catheter is inserted into the

NEEDLES AND CATHETERS FOR PERIPHERAL LINES

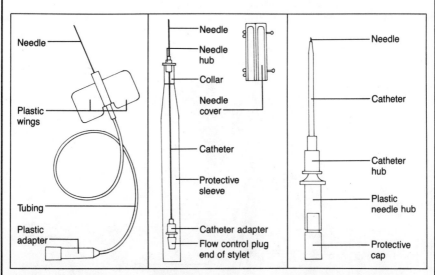

Winged infusion set
Purpose: short-term therapy for any cooperative adult patient; therapy of any duration for an infant or child or for an elderly patient with fragile or sclerotic veins.
Advantages: lower incidence of infection and phlebitis than with catheters; easy to insert and secure.
Disadvantage: risk of irritation or puncture of vein from movement.

Inside-the-needle catheter
Purpose: long-term therapy for the active or agitated patient; also used for central venous insertion.
Advantages: puncture of vein less likely than with a needle; more comfortable for the patient once it is in place; available in many lengths; most plastic catheters contain radiopaque thread, permitting easy location.
Disadvantages: greater incidence of infection and phlebitis than with a needle or shorter over-the-needle catheter; some hospitals may not allow nurses to insert it; catheter easily severed; kinking possible due to joint flexion.

Over-the-needle catheter
Purpose: long-term therapy for the active or agitated patient.
Advantages: puncture of vein less likely than with a needle; more comfortable for the patient once it is in place; contains radiopaque thread for easy location; easy to insert; some units come with a syringe attached that permits easy checking for blood return and prevents air from entering the vessel upon insertion.
Disadvantages: greater incidence of infection and phlebitis than with a needle; kinking possible due to joint flexion.

CATHETER POSITION

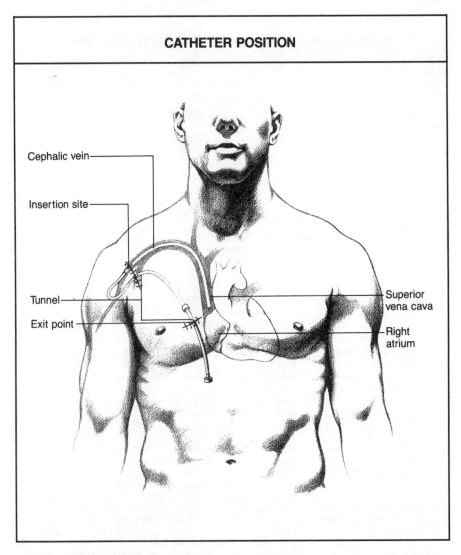

jugular, subclavian, cephalic, thyroid, or facial vein and is then tunneled so that the exit site is lateral to the xiphoid process. (See *Catheter Position.*) Firm tissue ingrowth into a Dacron cuff, with secondary catheter fixation, occurs in 2 to 3 weeks. The cuff then serves as a mechanical barrier against bacterial and fungal invasion. Many implanted catheters have remained in place several years. The location of the catheter exit site enables the knowledgeable and capable patient to care for his own catheter.

Occasionally, the catheter is inserted into the brachial vein in the antecubital fossa or into one of the internal or external jugular veins. However, the catheter tip is always positioned in the superior vena cava.

Each type of silastic catheter is chosen for its particular merits.
• The Hickman catheter is a single-lumen catheter with a Dacron cuff 30 cm from the hub. It is most frequently used for oncology patients and others who require frequent infusions or blood sampling.

- The Broviac catheter is also a single-lumen catheter, but its internal diameter is smaller than the Hickman's. It is often used in pediatric and neonatal patients.
- The Groshong catheter is a single-lumen catheter with a two-way valve in the tip. This permits fluid infusion or blood withdrawal and decreases the chance of air intake or blood backup in the line.
- The Hickman/Broviac catheter is a double-lumen catheter that is a fusion of the Hickman and Broviac catheters with a single Dacron cuff. The smaller lumen (Broviac) is used for the infusion of solutions; the larger lumen (Hickman) is used for blood sampling and for additional venous access.
- The Arrow-Howes catheter is a triple-lumen polyurethane catheter. Such multilumen catheters are recommended for patients who require multiple venous access routes and whose peripheral veins have been overused. The proximal lumen has the longest pigtail; it is used for blood sampling and blood and medication administration. The middle lumen has a medium-length pigtail; it is used for TPN or for medications if TPN is not used or anticipated. The distal lumen has the shortest pigtail and is used for central venous pressure monitoring, blood administration, high-volume fluids, and colloid and medication administration. For more information on the routine care and maintenance of silastic catheters, see Chapter 14, Maintaining I.V. Therapy.

Implantable infusion ports

An implantable infusion port is a device that consists of catheter tubing attached to an injection port, which has a self-sealing entry septum. The device is implanted under the skin surgically, using local anesthesia. The catheter is then tunneled to a central vein leading into the right atrium. These infusion devices are also available for arterial, peritoneal, and epidural use. The devices come with catheters of varying lumen sizes, and usage of the port determines which size is chosen. Currently available devices include Infuse-A-Port, Port-A-Cath, MediPort and Chemoport (single and double lumen).

Implantable infusion ports are used for older children and adult patients who require long-term venous access for chemotherapy, other I.V. medications, fluids, or blood products and for patients in whom external protrusion of the catheter is undesirable. They can also be used for blood sampling.

The advantages of the implantable infusion device over other catheters are that it needs no dressing changes, needs only monthly heparinization, and causes less restriction of everyday activity. It also reduces the impact on body image and the risk of infection. For a complete discussion of these devices, refer to "Infusing a drug through an implantable infusion port" in Chapter 8.

Selecting a venipuncture site

Selection of the best possible venipuncture site is an important factor in the success of I.V. therapy, and in the preservation of sites for future therapy. The most important considerations in selecting an appropriate vein include location, condition of the vein, purpose of the infusion, duration of therapy, previous I.V. therapy, cooperation required by the patient, and when possible, patient preference.

Peripheral sites

Peripheral veins are best suited for isotonic fluids, most medications, and TPN solutions with a concentration of less than or equal to 12.5%. Therapy is usually short-term (less than 3 weeks) or intermittent. Patient cooperation is required for insertion and maintenance of the I.V. line, and the site should allow adequate stabilization. See Chapter 14, Maintaining I.V. Therapy.

In choosing a peripheral vein, both arms should be assessed. Accessibility must be considered, but the most prominent vein is not necessarily the best. A vein may be prominent because it is sclerosed, or it may be in an unsuitable location. Select a vein in the nondominant arm, preferably, but never one in an edematous or impaired arm or leg.

For fluid replacement, choose a small vein unless a large vein will be needed for subsequent therapy. This leaves the large veins available for emergency infusion. If long-term therapy is anticipated, start with a vein at the most distal site so you can move upward as needed for additional insertion sites. For infusion of a caustic medication, choose a site away from joints, with

PERIPHERAL VENIPUNCTURE SITES

SITE	LOCATION/ APPROACH	REASONS FOR SELECTION	CONSIDERATIONS
Hand			
Digital veins	• Run along lateral and dorsal portions of fingers.	• May be used for short-term therapy. • May be used when other means are not available.	• Fingers must be splinted with a tongue blade, decreasing ability to use hand. • Infiltration occurs easily. • Uncomfortable for patient. • Insertion of a small-gauge catheter permits greater flexibility.
Metacarpal veins	• On dorsum of hand; formed by union of digital veins, between the knuckles.	• Veins easily accessible. • Lie flat on the back of the hand.	• In adult or larger child, bones of hand act as splint. • A short catheter should be used, so it does not decrease wrist movement. • Firm taping is necessary.
Arm			
Accessory cephalic vein	• Runs along the radial bone, as a continuation of the metacarpal veins of the thumb.	• Large vein excellent for venipuncture. • Readily accepts large-gauge needles. • Does not impair mobility.	• Most commonly used. • Sometimes difficult to position catheter "flush" with skin. • Does not require an armboard in an older child or adult.
Cephalic vein	• Branches off the accessory cephalic vein on the inside of the forearm, just above the elbow.	• Large vein excellent for venipuncture. • Readily accepts large-gauge needles. • Does not impair mobility.	• Proximity to elbow may decrease joint movement.
Median antebrachial vein	• Arises from palm and runs along ulnar side of inner forearm.	• Vein holds butterfly needles well. • A last resort when no other means are available.	• Many nerve endings in area may cause painful venipuncture or be damaged by infiltration. • Infiltration occurs easily in this area.
Basilic vein	• Runs up along ulnar bone from dorsal venous network and empties into the antecubital fossa.	• Will take a large-gauge needle easily.	• Uncomfortable position for patient during insertion. • Site is painful for venipuncture due to penetration of dermal layer of skin where nerve endings are located.
Antecubital veins	• Located in antecubital fossa. • Median cephalic—radial side. • Median basilic—ulnar. • Median cubital—rises in front of elbow joint.	• Large veins facilitate drawing blood. • Often visible or palpable in children when other veins will not dilate. • May be used in an emergency or as a last resort.	• Difficult to splint elbow area with armboard. • Median cephalic crosses in front of brachial artery. • An I.V. started in this area should be changed as soon as possible to a better location.

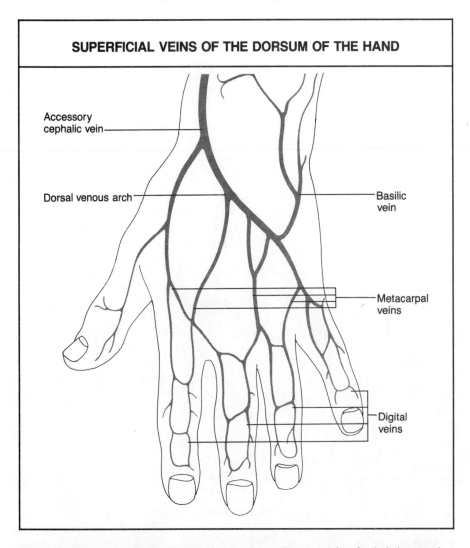

SUPERFICIAL VEINS OF THE DORSUM OF THE HAND

plenty of subcutaneous tissue. Be sure the vein can accommodate the cannula used.

For information on the advantages and disadvantages of specific peripheral sites, see *Peripheral Venipuncture Sites*. To locate these sites, see illustrations on pp. 189 and 190.

Central sites

Central veins carry an increased risk of infection, but they are usually chosen when therapy requires infusion of a great volume of fluid, hypertonic fluids, irritating drugs, or high-calorie TPN solutions with a concentration greater than 12.5%. Central veins are also used in emergency situations, when a peripheral vein is inaccessible, or when long-term or home therapy is planned.

The physician will choose the venipuncture site (see p. 190), but the nurse assists in the venipuncture (see Chapter 13, Performing I.V. Therapy Procedures), maintains the site (see Chapter 14, Maintaining I.V. Therapy), and teaches the patient his responsibilities and restrictions (see Chapter 14).

The tip of a central venous catheter usually lies at or near the junction of the right atrium and superior vena cava. (See *Catheter Position*, p. 186.) It may be reached from

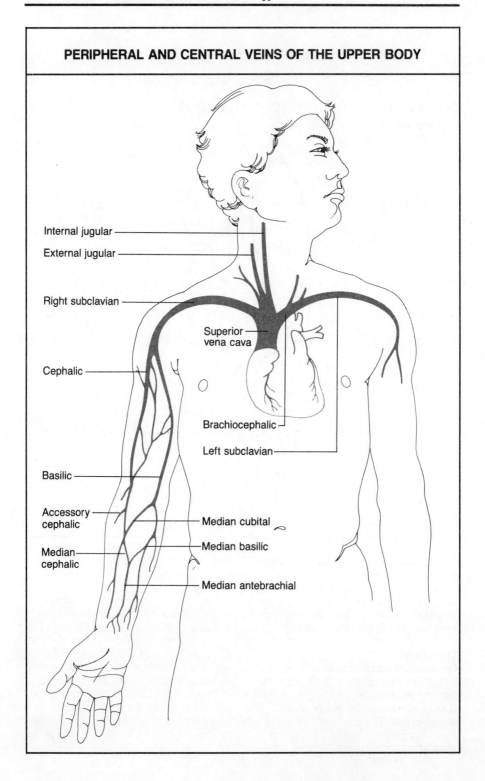

CENTRAL VENIPUNCTURE SITES

Site	Location/Approach	Reason for Selection	Considerations
Subclavian vein	• Approached under clavicle, usually left side first	• Easily accessed	• Close proximity to lungs, arteries, and lymph nodes increases the chance of complications.
Jugular veins (internal and external)	• Located on lateral sides of neck between ear and clavicle	• More accessible than subclavian in babies and young children	• Internal jugular is more difficult to reach, but is a more direct route to central locale. • Difficult to dress site because of natural folds of neck.
Femoral vein	• Anterior groin area, in the fold where the thigh meets the pelvis	• Useful in emergencies and/or if upper chest and neck are not available	• Difficult to keep area clean and infection-free, especially in babies and young children.

a variety of sites, using an appropriate length and type of central line catheter. The most commonly used sites are listed in *Central Venipuncture Sites*.

Preparing the patient for I.V. therapy

Although I.V. therapy is a common treatment modality, the patient may view it as a new experience. He may also be apprehensive about the procedure and concerned that his condition has worsened. If the patient is a child, his fears may be completely unrealistic. For example, he may think he is about to be poisoned, or that the needle will never be removed. Help the patient relax. Take the mystery out of venipuncture and I.V. therapy by providing information and anticipating and answering questions.

Assess the patient's previous experience, his expectations, and his current knowledge of venipuncture and I.V. therapy. Offer teaching appropriate to the patient's needs and ability to learn; use preprinted pamphlets, sample catheters and I.V. equipment, slides, videotapes, and information provided by other patients, if appropriate. Explain why I.V. therapy is needed, how the venipuncture is performed, how I.V. therapy will limit his activities, and how he can help maintain proper infusion flow.

Provide reassurance. Caregivers should be highly skilled in venipuncture technique so that multiple punctures are avoided. Allow the patient to express his concerns and voice his fears. Have him use stress-reduction techniques such as deep, slow breathing. Allow the patient and his family to participate in his care as much as possible.

If the patient is agitated, try to postpone the procedure until he is calmer. Since tension makes the veins constrict, his cooperation is important. If he is still anxious despite your efforts to quiet him, a mild sedative may help. Occasionally, the physician may have to order restraints (for example, when a patient is combative).

When the patient is as calm as possible, put him in a supine position with his head slightly elevated. Make sure the room is quiet and well lighted. This will help your patient relax and will increase your ability to concentrate.

Documentation of I.V. therapy

I.V. therapy may be documented on progress notes, a special I.V. therapy sheet or flow sheet, or a nursing care plan on the patient's chart. It is also documented on the intake and output sheet.

Documentation of *I.V. device insertion or the initiation of therapy* should specify:
- size and type of device used (also label on I.V. site)
- inserter (also label on I.V. site)
- date and time (also label on I.V. site)
- I.V. site
- type of solution
- any additives
- complications, patient response, and nursing interventions
- patient teaching.

For example, the nurses' notes for a 20-year-old patient receiving a continuous aminophylline drip might read:
Date: (specify)
Time: (specify)
S: "I've had I.V.'s before," patient.
O: Patient assisted with choice and preparation of I.V. site. Veins visible and palpable on both extremities.
A: Need for initiation of I.V. for continuous medication administration.
P: 20G catheter inserted in left supplementary cephalic vein. Catheter secured with tranparent dressing, after flushing with 2 ml sterile saline for injection to assure patency. Aminophylline infusion (250 mg aminophylline in 250 ml D_5W) hung, running via infusion pump at ordered rate. Patient verbalized that he would notify nurse if I.V. started to hurt, and would keep the site dry.
Signature, RN

Documentation of *I.V. therapy maintenance* should specify:
- condition of the site
- dressing changes
- site changes
- site care
- tubing and solution changes.

(For more information, See Chapter 14, Maintaining I.V. Therapy.)

Documentation of *discontinuation of I.V. therapy* should specify:
- time and date
- reason for discontinuing
- patient reactions, complications, and nursing interventions

- follow-up actions (for example, Band-Aid applied to site, I.V. restarted in another extremity).

For example, nurses' notes for discontinuation of I.V. therapy might read:
Date:
Time:
S: "This is sore," patient pointing to I.V. site.
O: Last dose of medication running via 20G catheter in right basilic vein. 2-cm red area proximal to I.V. site, tender and cordlike on palpation. No evidence of exudate.
A: Altered skin integrity; phlebitis.
P: I.V. discontinued, sterile dressing applied to site. Physician notified.
Signature, RN

The following guidelines should be considered when documenting I.V. therapy on the intake and output sheet:
- Fluid levels on I.V. bottles and bags are read hourly in children, and less often (but at least once in every shift) in adults.
- Hourly intake is kept of all I.V. infusions, including fluids, medications, flush solutions, blood and blood products, and TPN.
- Totals of amounts of each infusate are documented, as well as grand totals of all infusions, so fluid balance may be monitored.
- Output is also indicated, either hourly or less often, including urine, stool, vomitus, and gastrointestinal drainage.
- Fluid levels are "read" from the glass container, plastic container (you may need to "pull" the bag taut for more accurate reading), or volume control set. The levels are used as a rough indicator of the amount infused or remaining to be infused.

Review Questions

1. The following solution may not be administered by peripheral I.V. line:
   A. D_5W
   B. Aminophylline drip
   C. $D_{20}W$
   D. $D_{12}W$

2. I.V. access is used to:
   A. Provide nutrition
   B. Maintain fluid/electrolyte balance
   C. Withdraw blood samples
   D. All of the above

3. The following is a complete I.V. order:
Date: 7/7/87
Time: 1300
Infuse D_5W at 50 ml/hour.
Signature, MD
True or false?

4.-5. Indicate tonicity of the following solutions:
D_5W _____
Peripheral hyperalimentation solution of $D_{10}W$ _____

6.-10. Match the solution to the indication:

Solution	Indication
A. D_5W	____ 6. Compatible with blood products
B. 0.9 NaCl or NSS	____ 7. Severe hyponatremia
C. LR	____ 8. Burns
D. 3% NaCl	____ 9. Sickle cell crises
E. $D_5$45 NaCl	____ 10. Medication vehicle

11. Calculate the rate in drops/minute if the order reads: Give 250 ml over 3 hours via microdrip set.

12. A _____ infusion set should be used with an evacuated glass I.V. bottle.

13. A _____ micron filter is the most commonly used in-line I.V. filter for giving fluids and hyperalimentation.

14. All the air is primed out of the I.V. tubing after the set has been connected to the patient. True or false?

15.-16. Choose the infusion control device you would use to infuse the following therapies:
   Routine fluid replacement in a 50-year-old man   15. _____
   Transfusion of packed red blood cells to a 7-year-old leukemia patient   16. _____

17. An arm board must be used when inserting an I.V. line in the forearm of an adolescent. True or false?

18.-19. Choose the I.V. device best suited for the following patients:
   Blood transfusion to a 5-year-old in the short procedure unit   18. _____
   Periodic chemotherapy on a 25-year-old woman, for 1 year of therapy   19. _____

20. A nursing documentation of I.V. insertion should contain the following:
A. Inserter
B. Date/Time
C. Site
D. I.V. cannula type/gauge
E. All of the above

Selected References

Acevedo, M. "Electronic Flow Control," *National Intravenous Therapy Association* 2:105-06, 1983.

Boomus, M. "Intravenous Filtration: Why and How," *National Intravenous Therapy Association* 4:187-92, 1982.

Coggin, S. "The Selection and Use of Intravenous Pumps and Controllers: The Nursing Viewpoint," *National Intravenous Therapy Association* 1:16-22, 1981.

Crudi, C., and Larkin, M. *Core Curriculum for Intravenous Nursing, National Intravenous Therapy Association.* Philadelphia: J.B. Lippincott Co., 1984.

Feeney, L. "Documentation of I.V. Therapy," *National Intravenous Therapy Association* 1:8-10, 1979.

Gibson, J. "Arterial Line Placement, Monitoring and Maintenance," *National Intravenous Therapy Association* 2:140-41, 1981.

Grilli, E. "Getting Down to Basics: Intravenous Infusion Therapy," *National Intravenous Therapy Association* 1:48-51, 1979.

Huey, F., "What's on the Market? A Nurse's Guide," *American Journal of Nursing* 902-10, June 1983.

"Intravenous Nursing Standards of Practice," *National Intravenous Therapy Association,* November 1981.

Labry, J. "Infusion Monitoring Devices," *National Intravenous Therapy Association* 5:366-67, 1981.

Larkin, M. "Heparin Locks," *National Intravenous Therapy Association* 1:18-19, 1979.

Lorenzon, B. "Final Filtration," *National Intravenous Therapy Association* 5:322-27, 1981.

Masoorlie, S. "Trouble Free I.V. Starts," *Registered Nurse* 44:20-27, February 1981.

Piercy, S. "Children on Long-Term I.V. Therapy," *Nursing81* 11:66-69, September 1981.

Plummer, A. *Principles and Practice of Intravenous Therapy*, 3rd ed. Boston: Little, Brown & Co., 1982.

Sager, D.P., and Bomar, S.K. *Intravenous Medications*. Philadelphia: J.B. Lippincott Co., 1980.

Steel, J. "Too Fast or Too Slow: The Erratic I.V.," *American Journal of Nursing* 898-901, June 1983.

Umlas, J. "The Effect of Thin-Walled Intravenous Catheters on Transfusion Flow Rates, Cellular Integrity, and Apheresis Procedures," *Plasmather Transfusion Technology* 5:229-35, 1984.

Warwick, R., and Williams, P. *Gray's Anatomy*. Philadelphia: W.B. Saunders Co., 1973.

Webb, J. "Contemporary Comments on Infusion Pumps," *National Intravenous Therapy Association* 1:9-14, 1981.

Weinstein, S. "Nursing Considerations: Flow Control," *National Intravenous Therapy Association* 6:422-25, 1981.

Wetmore, N. "Nursing Responsibilities with Arterial Access," *National Intravenous Therapy Association* 6:428-30, 1981.

Wilkes, G., et al. "Long-Term Venous Access," *American Journal of Nursing* 85:793-96, July 1985.

Wilson, J.M. "Right Atrial Catheters (Broviac and Hickman): Indications, Insertion, Maintenance and Protocol for Home Care," *National Intravenous Therapy Association* 6, January/February 1983.

Performing I.V. Therapy Procedures

I.V. therapy encompasses a wide variety of procedures, all of which require fundamental knowledge of anatomy and physiology, aseptic technique, and the same basic equipment. This chapter discusses the most common I.V. procedures seen in both hospital and home-care settings.

Inserting a peripheral line

Insertion of a peripheral line must be done using aseptic technique to avoid introducing pathogens into the circulatory system. Doing a venipuncture is basic to this and other forms of I.V. therapy. The technique is not a difficult one if certain principles and basic steps are followed. There are both indications and contraindications for venipuncture. The most favorable venipuncture sites are the cephalic, basilic, and antebrachial veins in the lower arm and the veins in the dorsum of the hand. The least favorable are the leg and foot veins because of the increased risk of thrombophlebitis. The antecubital fossa also should be avoided, since this is the preferred site of venipuncture for drawing blood and for peripheral access to a central line.

Equipment and materials
You will need an alcohol sponge, povidone-iodine sponges and ointment, a tourniquet (soft rubber tubing or blood pressure cuff), two I.V. needles (angiocaths, wing-tipped, or cannulas), sterile 2" x 2" gauze sponges, 1" nonallergenic tape, I.V. solution with attached and primed administration set, and an I.V. pole. You may need an armboard, 2" roller gauze or elasticized gauze, and a small adhesive bandage.

Steps
• Confirm the identity of the patient by checking the name, room number, and bed number on his wristband. *Do not rely on the patient's response to the name you pronounce on entering the room.*
• Place the I.V. pole in the proper slot in the patient's bed. If you are using a portable I.V. pole, position it close to the patient.
• Hang the I.V. solution with attached primed administration set on the I.V. pole.
• Explain the procedure to the patient to ensure cooperation and reduce anxiety, which can cause a vasomotor response resulting in venous constriction.
• Also explain why I.V. therapy is needed, how much discomfort he can expect, how therapy will limit his activities, and how he can help keep the infusion flowing properly.
• Wash your hands thoroughly to prevent infection.
• Select the puncture site—preferably a vein in the nondominant arm, but never one in an edematous or impaired arm or leg. *For fluid replacement,* choose a small vein unless a large vein will be needed for subsequent therapy. This leaves the large veins available for emergency infusion. *If long-term therapy* is anticipated, start with a vein at the most distal site so you can move upward as needed for additional insertion sites. *For infusion of a caustic medication,* choose a site away from joints, with plenty of subcutaneous tissue. Be sure the vein can accommodate the needle or cannula being used.
• Wrap the tourniquet 4" to 6" (10 to 15 cm) above the intended puncture site to dilate the vein. Check for distal pulse. If it is not present, release the tourniquet and reapply with less tension to prevent arterial occlusion.

GUIDE TO COMMON SKIN PREPARATIONS

Antiseptic	Advantages	Disadvantages	Special considerations
Iodine tincture 1% to 2%	• Inexpensive and reliable • More effective than iodophors	• May burn or chap skin • May cause an allergic reaction • Discolors skin	• Always ask the patient if he has any allergies before applying. • Use moderate friction when applying. • Wash off the iodine with 70% alcohol after 30 to 60 seconds. • Do not cover the skin before the iodine is washed off. • Do not mix iodine with hydrogen peroxide. • Sodium thiosulfate is the antidote of choice for accidental ingestion.
Povidone-iodine (water-soluble complexes of iodine and organic compounds; also called iodophors) Betadine*, Proviodine**, Sepp	• Less irritating than iodine tinctures • Does not stain skin as much as iodine • Available in form of prep pads, applicator sticks, and crushable capsules	• Less effective than regular iodine solutions • May be absorbed through the skin during prolonged use • May cause an allergic reaction	• Always ask the patient if he has any allergies before applying. • Do *not* wash it off—use full strength. • Allow it to dry 2 to 4 minutes before insertion.
Alcohol isopropyl 70%	• Effective as a germicidal when used in concentrations of 70% to 80% • May be used as a substitute prep when the patient is allergic to iodine	• Not effective against spore-forming organisms, viruses, or tubercle bacilli • Evaporates quickly • Flammable and explosive • Dries skin excessively	• Apply with moderate friction for at least one minute.

*Available in the United States and in Canada.
**Available only in Canada.

- Lightly palpate the vein with your index and middle fingers. If it rolls or feels hard or ropelike, select another vein.
- If the vein is easily palpable but not sufficiently dilated, one or more of the following techniques may help raise the vein: Tap gently with your finger over the vein, or place the extremity in a dependent position for several seconds. If you have selected a vein in the arm or hand, tell the patient to open and close his fist several times.
- When excessive hair covers the selected site, clip the hair rather than shave it. Shaving may cause microabrasions and nicks that expose underlying tissues to bacterial invasion.
- If necessary, wash the area with soap and water before cleansing with antiseptic solution.
- Cleanse the venipuncture site with an alcohol sponge and then povidone-iodine, working in a circular motion outward from the site to a diameter of 2" to 4" (5 to 10 cm) to remove skin bacteria that would otherwise be introduced into the vascular system with the venipuncture. Allow the povidone-iodine to dry. (See *Guide to Common Skin Preparations* for information on other antiseptic solutions.)
- Once the skin has been cleansed, *do not touch the site*. If the site must be palpated to relocate the vein, the skin must be cleansed again.
- Position yourself in front of the limb, with your dominant hand in alignment with the vein to be punctured. The needle or catheter should always be in your dominant hand.

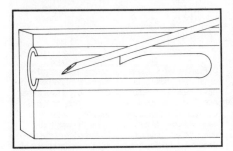

- Grasp the needle or catheter. If you are using a *winged infusion set*, hold the short edges of the wings between your thumb and forefinger, with the bevel facing upward. (See illustration above.) Then, squeeze the wings together. (See illustration above right.) If you are using an *over-the-needle catheter*, grasp the plastic hub with your dominant hand, remove the cover, and examine the catheter tip. If the edge is not smooth, discard and replace the device. If you are using an *inside-the-needle catheter*, grasp the needle hub with one hand, and unsnap the needle cover. Then, rotate the catheter device until the bevel faces upward.
- Using the thumb of your opposite hand, stretch the skin taut below the puncture site to stabilize the vein.

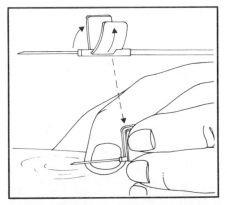

- Hold the needle at a 45-degree angle ½" below and slightly to one side of the puncture site (see illustration above).
- Tell the patient you are about to insert the needle, and push the needle through the skin until you meet resistance. Lower the needle to a 15° to 20° angle, and slowly pierce the vein; you should feel it pop when it enters the vein.
- When you observe blood flashback behind the needle, you can be certain the needle is in the vein. Tilt the needle slightly upward and advance it farther into the vein to prevent puncture of the posterior vein wall.
- If you are using a *winged infusion set*, advance the needle fully, if possible, and hold it in place. Release the tourniquet, open the administration set clamp slightly, and check for free flow or infiltration. Then tape the winged infusion set and tubing in place, using the chevron method (see *Methods of Taping a Venipuncture Site*, p. 198) to prevent movement of the needle, which could cause irritation and phlebitis.
- If you are using an *over-the-needle catheter*, pull back on the needle with one hand and advance the catheter fully with your opposite hand. Then, apply pressure to the vein

METHODS OF TAPING A VENIPUNCTURE SITE

Chevron method

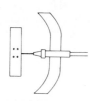

1. Cover the venipuncture site with an adhesive strip or a 2"x 2" sterile gauze pad. Then, cut a long strip of ½" tape. Place one strip, sticky side up, *under* the needle, parallel to the short strip of tape.

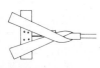

2. Cross the end of the tape over the opposite side of the needle, so the tape sticks to the patient's skin.

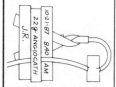

3. Apply a piece of 1" tape across the two wings of the chevron.
  Loop the tubing and secure it with another piece of 1" tape. On the last piece of tape you apply, write the date and time of insertion, type and gauge of needle or catheter, and your initials.

U method

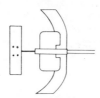

1. Cover the venipuncture site with a 2"x 2" sterile gauze pad or an adhesive strip. Then, cut three strips of ½" tape. With the sticky side up, place one strip under the tubing.

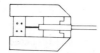

2. Bring each side of the tape up, folding it over the wings of the needle, as shown here. Press it down, parallel to the tubing.

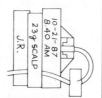

3. Loop the tubing and secure it with a piece of 1" tape. On the last piece of tape you apply, write the date and time of insertion, type and gauge of needle or catheter, and your initials.

Two-tape method

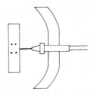

1. Cover the venipuncture site with an adhesive strip or a 2"x 2" gauze pad. Then, place a 2" strip of ½" tape, sticky side up, *under* the needle.

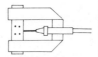

2. Fold the tape ends over and affix them to the patient's skin in a U-shape, as shown here.

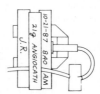

3. Place a second strip of ½" tape, sticky side down, over the needle hub. On the last piece of tape you apply, write the date and time of insertion, type and gauge of needle or catheter, and your initials.
  With this method, you can remove the upper strip of tape to check the insertion site while the lower strip anchors the needle.

H method

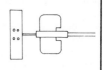

1. Cover the venipuncture site with a 2"x 2" sterile gauze pad or an adhesive strip. Then cut 3 strips of 1" tape.

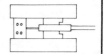

2. Place one strip of tape over each wing, keeping the tape parallel to the needle.

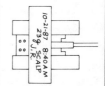

3. Now, place another strip of tape perpendicular to the first two. Either put it directly on top of the wings, or put it just below the wings, directly on top of the tubing. On the last piece of tape, write the date and time of insertion, type and gauge of needle or catheter, and your initials.

beyond the catheter tip to prevent blood leakage, and remove the needle. Release the tourniquet, and attach the administration set to the catheter hub. Then, open the administration set clamp slightly, and check for free flow or infiltration. Using the chevron method, tape the catheter, attaching the tape to the catheter hub.

• If you are using an *inside-the-needle catheter*, remove the tourniquet, hold the needle in place with one hand, and with your opposite hand grasp the catheter through the protective sleeve. Then, slowly thread the catheter through the needle until the hub is within the needle collar. *Never* pull back on the catheter without pulling back on the needle, to avoid severing and releasing the catheter into the circulation, causing an embolus. Then, withdraw the metal needle, and cover it with the protector, if one is present. Remove the stylet and protective sleeve, and attach the administration set to the catheter hub. Open the administration set clamp slightly, and check for free flow or infiltration. Use the chevron method to tape the catheter, attaching the tape to the needle hub.

• Apply povidone-iodine or antimicrobial ointment at the insertion site, and cover with a sterile gauze sponge, small adhesive bandage, or transparent occlusive dressing, which allows examination of the insertion site without removal of the dressing.

• Loop the I.V. tubing (see *Methods of Taping a Venipuncture Site*) on the extremity, and secure the tubing with tape. The loop allows some slack to prevent tension on the line, which could dislodge the catheter.

• Label a piece of tape with the type and gauge of needle or catheter, the date and time of insertion, and your initials. Place it over the insertion site.

• If the puncture site is near a movable joint, secure an armboard with roller gauze, elasticized gauze, or tape over the joint to provide stability. Excessive movement can dislodge the needle or catheter and increase the risk of thrombophlebitis.

• Document in the nurses' notes the type and gauge of needle or catheter, the location of the insertion site, the type and flow rate of the I.V. solution, the name and amount of medication in the solution (if any), and the date and time.

Nursing considerations

• If routine methods fail to dilate the vein sufficiently, apply warm, moist compresses for 5 to 10 minutes.

• If you are penetrating a large vein and institutional policy permits, inject 0.1 to 0.3 ml of lidocaine with a tuberculin syringe around the site. This causes a wheal, which may obscure a smaller vein, but increases patient comfort. Then, hold the needle at a 15° to 20° angle directly over the vein, and pierce the skin and vein in one motion.

• If you fail to see blood flashback after entering the vein, the needle or catheter may be pressed against the opposite wall of the vein. Pull the needle or catheter back slightly and observe for flashback. If no flashback appears, remove the needle or catheter and try again.

• A new needle or catheter should be used for each venipuncture attempt, and you should not make more than two attempts to initiate I.V. therapy. Ask another nurse to perform the venipuncture, after the second attempt fails. (Note: Absence of blood flashback may also be due to extreme dehydration or hypovolemia.)

• If a slight blood flashback appeared at first and then disappeared, the needle or catheter probably passed through the opposite wall of the vein. Withdraw and begin again.

• If blood flashback is present but the I.V. solution flow rate is sluggish, the tip of the catheter may be up against a valve. Notify the physician, who may reposition it.

• Peripheral line complications can result from the needle or catheter or from the solution. See *Local Complications of Peripheral I.V. Therapy*, pp. 222-223, and *Systemic Complications of Peripheral I.V. Therapy*, pp. 224-225, for more information.

• If an I.V. site infiltrates or becomes irritated, the peripheral line is removed. See *Removing a Peripheral I.V. Line*, p. 200.

• Inside-the-needle catheters should not be used for routine peripheral I.V. lines, because their placement has been associated with more local trauma and bacterial colonization than other catheters.

• In an emergency, when the skin has not been prepared adequately, a second line should be started after the patient has been

---

REMOVING A PERIPHERAL I.V. LINE

A peripheral I.V. line should be removed when the I.V. infiltrates, the site becomes irritated, or the needle or catheter is changed to a new site, usually every 48 to 72 hours. To remove the line, follow the steps below:
- Gather supplies (sterile gauze pad, tape, Band-Aid).
- Wash your hands.
- Clamp the I.V. tubing to stop the infusion.
- Gently remove all the tape from the needle or catheter and the skin.
- Open the supply packages.
- Hold the sterile gauze pad over the insertion site and withdraw the needle or catheter with a gentle, brisk movement, keeping it parallel to the skin. (This prevents damage to the posterior wall of the vein, which may result in thrombus formation.)
- Raise the extremity to prevent hematoma formation and apply pressure over the site for 30 to 60 seconds, or until bleeding has stopped. Do not rub the site. (Alcohol should not be used to remove an I.V. because it prevents hemostasis at the site.)
- Cover the site with a sterile gauze pad and tape, or apply a Band-Aid.
- Document in the nurses' notes the time of removal, reason for removal, catheter length and integrity, condition of the site, how the patient tolerated the procedure, and any necessary nursing interventions.

---

stabilized. The emergency line should then be removed, and the previous site observed for 48 hours.

Inserting a heparin lock

A heparin lock consists of a winged-tip needle with tubing ending in a resealable rubber injection port. Filled with dilute heparin to prevent blood clot formation, the device maintains venous access in patients receiving I.V. medication regularly or intermittently but not requiring continuous infusion of fluids. It proves superior to a keep-vein-open line because it minimizes the risk of fluid overload and electrolyte imbalance, cuts costs, reduces the risk of contamination by eliminating I.V. solution containers and administration sets, increases patient comfort and mobility, reduces patient anxiety, and allows collection of blood samples without repeated venipuncture.

Use of a heparin lock is contraindicated in patients with clotting disorders or uncontrolled bleeding.

Equipment and materials

You will need a heparin lock, dilute heparin solution in a 1-ml syringe, a 25G needle of appropriate length, povidone-iodine sponges, alcohol sponges, a tourniquet, a dressing, and tape.

Some facilities use a 100 U/ml heparin flush; others use 10 U/ml; and still others use normal saline solution in place of heparin. Prefilled heparin cartridges are available in both dosages for use in a syringe cartridge holder.

Steps
- Confirm the identity of the patient by checking the name, room number, and bed number on his wristband.
- Explain the procedure to the patient, and describe the purpose of the heparin lock.
- Wash your hands thoroughly to prevent contamination of the venipuncture site.
- Remove the set from its packaging, wipe the port with an alcohol sponge, and inject a dilute heparin solution to fill the tubing and needle. This removes air from the system, preventing formation of an air embolus.
- Select a venipuncture site (see "Selecting a venipuncture site," p. 187), and cleanse it first with alcohol and then with povidone-iodine sponges, wiping outward from the site in a circular motion.
- Perform the venipuncture, and ensure correct needle placement in the vein. Then, release the tourniquet.
- Tape the set in place, using the chevron method or an accepted alternative (see *Methods of Taping a Venipuncture Site*, p. 198). Loop the tubing so the injection

CONVERTING AN I.V. LINE INTO A HEPARIN LOCK

Male adapter plugs allow conversion of an existing I.V. line to a heparin lock for intermittent infusion of a medication. To convert, prime the male adapter plug with dilute heparin. Then, clamp the I.V. tubing, remove the administration set from the catheter or needle hub, and insert the male adapter plug. Next, inject the remaining dilute heparin to fill the line and to prevent clot formation.

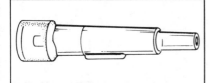

This long male adapter plug slides into place.

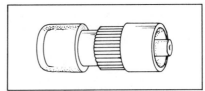

This short male adapter plug twists into place.

---

port is free and easily accessible. Some facilities use an elastic net dressing over the top of the heparin lock and sterile dressing, leaving the port exposed.
• Apply a sterile dressing. On the last piece of tape used to secure the dressing, write the time, date, and your initials.
• Flush the set with the remaining heparin to prevent clot formation.
• Inject 1 ml of dilute heparin solution every 6 to 12 hours, or according to the physician's orders, to maintain patency of the heparin lock.
• Record the date and time of insertion and the type and gauge of needle in the nurses' notes.

Nursing considerations
• If ordered, obtain a blood sample for activated partial thromboplastin time before inserting the heparin lock, because small amounts of heparin can alter the results of this test.
• If the patient feels a burning sensation during injection of heparin, stop the injection and check needle placement. If the needle is in the vein, inject the heparin at a slower rate to minimize irritation.
• Flush the heparin lock to maintain patency. Follow institutional policy regarding the type of solution and the frequency of flushing.

• Change the sterile dressing every 24 hours, and the heparin lock every 72 hours, using a new venipuncture site. Some facilities use a transparent occlusive dressing to cover the entire device. This allows more patient freedom and easier observation of the injection site.
• Use of a heparin lock has the same potential complications as the use of a peripheral I.V. line. See *Local Complications of Peripheral I.V. Therapy*, pp. 222-223, and *Systemic Complications of Peripheral I.V. Therapy*, pp. 224-225, for further information.
• If the patient has an I.V. infusion running and the physician orders it discontinued and a heparin lock inserted in its place, the existing line can be converted into a heparin lock. Most I.V. needles and cannulas can be converted by disconnecting the I.V. tubing and inserting a male adapter plug into the cannula. See *Converting an I.V. Line into a Heparin Lock*.

Assisting with a venesection (cutdown)

Performed by a physician with a nurse assisting, venesection (or cutdown) is the sterile insertion of a catheter into the basilic or cephalic veins of the antecubital fossa—or, less frequently, into the femoral and saphenous veins because of the risk of phlebitis and emboli—after surgical exposure and incision. After insertion, the catheter is used for the same purposes as a peripheral I.V. line.

Venesection is indicated when a vein cannot be entered percutaneously because of obesity, venous collapse or sclerosis, or peripheral vasoconstriction from massive, rapid blood loss.

Equipment and materials
You will need a cutdown tray and cutdown catheter; povidone-iodine sponges and ointment; sterile gown, gloves, and mask for the physician; a sterile drape; alcohol sponges; a 3-ml syringe with a 25G needle of appropriate length; 1% or 2% lidocaine injectable; I.V. solution and administration set ready for use; a silk-suture pack; and sterile gauze sponges, sterile roller gauze, and 1" adhesive tape. (Most institutions have prepared cutdown trays. These usually include scalpel, blades, scissors, curved and straight hemostats, and retractors.)

Steps
- Confirm the identity of the patient by checking the name, room number, and bed number on his wristband.
- Supplement the physician's explanation of the procedure, as necessary, to reduce the patient's anxiety and ensure his cooperation. Make sure the patient has signed a consent form.
- Wash your hands thoroughly to reduce the risk of bacterial contamination of the sterile field.
- Position the patient so the surgical site is fully exposed and accessible. Then, place a linen-saver pad under the limb to prevent blood leakage onto the bed.
- Place the cutdown tray on a table in the position preferred by the physician, and open the exterior wrap without touching the inside.
- Assist the physician to put on a gown, gloves, and mask.
- Swab the top of the local anesthetic container with an alcohol sponge, and invert it so the physician can fill the syringe. He then injects the anesthetic and prepares and drapes the area.

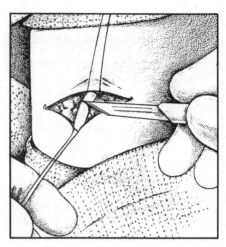

- The physician makes an incision into the skin, exposes the vein, and then makes a small incision in the vein, as shown in the illustration above.
- Open the catheter package using sterile technique and, when requested, present the package to the physician so the catheter can be removed.
- After the physician inserts the catheter, attach the primed I.V. line to the hub and allow the solution to flow freely for a few minutes to flush blood from the catheter and prevent clot formation. The physician then sutures the incision and the catheter.
- Put on sterile gloves and apply povidone-iodine ointment to the insertion site, as shown below.

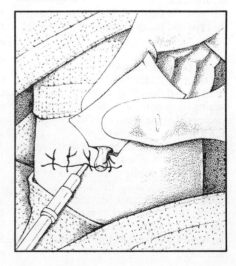

- Tape the catheter in place to prevent stress on the sutures.
- Place a 4" x 4" gauze sponge over the site, wrap with roller gauze, and tape the edge of the gauze to secure the dressing.
- Label the last piece of tape "cutdown," and indicate the size of the catheter, the time, and the date, as shown below.

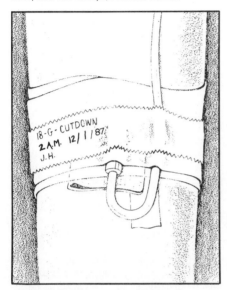

- Adjust the I.V. flow rate, as ordered.
- Record in the nurses' notes the time and date of the procedure, the physician's name, the type and gauge of catheter, and the type of solution and rate of infusion.

Nursing considerations
- If the insertion site is the antecubital fossa, immobilize the extremity with an armboard, as necessary.
- Check distal pulses, skin temperature, and nail-bed color to detect blood flow obstruction.
- Observe the puncture site for redness, inflammation, and drainage; if present, notify the physician.
- If venesection was performed on a lower extremity, watch for signs of phlebitis or pulmonary emboli, because this area is more vulnerable to infection and clot formation.
- If the patient experiences pain at the incision site after the local anesthetic wears off, offer an analgesic, if ordered.
- Phlebitis, infection, infiltration, and thrombus formation are the most common complications of venesection. See also *Removing a Cutdown Catheter*, p. 204.

Assisting with insertion of a central venous line

Performed by a physician, insertion of a central venous line is the sterile threading of an inside-the-needle catheter through the subclavian vein or, less commonly, the jugular vein, into the superior vena cava. (See *Central Venipuncture Sites*, p. 191. Once in place, the central venous line allows monitoring of vena cava blood pressure, which indicates blood volume or pump efficiency, and aspiration of blood samples for diagnostic tests. It also allows administration of I.V. fluids when decreased peripheral circulation causes peripheral venous collapse, when prolonged I.V. therapy reduces the number of usable peripheral veins, and when adequate dilution is necessary (for large fluid volumes or for irritating or hypertonic fluids, such as hyperalimentation solutions).

Equipment and materials
You will need a shave preparation kit, if necessary; sterile gloves, sterile drapes, and masks; povidone-iodine sponges and ointment; alcohol sponges; a 3-ml syringe with a 25G 1" needle; 1% or 2% lidocaine injectable; two radiopaque inside-the-needle catheters; a 10-ml syringe with Luer-Lok tip; I.V. solution with administration set prepared for use; sterile 4"x 4" gauze sponges; 1" adhesive tape; and sterile scissors.

Some institutions have prepared trays containing most of the equipment necessary for insertion.

Steps
- Confirm the identity of the patient by checking the name, room number, and bed number on his wristband.
- Before insertion of a central venous line, confirm catheter size with the physician. Usually, a 14G or 16G catheter is selected. Set up the I.V. solution and prime the administration set. As ordered, notify the ra-

> **REMOVING A CUTDOWN CATHETER**
>
> If institutional policy permits you to remove a cutdown catheter, you can follow almost the same procedure you would use to remove a central line. However, keep these important differences in mind:
> • In the cutdown procedure, remove only the retaining sutures the physician may have used to secure the catheter. Take care not to nick the catheter or cut any skin sutures.
> • After you have removed the catheter, press a 2"x2" sterile gauze pad to the site to stop the bleeding. Then, apply antimicrobial ointment, and firmly tape another 2"x2" sterile gauze pad over the site. You will not need a pressure bandage, because the skin sutures will hold the incision closed.
> Document the date and time of catheter removal in the nurses' notes.

diology department that a portable X-ray machine will be needed.
• Reinforce the physician's explanation of the procedure, and answer the patient's questions. Ensure that the patient has signed a consent form, if necessary, and check his history for hypersensitivity to local anesthesia.
• Wash your hands thoroughly.
• Establish a sterile field on a table, using a sterile towel or the wrapping from the instrument tray.
• Place the patient in the Trendelenburg position to dilate veins and reduce the risk of air embolism.
• *For subclavian insertion,* place a rolled blanket lengthwise between the shoulders to increase venous distention. *For jugular insertion,* place a rolled blanket under the opposite shoulder to extend the neck, making anatomic landmarks more visible.
• Place a linen-saver pad under the appropriate area to prevent soiling the bed.
• Turn the patient's head away from the site to prevent possible contamination from airborne pathogens and to make the site more accessible. Or, if dictated by institutional policy, mask the patient unless this increases his anxiety or is contraindicated because of respiratory status.
• Cleanse the insertion site with soap and water to remove dirt and body oils. If necessary, shave the area. Then, put on a mask and gloves and cleanse the area around the insertion site with povidone-iodine, working in a circular motion outward from the site to avoid reintroducing contaminants.
• After the physician puts on a sterile mask and gloves and drapes the area to create a sterile field, open the packaging of the 3-ml syringe and present it to him using sterile technique.
• Wipe the top of the lidocaine vial with alcohol and invert it. The physician then fills the 3-ml syringe and injects the anesthetic into the site.
• Open the packaging of the catheter and the 10-ml syringe and present them to the physician using sterile technique. He then attaches the catheter needle to the syringe, punctures the skin, and inserts the catheter. During this time, prepare the I.V. administration set for immediate attachment to the catheter hub.
• Ask the patient to perform Valsalva's maneuver while the physician attaches the I.V. line to the catheter hub. *This increases intrathoracic pressure, reducing the possibility of an air embolus.*
• After the physician attaches the I.V. line to the catheter hub, set the flow rate, as ordered. The physician then sutures the catheter in place.
• As ordered, put on sterile gloves, apply povidone-iodine ointment over the site, and apply a sterile 4"x 4" gauze dressing.
• After an X-ray confirms correct catheter placement, secure the catheter with tape, reapply the sterile dressing, or cover the site with a transparent occlusive dressing.
• Label the dressing with the time and date of catheter insertion and catheter length (if not imprinted on the catheter).
• Record in the nurses' notes the time and date of insertion, the length and location of the catheter, the solution infused, the physician's name, and the patient's response. Also document the time of the X-ray, its results, and your notification of the physician about X-ray results.

Nursing considerations
- As soon as possible after insertion, catheter placement should be checked by X-ray. If hyperalimentation fluid is ordered, begin this infusion only after an X-ray confirms correct catheter placement. When catheter placement is in doubt, infuse another solution such as 10% dextrose in water until correct placement is ensured.
- Be alert for signs of air embolism, such as sudden onset of pallor, cyanosis, dyspnea, coughing, and tachycardia, progressing to syncope and shock. If any of these signs occur, place the patient on his left side in the Trendelenburg position, and notify the physician.
- Watch for signs of pneumothorax: shortness of breath, tachycardia, and chest pain. Notify the physician immediately if such signs appear.
- Change the dressing and tubing every 24 hours or according to institutional policy, but change it immediately if the dressing becomes soiled, wet, or loose.
- Dressing changes for a central venous line should be done using sterile technique. This is especially important when hyperalimentation solution is being infused. (See "Regular maintenance of I.V. sites and systems," p. 215.)
- With subclavian vein insertion, pneumothorax is the most common complication. With jugular vein insertion, the catheter may be misdirected toward the brain instead of into the vena cava; a chest X-ray will show this. At either site, air embolism is a possible complication. Other complications are those associated with peripheral lines and inside-the-needle catheters. (See *Local Complications of Peripheral I.V. Therapy,* pp. 222-223; and *Systemic Complications of Peripheral I.V. Therapy,* pp. 224-225.)

Removing a central venous line

Removal of a central venous line on completion of therapy or onset of complications is a sterile procedure and often requires suture removal. If infection is suspected, the procedure includes collection of a specimen of the catheter tip for culture.

Equipment and materials
You will need a sterile suture-removal set, sterile gloves, two masks (if necessary for suspected infection), a sterile drape, alcohol sponges, povidone-iodine ointment, sterile 4"x 4" gauze sponges, a sterile plastic adhesive-backed dressing, and a sterile culture tube and sterile scissors for a culture, if necessary.

Steps
- Confirm the identity of the patient by checking the name, room number, and bed number on his wristband.
- Explain the procedure to the patient, and wash your hands.
- Note the length of the catheter, which should be imprinted on the catheter or written on the dressing. Open the suture-removal set, and use the inside surface of the wrap to establish a sterile field.
- Using sterile technique, open two gauze sponges and one alcohol sponge and drop them onto the sterile field. Squeeze povidone-iodine or antimicrobial ointment onto one gauze sponge. Then, loosen and carefully remove the dressing. If a culture of the catheter is to be taken because of suspected infection, put masks on yourself and the patient before dressing removal to prevent contamination by airborne organisms.
- Close the flow clamp on the I.V. tubing, and put on sterile gloves.
- Remove any sutures securing the catheter, *taking care not to cut the catheter.* If you are removing a cutdown catheter, avoid cutting any skin sutures.
- Ask the patient to perform Valsalva's maneuver to reduce the possibility of an air embolism as you grasp the needle or catheter hub and slowly and carefully withdraw it from the vein. If the catheter cannot easily be retracted, allow the patient to relax; then try again. Avoid forceful retraction, because venous spasm may be causing the resistance. If resistance continues, tape the catheter in place and notify the physician.
- After you have removed the catheter, apply pressure with a gauze sponge to stop bleeding. Carefully inspect the tip of the catheter, taking care to prevent contamination. The tip should appear round and smooth. If it is ragged or damaged, notify the physician immediately, because a severed catheter can cause an embolus. If the catheter appears severed, place it on the sterile field and measure its length.

- After bleeding stops, inspect the insertion site for signs of infection, and collect a specimen of any drainage for culture. Cleanse the area around the insertion site with an alcohol sponge to remove dried blood and adhesive, then apply povidone-iodine or an antimicrobial ointment to the area. Apply a sterile plastic adhesive-backed dressing to prevent exposure of the incision to air.
- A sterile occlusive dressing should be placed over the catheter insertion site for at least 48 hours or the length of time it takes for the site to heal.
- If a culture specimen from the catheter is required, prepare the site with alcohol before catheter removal, as ordered, and use sterile scissors to cut a 1" (2.5-cm) segment from the tip of the removed catheter. Then, place the specimen in the sterile culture tube, and send it to the laboratory immediately.
- After removing the central venous line, record in the nurses' notes the time and date of removal and the type of antimicrobial ointment and dressing applied. Also record the condition of the catheter insertion site and the collection of a culture specimen.

Assisting with insertion of an arterial line

Insertion of an arterial line is a sterile procedure performed by a physician. During insertion, a catheter is introduced into the brachial, the radial, or occasionally the femoral artery. The brachial site, which is easily observed and maintained, may provide more accurate blood pressure readings than the radial site, because it is closer to the heart. However, use of this site necessitates splinting the elbow to stabilize the catheter. Use of the radial site, also easily observed, may result in difficult and painful catheter insertion because of the artery's small lumen. Catheter insertion into the femoral artery, the easiest to locate and puncture in an emergency, carries a high risk of thrombosis. Once in place at any of these sites, an arterial line allows frequent monitoring of blood pressure and sampling of arterial blood for blood gas determination.

The patency of an arterial line is maintained by a continuous flush of heparinized saline solution, administered under pressure to reduce the risk of clot formation. Because an arterial line carries the risk of bleeding and thrombosis, its insertion is contraindicated in patients with severe coagulopathy, unless the potential benefits outweigh the risks.

Equipment and materials

You will need an I.V. pole and a 500-ml bag of normal sterile saline solution; heparin; 1 to 2 units/ml of saline solution; a pressure bag; a medication-added label; two 3-ml syringes, one with a 21G to 25G 1" needle for heparin injection into the saline solution and one with a 25G 1" needle for the physician to use for injection of local anesthetic; alcohol sponges; a nonvented I.V. administration set with microdrip chamber; 6" extension pressure tubing; a continuous flush device; a three-way stopcock and dead-end stopcock caps; povidone-iodine sponges and ointment; sterile gloves (for the physician); 1% or 2% lidocaine injectable; a linen-saver pad; a sterile towel; a 16G to 20G catheter (type and length depend on site, patient's size, and other possible uses of the line); and a sterile adhesive bandage, sterile 4" x 4" gauze sponges, and 1" adhesive tape.

You may need suture material, sterile scissors, and a splint or armboard.

Most institutions use prepackaged arterial line sets containing dead-end caps, connected extension pressure tubing, a continuous flush device, and a stopcock.

Steps

- Confirm the identity of the patient by checking the name, room number, and bed number on his wristband.
- Reinforce the physician's explanation of the procedure, as needed. Check the patient's history for hypersensitivity to the local anesthetic or to iodine.
- Wash your hands thoroughly, and maintain asepsis when setting up the equipment.
- Confirm the insertion site with the physician, and position the patient so the site is well lighted and accessible. Before the radial site is chosen, the Allen's test is per-

HOW TO PERFORM THE ALLEN'S TEST

Before drawing blood from a radial artery or inserting an arterial line, perform the Allen's test to determine whether the patient will receive enough blood through the ulnar artery to supply the hand if occlusion of the radial artery occurs.

First, have the patient rest his arm on the mattress or bedside stand, supporting his wrist with a rolled towel. Ask him to clench his fist. Then, apply pressure on both the radial and ulnar arteries and hold the position for a few seconds.

Maintaining pressure, ask the patient to unclench his fist and to hold his hand in a relaxed position. The palm will be blanched, because normal blood flow to the fingers is being impaired.

Release the pressure on the ulnar artery. If the hand becomes flushed, indicating the rush of oxygenated blood to the hand, a radial artery puncture may be performed. If it does not become flushed, repeat the test on the other arm. If neither arm produces a positive result, choose another site.

---

formed to assess blood supply to the hand (see *How to Perform the Allen's Test*).
- Place a linen-saver pad and sterile towel under the arm or leg to create a sterile field and to prevent blood from soiling the area.
- After the physician puts on sterile gloves, open the wrapping of a povidone-iodine sponge and an alcohol sponge, using sterile technique. The physician takes the sponges and cleanses the insertion site.
- Open the packaging and present the 3-ml syringe to the physician, maintaining sterile technique. Then, wipe the rubber stopper of the lidocaine bottle to allow the physician to withdraw the anesthetic. He then injects the anesthetic into the site.
- Open the catheter packaging, using sterile technique. The physician grasps the catheter, flushes it with saline solution, inserts it into the artery, and attaches the administration set.
- Open the flow clamp and activate the fast-flush release to flush blood from the catheter.
- If the physician intends to suture the catheter, temporarily tape the tubing to the patient's arm to keep it in place during suturing. If he does not suture the catheter, tape it securely in place.
- Apply povidone-iodine ointment to the insertion site and cover it with a dressing.
- If necessary, apply an armboard or splint to immobilize the insertion site.
- Tape the solution tubing to the patient's arm.

- After insertion, record in the nurses' notes the time, date, physician's name, insertion site, and the type, gauge, and length of catheter.

Nursing considerations
- After insertion of an arterial line, observe the patient for complications (see *Arterial Line Complications*, p. 229).
- Check the arterial line for mechanical problems on a regular basis, and be sure that all connections are tight, because a patient with normal cardiac output can lose 300 to 500 ml of blood/minute from an 18G catheter.
- Avoid obscuring the catheter hub connection with the dressing. The connection must be visible and accessible at all times.
- Flush the line every hour or according to institutional policy.
- Check the pressure bag to ensure a constant reading of 300 mmHg.
- Check pulses distal to the insertion site every 2 hours to detect circulatory impairment.
- Change the dressing, tubing, continuous flush device, and I.V. bag every 24 to 48 hours, according to institutional policy.

Assisting with removal of an arterial line

Removal of an arterial line is usually performed on completion of therapy or onset of complications. This is a sterile procedure performed primarily by a physician.

Equipment and materials
You will need two sterile 4"x 4" gauze sponges, povidone-iodine ointment, an adhesive bandage, and alcohol sponges. You may need a sterile suture removal set, a small sandbag (for removal from a femoral artery), a sterile container, and sterile scissors.

Steps
• Confirm the identity of the patient by checking the name, room number, and bed number on his wristband.
• Wash your hands and explain the procedure to the patient. The physician gently removes the dressing to avoid dislodging the catheter, and removes any sutures.
• Turn off the flow clamp to prevent fluid leakage, and open the sterile gauze sponge using sterile technique.
• The physician withdraws the catheter with a gentle, steady motion, keeping it parallel to the artery to reduce the risk of trauma. The physician or nurse then immediately applies pressure with a gauze sponge for at least 7 minutes to a brachial site, 5 minutes to a radial site, and 10 minutes to a femoral site or until bleeding ceases.
• Apply povidone-iodine ointment to the site, fold a gauze sponge in half, place it over the site, and cover it with an adhesive bandage to apply pressure. Check the distal pulse to detect arterial obstruction from an overly tight bandage.
• Periodically check the site for hematoma or bleeding.
• Place a small sandbag, covered with a washcloth or pillowcase, over a femoral site to prevent delayed bleeding. Check for bleeding under it at least every 15 minutes for the first hour, every 30 minutes for the second hour, and then every hour for 6 hours.
• Watch for changes in pulse intensity, skin color, and temperature of the arm or leg. These changes can indicate thrombus formation.
• Observe for signs and symptoms of pulmonary embolus: dyspnea, chest pain, tachycardia, coughing, or blood-tinged sputum, and notify the physician immediately if these occur.

• Change the pressure dressing to an adhesive bandage after 2 hours for a brachial or radial site and after 8 hours for a femoral site.
• Document in the nurses' notes the date and time of arterial line removal, the name of the physician who removed it, condition of the insertion site, and any catheter specimens sent for culture.

Nursing considerations
• If you suspect infection, cleanse the insertion site with an alcohol sponge before catheter removal. After the catheter is removed, cut off the tip using sterile scissors, place it in a sterile container, and send it to the laboratory for culture.

Review Questions

1. State five possible reasons for performing a venipuncture.

2. How do you positively establish a patient's identity before a venipuncture?
   A. Say his name out loud
   B. Check his bracelet for name and identification number
   C. Check the name tag on his bed
   D. All of the above

3. Which technique is used for the following procedures, sterile or aseptic?
   A. Insertion of a peripheral line
   B. Removal of a peripheral line
   C. Insertion of a heparin lock
   D. Conversion of an I.V. line to a heparin lock
   E. Cutdown
   F. Removal of a cutdown catheter
   G. Insertion of a central venous line
   H. Removal of a central venous line
   I. Insertion of an arterial line
   J. Removal of an arterial line
   K. Culturing a removed central venous or arterial catheter

4. With what procedure should an X-ray be taken immediately afterward to check catheter placement?

5. What are some of the pros and cons of shaving a venipuncture site?

6. What is the name of the test performed before an I.V. line is inserted into the radial artery, and what is its purpose?

7. What are some of the most common complications associated with the following?
   A. Subclavian vein insertion
   B. Jugular vein insertion
   C. Arterial insertion

8. What four pieces of information should appear on the last tape placed at the arterial or venous insertion site?

9. What is the purpose of priming the heparin lock with heparin flush before insertion?

10. Why is it important to check the connections in an arterial line on a regular basis?

Selected References

Allen, J.R. "Guidelines for Changing Administration Sets for Intravenous Fluid Therapy," *National Intravenous Therapy Association* 3(5):175, 1980.

Brunner, L.S., and Suddarth, D. S. *Lippincott Manual of Nursing Practice*, 3rd ed. Philadelphia: J.B. Lippincott Co., 1982.

Hauer, J.M., et al. "Autotransfusion," in *Proceedings of the First International Autotransfusion Symposium*. Amsterdam: Elsevier-North Holland, 1981.

"Intravenous Standards of Nursing Practice," *National Intravenous Therapy Association*, 1981.

Managing I.V. Therapy. Nursing Photobook Series. Springhouse, Pa.: Springhouse Corp., 1983.

Plummer, A. *Principles and Practices of Intravenous Therapy.* Boston: Little, Brown & Co., 1982.

Procedures. Nurse's Reference Library. Springhouse, Pa.: Springhouse Corp., 1983.

Sager, D.P., and Bomar, S.K. *Intravenous Medications.* Philadelphia: J.B. Lippincott Co., 1980.

Weinstein, S. *Memory Bank for I.V.s.* Baltimore: Williams & Wilkins Co., 1986.

Wong, E.S., et al. "Guidelines for the Prevention and Control of Nosocomial Infections," *Infection Control* 2:119, March/April 1981.

Maintaining I.V. Therapy

For the patient to receive maximum benefit from I.V. therapy, you must be familiar with the requirements of maintenance, which are covered in this chapter. These include closely monitoring the flow rate, maintaining line patency, and preventing complications. (See Chapter 6 for information on preparing medications for I.V. administration and Chapters 8 and 12 for information on procedures.)

Team concept

I.V. therapy is developing into a nursing subspecialty. Recent studies have shown that fewer complications develop when the same nurse consistently manages a patient's I.V. therapy. The Centers for Disease Control recommend use of intravascular therapy teams. In some institutions this team concept has been revived, and designated nurses manage specific aspects of the therapy. This system offers the advantage of continuity of care and allows the staff nurse to concentrate on the patient's other needs.

Factors affecting flow rate

The staff nurse is usually responsible for maintaining I.V. flow rate. At many institutions, policy calls for routine checks of I.V. solution, rate, and site at the beginning of every shift. This may be accomplished during the walking report or I.V. "rounds." Several factors affect flow rate, including characteristics of the fluid being infused, the height at which the container is hung, the type of administration set, and the size, thickness, and position of the cannula.

The fluid
Viscous or "thick" fluids such as blood products, colloids (such as albumin), suspensions (such as amphotericin B), and highly osmolar solutions may infuse with difficulty. These solutions may be diluted with compatible fluid or infused using an infusion control device (a pump or controller) to facilitate maintenance of correct flow rate. Admixtures, such as antibiotics, must be completely diluted when reconstituted, and the container must be agitated after admixing a medication. This ensures uniformity of the solution, aids the flow, and prevents a bolus effect. Blood products such as red blood cells and platelets are often agitated *gently* during flow because denser cells may clump in the bottom of the container.

Container height
The type of I.V. solution container does not usually affect flow rate; however, container height can easily alter it. The I.V. container should always be above the patient's heart to adequately overcome normal blood pressure. A distance of 30" to 36" (76 to 91 cm) between a *peripheral* I.V. site and the container is usually adequate. For *central* lines, the container may have to be kept higher, or an infusion control device may be needed to overcome higher venous pressure. For *arterial* lines, use of an infusion pump or a pressure bag (kept around the fluid container at between 150 to 300 mm Hg) is usually necessary to overcome arterial pressure. Infusion pump pressures are usually measured in pounds per square inch (psi). (See *Pressures* table opposite for information on the relationship between mm Hg and psi.)

PRESSURES	
Peripheral venous	10 to 30 mm Hg
Central venous	15 to 30 mm Hg
Arterial	150 to 250 mm Hg
Volumetric infusion pumps	10 to 25 psi = 520 to 1,290 mm Hg
Gravity to infuse I.V. fluid at 36" above I.V. site	1.3 psi = 70 mm Hg

*1 psi = 50 mm Hg

Administration sets

Gravity infusion sets are manufactured in many different configurations, including straight drip sets (usually macrodrip, 15 or 20 drops/ml) and volume control sets (usually microdrip, 60 drops/ml). A macrodrip set is usually sufficiently accurate for maintenance infusions in adults; however, fluid viscosity may alter drop size, creating slight alterations in volume delivered. Microdrip sets, used for pediatric patients, deliver fluid at a more accurate rate because drop size does not vary significantly.

Vented sets should be used for evacuated glass containers. Flow rate will otherwise be hampered because air cannot enter the bottle to displace the fluid.

Vented or nonvented sets may be used with bags of fluid. A vented set may leak, however, necessitating the capping of the vent with the spike cover (or other sterile cap) to prevent leakage of the solution. Many manufacturers recommend this procedure in their instructions for use.

Flow control clamps on infusion sets vary with the manufacturer. Usually a roller clamp, with a wheel that is tightened or loosened around the I.V. tubing, is used to adjust gravity flow. Also available are slide clamps, which can be moved horizontally to open or close the I.V. line; however, fine adjustment of flow is not possible with this type of clamp. Another type of flow control clamp is a rate minder, which usually is added on to the I.V. tubing. This device is labeled with numbers indicating flow rate in milliliters per hour; it can be set to the desired flow rate. Rate minders provide accurate flow only with certain I.V. cannulas in place (usually 20G or larger) and do not normally deliver infusions at rates lower than 5 to 10 ml per hour. They are used mainly in adult patients for this reason.

I.V. device

The size of the I.V. cannula, needle, or catheter—as well as the size of the vein in which it is inserted—may also affect flow rate. I.V. devices vary in size from the smallest butterfly (27G) to the largest I.V. catheter (14G). The smaller the I.V. cannula, the slower the infusion will flow, and you should choose the smallest cannula available for the size of the vein and the viscosity of the solution.

Thin-walled, small-gauge I.V. catheters offer flow rates comparable to thicker-walled, larger-gauge catheters because they have lumens of comparable size. (Even blood products and colloids can be infused through 24G thin-walled catheters without damage.) Infusion control devices are often used with small-gauge catheters for pediatric and geriatric patients.

Cannula position may also affect flow rate. If the catheter is against the wall of the vein or near a valve, the flow can diminish or stop.

Maintaining flow rate

Checking flow rate

National Intravenous Therapy Association (NITA) standards require checking flow rate at least every 8 hours or every shift. Many nurses, however, check flow rate every time they are in the patient's room and after the patient's position has been changed.

The practice of checking flow rate is modified for special-care patients, such as those in intensive care and pediatrics, or for patients receiving a drug that is dangerous

WHAT TO DO WHEN AN INFUSION STOPS

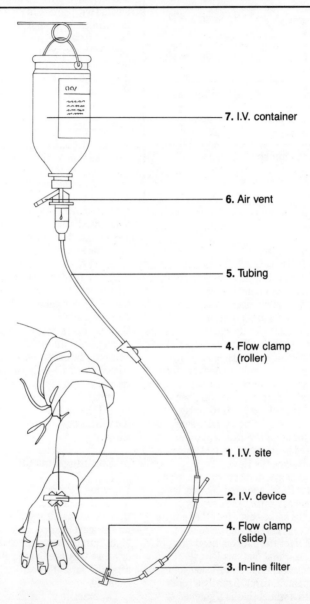

- 7. I.V. container
- 6. Air vent
- 5. Tubing
- 4. Flow clamp (roller)
- 1. I.V. site
- 2. I.V. device
- 4. Flow clamp (slide)
- 3. In-line filter

In a systematic fashion, assess the I.V. system from the patient to the fluid container, looking for potential trouble areas:
1. Check the I.V. site. Infiltration or phlebitis may slow or stop the flow rate.

2. Check the I.V. device for patency. Patency may be affected by a variety of factors, some of which may be easily remedied.
• The position of the patient's limb may

cause flow stoppage by increased blood pressure if the limb is positioned too high, or by vein occlusion if the limb is flexed or lying directly on the I.V. site itself. Reposition if necessary.
- The tip of the needle may be against the wall of the vein or a valve. Lift up or pull back the cannula to facilitate adequate flow rates.
- Encircling the arm with tape may create a "tourniquet effect" and decrease flow rate, as will taping the I.V. site too tightly. Release or remove tape and reapply as necessary.
- Smaller cannulas may kink or "accordion fold" and impede flow. Pull back the cannula to reestablish flow.
- Local edema and/or poor tissue perfusion resulting from disease can block venous flow. Move the I.V. line to an unaffected site.
- Infusion of incompatible fluids or medications may result in formation of a precipitate that may block the I.V. tubing and cannula, and may even expose the patient to a life-threatening embolism. Always check the compatibility of medications and I.V. solutions prior to administration. Replace the cannula if it is occluded.

3. Check the in-line filter (if one is being used). Verify that the proper size and type of filter is attached. I.V. fluids are usually run through a 0.22- or 0.45-micron filter that eliminates air from the system as well as microorganisms. Single-use filters should not be used for in-line filtration, only for drawing up a medication or administering a bolus dose. If the wrong size or type of filter is used, it may not allow the solution to pass through and the filter may become blocked. For example, drugs such as amphotericin B and Atgam are made up of molecules too large to pass through a 0.22-micron filter; they would rapidly block the filter and cause flow stoppage. Replace the filter if necessary.

Filters used beyond the recommended time are subject to blockage by minute particles and microorganisms, resulting in flow stoppage or exposure of the patient to bacterial toxins and sepsis. The interval between filter changes usually ranges from 24 to 48 hours, depending on manufacturer's instructions. Change the filter if necessary.

4. Check the flow clamp(s). Check to be sure all clamps are open, including the roller clamp, and any lower clamps or those on secondary sets, such as a slide clamp on a filter. A roller clamp may also become jammed if the roller is pushed up too far.

5. Check the tubing. Check to see if the tubing is kinked, if the patient is lying on it, or, in the case of I.V. tubing that does not have "memory," check to see if the tubing remains crimped where the clamp may have been tightened around it. If the tubing is crimped, gently squeezing the crimped area between your fingers will usually "round out" the tubing to its original shape.

6. Check the air vents. If an evacuated glass container is used, an air vent is necessary to achieve solution flow. Insert one if it is not in place. With volume control sets, an air vent is usually located at the top of the calibrated chamber. If solution flow stops, patency of this vent and location of the vent clamp (if any) should be verified. Check the patency by following manufacturer's instructions.

7. Check the I.V. container. Check the fluid level in the container. If the container is empty, replace it as ordered. If the solution is cold, it may cause venous spasm and decrease flow rate. Warm compresses applied to the vein may relieve venous spasm and help increase flow rate. Make sure subsequent solutions are at room temperature. Finally, check to see if the spike at the end of the administration set has been pushed far enough into the container to allow passage of the solution.

If this system of checks does not identify the problem, the I.V. line should be removed and restarted in another location, with complete documentation of the situation in the patient's chart.

WHAT TO CHECK WHEN THE ALARM GOES OFF

When the alarm on an infusion control device goes off, check for the following:

Air in line	Make sure all air is out of the line during setup, including air trapped in Y sites, and that any connections are secure and the container is filled properly. Remove air by withdrawing it from a piggyback port with a syringe or using an air-eliminating filter initially. A wet air detector may also give a false reading; check for this.
Infusion complete	Reset the pump as ordered or discontinue the infusion. A slow keep-vein-open flow will usually run to keep the I.V. patent, as long as enough fluid remains in the container.
Empty container	Check for adequate fluid levels to be infused in the I.V. container and have another container available before the last one runs out.
Low battery	Battery life varies; keep the machine plugged in on A/C power as much as possible, especially while the patient is in bed. If the alarm rings, plug in immediately, or power may be totally lost for a time (usually a half hour to several hours).
Occlusion	Check that all clamps on the system are open, look for kinked tubing, and determine patency of the I.V. device.
Rate change	Check that the ordered rate is indicated on the infusion control device and that the patient or family has not tampered with the controls.
Open door	The door should be fully closed; it may not shut if the device is not properly set up (for example, if the cassette is not inserted fully).
Malfunction	Usually indicates mechanical failure that requires attention of biomedical engineering department or manufacturer. Remove the infusion control device from patient use and label it clearly with a "broken" sign and the specific problem indicated.

on extravasation (see *Infusions with Increased Potential for Extravasation Injury,* p. 218). With each check, the I.V. site should be assessed for complications, and the patient's response to therapy should be assessed.

Determine flow rate by counting the number of drops per minute, using the second hand on a watch held up to the drip chamber. For infusions that are potentially toxic, flow should be timed a full minute for accuracy; otherwise, you can time for 15 seconds and multiply by 4. If the flow has slowed or stopped, see *What to Do When an Infusion Stops,* pp. 212 and 213.

An infusion control device or rate minder should also be timed once per shift, since these mechanical devices have an error rate ranging from 2% to 10%. Double checking verifies accuracy of fluid delivery.

Maintaining flow rate with infusion control devices
As with any machine, an infusion control device is only as good as the user allows it to be. Therefore, you should be thoroughly familiar with the features, setup, and troubleshooting of the system in use. This can be accomplished through inservice instruction and return demonstration until competency is achieved. (See *What to Check When the Alarm Goes Off* for general information on infusion control devices.)

Maintaining line patency

Maintaining the patency of the I.V. line is a primary nursing responsibility in I.V. therapy. If a needle or catheter becomes occluded, it must be removed and another venipuncture performed. This reduces the number of available venipuncture sites, which may be needed for future therapy, and causes unnecessary patient discomfort.

Maintaining peripheral line patency
• Use an I.V. pole during patient ambulation. This keeps the container high enough to maintain adequate flow.
• Tell the patient or assist him to keep his hand at waist level. A change in the position of the site may result in blood backflow or an increase in flow rate. Check the rate after the patient returns to bed.
• Change the I.V. solution container *before* it empties. This ensures that the flow will not stop, allowing blood backflow and clot formation.
• Check the flow rate at least once a shift, and preferably whenever entering the patient's room or changing his position, to ensure that flow has not slowed or stopped.
• If the peripheral line is being used for intermittent infusion of medication or I.V. solution, flush the I.V. device with heparinized saline solution according to institutional policy. Flushing is usually done with 1 to 2 ml of 10 or 100 units/ml of heparinized saline solution every 4 to 8 hours.
• Maintain positive pressure by keeping your thumb on the plunger of the syringe while withdrawing the needle after flushing. This prevents blood backflow in the line and potential clotting.

Maintaining central venous line patency
• If a central venous line is being used for intermittent infusion of medication or I.V. solution, flush the line with heparinized saline or plain sterile saline according to institutional policy. It is usually flushed with from 1 to 5 ml of 10 or 100 units/ml of heparinized saline or plain sterile saline for injection. Occasionally 1,000-unit heparin is used, but this is not common protocol.
• Maintain positive pressure by keeping your thumb on the plunger of the syringe while withdrawing the needle after flushing. This prevents blood backflow in the line and potential clotting.
• A central line catheter with a two-way valve (Groshong catheter) must be flushed with saline weekly or according to institutional policy.
• All lumens of a multi-lumen catheter (unless it is a Groshong catheter) must be flushed on a regular schedule with heparinized saline solution according to institutional policy.
• Implantable ports for venous access are flushed every 4 weeks, according to manufacturer's instructions.

Maintaining arterial line patency
• Check the pressure bag frequently to ensure a constant reading of 150 to 300 mm Hg, and maintain a continuous or hourly heparinized flush for arterial lines used for blood pressure monitoring.
• Implantable ports for arterial access are flushed weekly with heparinized saline, according to manufacturer's instructions.

Regular maintenance of I.V. sites and systems

Routine care during intravascular therapy, such as daily tubing changes and regular site rotation, helps prevent complications and is less costly and debilitating—and less time-consuming, in the long run—than treating complications. Daily site care and dressing changes permit observation of the insertion site for signs of inflammation or infection, the most common complications.

Catheter, dressing, tubing, and solution changes are performed on a regular basis according to institutional policy. (See *Regular Maintenance of I.V. Sites and Systems,* p. 216, for NITA guidelines on how often these procedures should be performed.)

Dressing changes
Changing a peripheral line dressing
• Gather the following equipment: povidone-iodine sponges and ointment, alcohol sponges, adhesive bandage, sterile

REGULAR MAINTENANCE OF I.V. SITES AND SYSTEMS

	Catheter change	Dressing change	Tubing/solution change
Peripheral	• Every 48 to 72 hours • Immediately if complication occurs	• Every 48 hours (or according to institutional policy)	• Tubing: every 24 to 48 hours or with change of I.V. device • Solutions hang for 24 hours or less
Arterial	• Every 48 to 72 hours • Immediately if complication occurs	• Every 48 hours (or according to institutional policy)	• Tubing: every 24 to 48 hours or with change of arterial catheter • Solution: every 24 hours
Central	• Polyvinylchloride or polyurethane catheters: every 30 days or more frequently if complication occurs • Silastic catheters (such as Broviac, Hickman, and Groshong): retained until patient no longer needs catheter or complication occurs	• Depends on protocol at each institution and type of dressing material used, as well as disease status of patient (may be daily in immunosuppressed patients) • Usual protocol is 3X weekly with tape dressings; 1 to 2X weekly if transparent dressings are used	• Tubing: every 24 to 48 hours or with change of catheter • Solutions hang for 24 hours or less

2"x2" gauze pad or transparent occlusive dressing, and 1" adhesive tape.
• Wash your hands.
• Hold the needle or catheter in place with your nondominant hand to prevent accidental movement or dislodgment, which could lead to infiltration. Then, gently remove the tape and the dressing.
• Assess the venipuncture site for signs of infection (redness and pain at the puncture site), infiltration (coolness, blanching, and edema at the site), and thrombophlebitis (redness, firmness, pain along the path of the vein, and edema). If such signs are present, apply pressure to the area with a sterile 2"x2" gauze pad and remove the catheter or needle. Maintain pressure on the area until the bleeding stops, and apply an adhesive bandage. Then, using new equipment, start the I.V. in another site.

• If there are no signs of complications at the puncture site, hold the needle or catheter at the hub and carefully cleanse around the site with a povidone-iodine or alcohol sponge. Work from the site outward to avoid introducing pathogens into the cleansed area.
• Apply povidone-iodine ointment and cover with an adhesive bandage or sterile 2"x2" gauze pad. Then, retape the site. (See *Methods of Taping a Venipuncture Site*, p. 198.)

Changing a central venous or arterial line dressing
• Gather the following equipment: povidone-iodine sponges and ointment, alcohol sponges, sterile 4"x4" gauze pads and 1" adhesive tape or transparent occlusive dressing, peroxide, sterile gloves and masks, and clean gloves and a paper bag for removal of the old dressing.

Maintaining I.V. Therapy

- Open the paper bag.
- Put on clean gloves or use clean hands to remove the old dressing, being careful not to pull the catheter.
- Inspect the old dressing for evidence of infection, and save it for culturing if discharge is present.
- Check the position of the catheter and the site for evidence of infection or infiltration.
- Put on sterile gloves and clean the skin around the catheter with alcohol or peroxide, moving from the insertion site outward. Do not pull on the catheter.
- Clean the site again using povidone-iodine, moving from the insertion site outward.
- When the area is completely dry, apply povidone-iodine ointment to the insertion site.
- If the catheter is taped (not sutured) to the skin, carefully replace soiled tape, using the chevron method and sterile tape. Unsoiled tape does not need to be replaced.
- Redress the site with sterile 4"x4" gauze pads and tape in place or use a transparent occlusive dressing.

Tubing and solution changes
Changing the solution
- Gather the following equipment: solution container and alcohol sponge.
- Wash your hands.
- If a *bottle* is to be replaced, remove the cap and seal from the new bottle, and swab its stopper with alcohol.
- Clamp the line, remove the spike from the old bottle, and quickly insert the spike into the new bottle. Then, hang the new bottle and adjust the flow rate.

Changing the tubing
- The tubing should be changed every 24 to 48 hours.
- Gather the following equipment: I.V. administration set, sterile 2"x2" gauze pad, adhesive tape, and hemostat (optional).
- Wash your hands.
- Reduce the I.V. flow rate, and remove the old spike from the container and place the cover of the new spike loosely over it.
- Keeping the old spike in an upright position above the patient's heart level, insert the new spike into the I.V. container and prime the system.
- Place a sterile gauze pad under the needle or catheter hub to create a sterile field.
- Disconnect the old tubing from the needle or catheter hub, being careful not to dislodge or move the I.V. device in the vein. If it is difficult to disconnect the old tubing, a hemostat may be used to hold the hub securely while the end of the tubing is twisted and removed. Do not clamp the hemostat shut because the tubing adapter, needle, or catheter hub may crack, necessitating a change of equipment and venipuncture site.
- Quickly attach the new, primed tubing to the I.V. device using aseptic technique.
- Adjust the flow to the prescribed rate.
- Label the new tubing with the date and time of tubing change.

Changing the tubing and solution
- Gather the equipment mentioned under tubing and solution changes.
- Wash your hands.
- Hang the new I.V. container and primed tubing on the I.V. pole.
- Stop the flow in the old tubing.
- Quickly disconnect the old tubing and connect the new tubing according to the steps under "Changing the tubing."

Documenting dressing, tubing, and solution changes
- Record dressing, tubing, and solution changes and the appearance of the venipuncture site in the nurses' notes. Also record if a specimen was obtained and sent to the laboratory for culture and sensitivity testing and the name of the physician notified.
- If an I.V. flow chart is being used, record the date, time, rate, type of solution and sequential solution container number as well as the date and time of dressing and tubing changes.

Preventing complications of I.V. therapy

The potential hazards of I.V. therapy range from minor to life-threatening complications, including infection, phlebitis, emboli, extravasation with or without tissue necrosis, and exsanguination. They may be associated with venipuncture, infusion, or the medication being administered. Any lapse of aseptic technique can introduce pathogens, a major cause of complications, into the circulatory system.

Complications may be local or systemic, or they may begin locally (infection at the venipuncture site) and become systemic (septicemia). Nursing actions are directed toward prevention or early detection of complications. (See *Local Complications of Peripheral I.V. Therapy*, pp. 222 and 223, *Systemic Complications of Peripheral I.V. Therapy*, pp. 224 and 225, *Central Venous Line Complications*, pp. 226 to 228, and *Arterial Line Complications*, p. 229.)

If complications occur, document the signs and symptoms, patient complaints, name of the physician notified, and treatment given.

Administering infusions with high risk of extravasation injury

Extravasation, or the infiltration of medication from the vein into surrounding tissue, occurs through a puncture in the vein wall or from leakage around the insertion site. Serious local tissue damage often results from such inadvertent infiltration of vesicant (blistering) drugs or fluids. This soft tissue damage may result in prolonged healing, potential infection, multiple debridements, cosmetic disfigurement, loss of function, and possibly amputation. Extravasation is the subject of many lawsuits because it is preventable in most cases and often results in serious consequences. (See *Patients at High Risk for Extravasation Injury* and *Infusions with Increased Potential for Extravasation Injury*.)

Preventing extravasation

When administering a vesicant, you must take precautions to prevent extravasation. Adhere strictly to proper I.V. therapy administration techniques and follow these guidelines:
- Do not use existing I.V. lines unless patency is assured. Perform a new venipuncture to ensure proper needle placement and vein patency.
- Select the site carefully. Distal veins that allow for successive proximal venipunctures are preferred to major veins. However, to preclude tendon and nerve damage through pos-

---

PATIENTS AT HIGH RISK FOR EXTRAVASATION INJURY

- Neonates or infants
- Geriatric
- Oncology
- Comatose or anesthetized
- Those who undergo CPR
- Those with peripheral or cardiovascular disease, diabetes mellitus, Raynaud's phenomenon, or disseminated intravascular coagulation
- Those treated using high-pressure infusion pumps
- In general, any patient undergoing therapy that involves infusion of irritant or vesicant drugs, or those too young or ill to verbalize discomfort caused by pain and pressure

---

INFUSIONS WITH INCREASED POTENTIAL FOR EXTRAVASATION INJURY

Medications
aminophylline, amphotericin B, arginine, barbiturates, calcium chloride, calcium gluconate, diazepam, dobutamine, dopamine, epinephrine, levarterenol, mannitol, metaraminol bitartrate, metronidazole, miconazole, nafcillin, nitroprusside sodium, norepinephrine phenytoin, potassium chloride, Renografin 60 (contrast dye), tetracycline, thiamylal, thiopental, vancomycin, vindesine
Fluids
dextrose 10% or greater, hyperalimentation
Chemotherapeutic agents
bisantrine, carmustine, chlorozotocin, dacarbazine, dactinomycin, daunorubicin, DHAD, doxorubicin, etoposide, fluorouracil, mechlorethamine or nitrogen mustard, methotrexate, mitomycin, mutamycin, plicamycin, streptozocin, vinblastine, vincristine

sible extravasation, try to avoid the dorsum of the hand. Avoid the wrist and digits, since they are difficult to immobilize. Avoid areas of previous damage or compromised circulation. If possible, keep a record of used sites to facilitate site rotation.
* If probing is necessary, the vein may be traumatized. Stop and start again at another site.
* Start the infusion with dextrose 5% in water or normal saline solution.
* Tape the needle securely, but do not cover the I.V. site. Use a transparent dressing so the site may be observed frequently for infiltration.
* Check for infiltration before starting the infusion. The most reliable way to do this is to apply a tourniquet above the needle to occlude the vein and see if the flow continues. If the flow stops, the vein is not infiltrated. If the flow continues, the vein may be infiltrated, and you should choose another site. Another way to check for infiltration is to lower the I.V. container and observe for blood backflow. This method is not completely reliable because the needle may have punctured the opposite vein wall yet still be partly in the vein.
* Flush the needle to ensure patency. If swelling occurs at the I.V. site, the solution is infiltrating and you should choose another site.
* Administer a vesicant by slow I.V. push through a running I.V. line or by small-volume infusion (50 to 100 ml), checking blood return every 0.5 ml.
* During administration, observe the infusion site for erythema or infiltration. Tell the patient to report burning, stinging, pain, itching, or temperature changes.
* Check needle placement by lowering the solution container to observe blood return.
* Follow drug administration with several milliliters of dextrose 5% in water or normal saline solution to rinse the drug from the vein and to preclude drug leakage when the needle is removed.
* Give irritating drugs last when multiple drugs are ordered.
* Avoid use of an infusion pump for administration of extravasating agents if possible. An infusion pump continues infusing the solution when infiltration is present until occlusion pressure is reached and an alarm goes off. Infiltration stops a gravity-drip infusion much sooner.

Treating extravasation injuries
Extravasation causes local pain and itching, edema, blanching, and decreased skin temperature in the affected extremity. Infiltration of a small amount of isotonic fluid or nonirritating drug usually causes only minor discomfort. However, infiltration of some drugs can severely damage tissue through irritative, sclerotic, vesicant, corrosive, or vasoconstrictive action. In these cases, immediate measures must be taken to minimize tissue damage, preventing the need for skin grafts or, rarely, amputation.

Treatment for extravasation of I.V. solutions and nonirritating drugs involves routine comfort measures, such as application of warm soaks. However, extravasation of corrosive drugs requires emergency treatment to prevent severe tissue necrosis. Treatment measures are controversial, and institutional policy must be followed. The following steps may be taken:
* Stop the I.V. flow and remove the I.V. line unless the needle is to be used as a path to infiltrate the tissue with the antidote.
* Estimate the amount of extravasated solution, and notify the physician.
* Administer the appropriate antidote following the physician's order and institutional policy. (See *Suggested Antidotes for Subcutaneous Treatment of Extravasation Injuries*, p. 220.)
* Elevate the extremity.
* Record the site of the extravasation, the patient's symptoms, the estimated amount of infiltrated solution, nursing treatment, the name of the physician notified, and the time he was notified. Continue to document the appearance of the infiltrated site and any associated symptoms.
* Follow institutional policy, and apply either ice packs or warm compresses to the affected area for a 20-minute period every 4 hours.
* If skin breakdown occurs, silver sulfadiazine cream and gauze dressings or wet-to-dry povidone-iodine dressings may be used as treatment.

SUGGESTED ANTIDOTES FOR SUBCUTANEOUS TREATMENT OF EXTRAVASATION INJURIES

Most of the following drugs are instilled either via the existing I.V. line, purposely infiltrating the area, or by use of a 1-ml Tuberculin syringe, injecting small amounts subcutaneously in a circle around the area where known infiltration of the extravasating drug has occurred. The needle is changed prior to each injection of antidote. Some of these drugs are used in combination with one another.

Antidote	Dosage	Extravasated drug
Hyaluronidase 15 units/ml (Mix a 150-unit vial with 1 ml normal saline for injection. Withdraw 0.1 ml and dilute with 0.9 ml saline to get 15 units/ml.)	0.2 ml × 5 subcutaneous injections around site	aminophylline calcium solutions contrast media dextrose 10% and above hyperalimentation solutions nafcillin potassium solutions vinblastine vincristine vindesine
Sodium bicarbonate 8.4%	5 ml	carmustine daunorubicin doxorubicin vinblastine vincristine
Phentolamine (Dilute 5 to 10 mg with 10 ml of sterile saline for injection.)	5 to 10 mg	dobutamine dopamine epinephrine metaraminol bitartrate norepinephrine
Sodium thiosulfate 10% (Dilute 4 ml with 6 ml sterile water for injection.)	10 ml	dactinomycin mechlorethamine mitomycin
Hydrocortisone sodium succinate 100 mg/ml (Usually followed by topical application of hydrocortisone cream 1%.)	50 to 200 mg 25 to 50 mg per ml of extravasate	doxorubicin vincristine
Ascorbic acid injection	50 mg	dactinomycin
Sodium edetate	150 mg	plicamycin

- With severe extravasation debridement, plastic surgery and physical therapy may be needed.

Home I.V. therapy

With patients being discharged from the hospital earlier, many procedures that were formerly done only in hospitals are now being done at home. I.V. therapy is one such procedure, and the frequency of home therapy is increasing rapidly. (For information on NITA policy standards, see *NITA Standards for Home I.V. Therapy*, pp. 22 and 23.)

Home I.V. therapy benefits both the patient and the hospital. Patients are more comfortable in the home environment, and they are able to perform daily activities between doses of medication. The cost of treatment is reduced for the patient, who pays only for the therapy, not for a hospital room. The cost is also reduced for the hospital if the patient is discharged early according to the DRG (diagnosis related group) rating for his illness.

The types of infusions commonly administered at home include fluids, antibiotics, antifungals, chemotherapy, insulin, chelating agents, total parenteral nutrition (TPN), and medications for pain control. More recently, some blood products have been given at home after at least the first infusion is given in the hospital.

Preparations commonly administered at home include I.V. drip medications mixed in 50- or 100-ml minibags and refrigerated or frozen until the patient is ready to use them, I.V. push medications that the patient can mix and administer, medications to be given via external or implanted pumps, and medications given by subcutaneous infusion.

Home care candidates are carefully selected according to the following criteria:
- The patient is willing and ready to learn.
- He is intellectually capable of learning how to administer I.V. therapy at home safely, as well as learning the potential complications and interventions, understanding asepsis, and ordering supplies.
- He has someone willing and able to help with the therapy, if help is required.
- He has the financial resources to cover the cost.
- His home environment permits safe, convenient administration of the therapy.

Instruction for home I.V. therapy usually begins in the hospital with a demonstration and discussion of the procedure. The patient, family member, or other caregiver involved must give a successful return demonstration and answer questions satisfactorily before the patient can be discharged.

Before the patient is discharged from the hospital, consider the following:
- He will need skilled nursing services for home I.V. therapy.
- He will need regular contact with a company that distributes supplies for home I.V. therapy. Some companies have a 24-hour hotline to address patient problems regarding equipment and supplies. Ideally, the company should be close enough to deliver supplies; it should be a national company if the patient will need supplies while traveling.
- If blood studies must be done during therapy, arrangements will have to be made for a nurse to go to the patient's home to draw blood or for the patient to go to a laboratory.
- The Visiting Nurse Association will have to be contacted if the patient needs general nursing services other than I.V. therapy services.

LOCAL COMPLICATIONS OF PERIPHERAL I.V. THERAPY

SIGNS AND SYMPTOMS	POSSIBLE CAUSES	NURSING ACTIONS	PREVENTION MEASURES
Hematoma (raised, discolored area caused by leakage of blood at venipuncture site)			
• Tenderness at venipuncture site • Area around site appears "bruised" • Inability to advance or flush I.V.	• Vein "blown" or punctured through other wall at time of venipuncture • Leakage of blood from needle displacement	• Remove I.V. device. • Apply pressure/warm soaks to affected area. • Recheck for bleeding. • Document.	• Do not advance needle further if resistance is met on venipuncture. • Choose a vein that can accommodate size of I.V. device.
Infiltration (leakage of I.V. fluid into surrounding tissues)			
• Swelling, tenderness above I.V. site that may extend along entire limb • Decreased skin temperature around site • Fluid continues to infuse even when vein is occluded • Backflow of blood absent • Flow rate slower or stopped	• Needle dislodged from vein or vein perforated	• Remove I.V. device. • Apply ice (early) or warm soaks (later) to aid absorption. • Elevate extremity. • Restart I.V. infusion above infiltration or in another limb. • Document. • See "Treating extravasation injuries," p. 219, for treatment of infiltration of vesicant drugs or fluids.	• Check I.V. site frequently (especially when using I.V. pump). • Do not obscure area above site with tape. • Restrict movement of limb by placing on armboard. • Teach patient to observe the I.V. site and report any pain, swelling, etc. • To confirm patency, apply a tourniquet above the I.V. site. Flow will continue if infiltration has occurred. Blood return is not always indicative of cannula patency; device may be partly in vein and have blood return, or small vein may be occluded by size of device.

(continued)

LOCAL COMPLICATIONS OF PERIPHERAL I.V. THERAPY (continued)

SIGNS AND SYMPTOMS	POSSIBLE CAUSES	NURSING ACTIONS	PREVENTION MEASURES
Phlebitis (irritation along vein)			
• Area along vein red, tender, and warm • Vein "hard" and cordlike when palpated • Decreased flow rate • Irritation increases with infusion	• Hypertonic, viscous medications or solutions • Repeated use of same vein for therapy • Movement of device in vein • Device too large or flow rate too rapid for size of vein • Clotting at tip of catheter (thrombophlebitis)	• Remove I.V. device. • Apply warm soaks. • Notify physician. • Restart I.V. infusion in a different limb. • Document.	• Use large or central veins for hypertonic solution infusion. • Choose smallest I.V. device for viscosity of infusate and size of vein. • Rotate I.V. sites frequently. • Verify drug compatibilities prior to infusion. • Stabilize the device to decrease movement in vein.
Site infection (local contamination of insertion site)			
• Redness, warmth, tenderness, and swelling at site • Possible exudate of purulent material	• Failure to maintain aseptic technique during insertion or site care • Duration of I.V. beyond recommended time • Immunosuppression	• Remove I.V. device. • Culture tip of device and site of I.V. • Clean site and apply bacteriostatic ointment. • Notify physician. • Restart I.V. infusion at a different site. • Document.	• Possibly use steel needles instead of catheters. • Maintain aseptic technique on I.V. insertion. • Change I.V. site and dressing frequently. • Educate staff regarding aseptic technique. • Monitor immunosuppressed patients closely.
Clotting (blockage at end of device in patient's vein)			
• Unable to flush I.V. easily • Tenderness at I.V. site • Sluggish flow rate	• I.V. rate too slow to maintain patency of device • I.V. not heparinized often enough • Activity or hematologic condition of patient causes increased backflow of blood	• Attempt to withdraw clot with syringe to clear I.V. line; if successful, flush as usual. • If clot cannot be withdrawn, remove I.V. device and restart in another area. • Document.	• Flush I.V. frequently or maintain constant flow rate. • Tightly secure all connections. • Assess patient status prior to insertion.

SYSTEMIC COMPLICATIONS OF PERIPHERAL I.V. THERAPY

SIGNS AND SYMPTOMS	POSSIBLE CAUSES	NURSING ACTIONS	PREVENTION MEASURES
Catheter embolism (all or part of I.V. device shears off into venous system)			
• Related to specific location of embolus: discomfort, decreased blood pressure, increased CVP, cyanosis, thready pulse, respiratory distress, unconsciousness	• Use of scissors near I.V. site (e.g., to remove tape) • Rethreading stylet into catheter (over-the-needle device) • Withdrawal of needle over catheter without care (inside-the-needle device) • Movement of patient on insertion or removal • Device not secured effectively	• Apply tourniquet above I.V. site to discourage further travelling of device in venous system. • Notify physician immediately. • Notify radiology department. • Document.	• Do not use scissors near I.V. site. • Withdraw device and stylet together if venipuncture is unsuccessful. • Be especially careful with removal of inside-the-needle devices.
Air embolism (air in the circulatory system; more common with central venous line)			
• Respiratory distress • Unequal breath sounds • Weak pulse • Increased CVP • Decreased blood pressure • Loss of consciousness	• Solution container empty • Disconnected I.V., which allows air to be sucked in • I.V. tubing that runs dry or is not purged of air properly	• Discontinue I.V. infusion. • Turn patient to left side, head down (to allow air to enter right atrium and be dispersed via pulmonary artery). • Administer oxygen. • Notify physician. • Document.	• Purge tubing completely of air before infusion. • Utilize air detection device on pump or air-eliminating filter proximal to I.V. site. • Secure connections.
Circulatory overload (more fluid volume than the circulatory system can manage)			
• Patient discomfort • Neck vein engorgement	• Roller clamp loosened to allow "run-on" I.V.	• Slow or stop infusion rate. • Raise head of patient's bed.	• Double-check I.V. rate ordered for size and condition of patient.

(continued)

SYSTEMIC COMPLICATIONS OF PERIPHERAL I.V. THERAPY (continued)

SIGNS AND SYMPTOMS	POSSIBLE CAUSES	NURSING ACTIONS	PREVENTION MEASURES
Circulatory overload *(continued)*			
• Increased blood pressure • Increased CVP • Fluid in lungs, rales, shortness of breath • Increased difference between fluid intake and output	• Set removed from pump, allowing run on of fluid • If pump used, infusion rate set too high • Miscalculation of fluid requirements	• Notify physician. • Administer medications, oxygen as ordered. • Document.	• Keep roller clamp out of patient's reach. • Monitor intake and output.
Systemic infection (septicemia or bacteremia caused by introduction of microorganisms into circulatory system)			
• Fever, chills without other apparent reason • Concomitant I.V. site infection • Nausea, vomiting • Malaise	• Contaminated I.V. device or infusate • Failure to maintain aseptic technique during insertion or administration • Immunosuppression • Device in vein longer than recommended	• Notify physician. • Identify other sources of infection. • Remove I.V. device. • Culture tip of I.V. device and infusate. • Restart infusion in another area. • Document.	• Examine fluid for cloudiness or turbidity, and container for cracks or leaks before infusion. • Monitor vital signs, especially temperature. • Maintain aseptic technique upon insertion or administration of I.V. therapy. • Secure all connections so equipment does not come apart and become contaminated. • Discard suspected contaminated material. • Change I.V. device and equipment at recommended interval. • Provide site care frequently. • Educate staff.

CENTRAL VENOUS LINE COMPLICATIONS

SIGNS AND SYMPTOMS	POSSIBLE CAUSES	NURSING ACTIONS	PREVENTION MEASURES
Pneumothorax (accumulation of air or gas in the pleural space); **hemothorax** (collection of blood in the pleural cavity); **chylothorax** (presence of chyle in the thoracic cavity); **hydrothorax** (collection of watery fluid in the pleural cavity)			
• Chest pain • Dyspnea • Cyanosis • Decreased breath sounds • With hemothorax, decreased hemoglobin because of blood pooling • Abnormal chest X-ray	• Puncture of lung with catheter during insertion or exchange over a wire • Puncture of large blood vessel with bleeding inside or outside of lung • Puncture of lymph nodes with leakage of lymph fluid • Infusion of solution into chest area through infiltrated catheter	• Notify physician. • Remove catheter or assist with removal. • Administer oxygen as ordered. • Set up for and assist with chest tube insertion. • Document.	• Position the patient head down (Trendelenburg) with a towel roll between the shoulder blades to dilate and expose vein as much as possible during insertion. • Assess for early signs of fluid infiltration, such as swelling in shoulder, neck, chest, and arm area. • Ensure immobilization of patient via adequate preparation for procedure and restraint during procedure; very active patients may need to be sedated or taken to the OR for central line insertion.
Air embolism (air in the circulatory system; more common with central lines)			
• Respiratory distress • Unequal breath sounds • Weak pulse • Increased CVP • Decreased blood pressure • Churning murmur over precordium • Loss of consciousness	• Intake of air into central venous system during catheter insertion, tubing changes; inadvertent opening, cutting, or breakage of catheter	• Clamp catheter immediately. • Turn patient on left side, head down (Trendelenburg), so air can enter right atrium and be dispersed via pulmonary artery, maintaining position for 20 to 30 minutes. • Administer oxygen. • Notify physician. • Document.	• Purge all air from tubing before hook-up. • Teach patient to perform Valsalva's maneuver during catheter insertion and tubing changes (bear down or strain and hold breath to increase CVP). • Use air-eliminating filters proximal to patient. • Use infusion control device with air detection capability. • Use Luer-Lok tubing, tape connections, or use locking devices for all connections.
Blockage of catheter lumen (tip or lumen of catheter inside patient becomes blocked)			
• Inability to flush catheter or infuse fluids without resistance	• Long-term catheterization • Improper flushing or failure to flush on schedule	• Attempt aspiration of clot (do not force clot). • Notify physician.	• Flush catheter routinely, maintaining positive pressure on plunger of syringe as needle is withdrawn. • Make sure all connections are securely tightened.

(continued)

CENTRAL VENOUS LINE COMPLICATIONS (continued)

SIGNS AND SYMPTOMS	POSSIBLE CAUSES	NURSING ACTIONS	PREVENTION MEASURES
Blockage of catheter lumen *(continued)*			
• Inability to withdraw blood from catheter or elicit backflow of blood • Formation of fibrin sheath on catheter tip (seen on X-ray)	• Increased blood clotting because of hematopoietic status of patient • Infusion of incompatible substances through catheter with resultant precipitate formation in lumen • Improper position of catheter in vein or tip of catheter against wall of vessel	• Possibly, infuse thrombolytic agents such as streptokinase or urokinase. • Possibly, remove catheter (may be repositioned in vein with verification by X-ray). • Reposition patient (lie on side of catheter insertion, cough, raise arm on side of insertion, lower head of bed, and check for flow). • Document.	• Use infusion pump if necessary to overcome venous pressure. • Assess hematologic status of patient. • Heparin may be added to some infusions, such as hyperalimentation solution. • Use in-line 0.22-micron filter for infusions. • Monitor frequent chest X-rays to assess catheter position.
Thrombosis *(formation of a thrombus)*			
• Edema at puncture site • Erythema • Ipsilateral swelling of arm, neck, face • Pain along vein • Fever, malaise • Tachycardia	• Sluggish flow rate • Composition of catheter material (some materials such as polyvinylchloride are more thrombogenic) • Hematopoietic status of patient • Preexisting limb edema • Infusion of irritating solutions • Repeated use of same vein or long-term use • Preexisting cardiovascular disease	• Notify physician. • Possibly, remove catheter. • Possibly, infuse anticoagulant doses of heparin. • Verify thrombosis with diagnostic studies. • Apply warm wet compresses locally. • Do not use limb on affected side for subsequent venipuncture. • Document.	• Maintain flow through catheter at steady rate with infusion pump, or flush at regular intervals. • Use catheters made of less thrombogenic materials or catheters coated to discourage thrombosis. • Dilute irritating solutions. • Use 0.22-micron filter on line.

(continued)

CENTRAL VENOUS LINE COMPLICATIONS *(continued)*

SIGNS AND SYMPTOMS	POSSIBLE CAUSES	NURSING ACTIONS	PREVENTION MEASURES
Local infection (local contamination of insertion or, for silastic catheters, exit site, or infection of subcutaneous tunnel for tunnelled catheters)			
• Redness, warmth, tenderness, swelling at site of insertion or exit • Possible exudate of purulent material • Local rash or pustules • Fever, chills, malaise	• Failure to maintain aseptic technique during insertion or care • Failure to comply with dressing change protocol • Wet or soiled dressing remaining on site • Immunosuppression • Irritated suture line	• Monitor temperature frequently. • Culture site. • Redress aseptically. • Possibly, use antibiotic ointment locally. • Treat systemically with antibiotics/antifungals, depending on culture results and physician order. • Catheter may be removed. • Document.	• Maintain strict aseptic technique. • Adhere to dressing change protocols. • Teach patient regarding swimming, bathing, etc. (patients with adequate white blood cell counts can do these activities at physician discretion). • Change dressing immediately if site becomes wet or soiled. • Change dressing more frequently if catheter is located in femoral area or near tracheostomy. • Complete ostomy care and wound dressings after catheter care.
Systemic infection (septicemia or bacteremia caused by introduction of microorganisms into the circulatory system; **primary**—from catheter itself; **secondary**—from other source, seeded to catheter)			
• Fever, chills without other apparent reason • Leukocytosis • Nausea, vomiting • Malaise • Elevated urine glucose level	• Contaminated catheter or infusate • Failure to maintain aseptic technique during solution hook-up • Frequent opening of catheter or long-term use of single I.V. access • Immunosuppression	• Draw central and peripheral blood cultures; if same organism, catheter is primary source of sepsis and should be removed. • If cultures do not match, but are positive, catheter may be removed or the infection may be treated through the catheter. • Treat patient with antibiotic regimen, as ordered. • Culture tip of device if removed. • Assess for other sources of infection. • Monitor vital signs closely. • Document.	• Examine fluid container for cloudiness, leaks, and turbidity before infusing. • Monitor urine glucose in TPN patients; if ($> 2+$), suspect early sepsis. • Use strict sterile technique for hook-up and disconnection of fluids. • Use 0.22-micron filter. • Catheter may be changed frequently to decrease chance of infection. • Violate catheter as little as possible, using closed system. • Educate staff and patient in aseptic technique.

ARTERIAL LINE COMPLICATIONS

SIGNS AND SYMPTOMS	POSSIBLE CAUSES	NURSING ACTIONS	PREVENTION MEASURES
Thrombosis (formation of a thrombus)			
• Loss or weakening of pulse below site • Loss of warmth, sensation, and mobility below site	• Arterial damage during catheter insertion or due to catheter movement • Sluggish rate of flush solution • Inadequately heparinized flush solution • Failure to flush catheter when necessary • Irrigation of clotted catheter with syringe	• Notify physician. • Possibly, set up for removal of line. • Possibly, set up for removal of clot by arteriotomy and Fogarty catheterization. • Document.	• Check distal pulse and flow rate hourly. • Tape the catheter securely, and splint the arm or leg. • Heparinize the flush solution. Flush the catheter hourly and after collecting blood samples. • Never irrigate an arterial catheter with a syringe.
Bleeding and hematoma (small, raised, discolored area caused by leakage of blood at venipuncture site)			
• Bloody dressing; blood flowing from disconnected line • Ecchymosis at the insertion site or of the limb	• Dislodged catheter • Disconnected line • Blood leakage around catheter	• If catheter is pulled out of the skin, apply direct pressure to the site. • If the line is disconnected, replace the contaminated equipment. • Notify physician. • Document.	• Frequently check the line connections and insertion site. • Tape the catheter securely, and splint the arm or leg.
Air embolism (air in the circulatory system)			
• Decreased blood pressure • Weak, rapid pulse • Cyanosis • Loss of consciousness	• Empty I.V. container • Air in the tubing • Loose connections • Stopcock turned wrong way	• Turn patient to his left side, so air entering the heart can be absorbed in the pulmonary artery. • Check the line for leaks. • Notify physician. • Monitor vital signs. • Administer oxygen, if ordered. • Document.	• Expel all air from the line before starting the infusion. • Secure all connections and check them routinely. • Change the I.V. container before it runs out.
Systemic infection (septicemia or bacteremia caused by introduction of microorganisms into circulatory system)			
• Sudden rise in temperature and pulse rate • Chills, shaking • Blood pressure changes • No other focus	• Poor aseptic technique • Contaminated equipment, solution, or medication • Immunosuppression	• Evaluate for other sources of infection. Collect samples of urine, sputum, blood, and I.V. solution for cultures, as ordered. • Notify physician. • Possibly, set up for removal of line. • Document.	• Change dressing regularly. • Use aseptic technique. • Avoid contaminating the site when bathing the patient. • If the line is accidentally disconnected, replace contaminated equipment.
Arterial spasm (contraction of arterial wall)			
• Intermittent loss or weakening of pulse below the insertion site	• Traumatic catheter insertion • Arterial irritation after catheter insertion	• Notify physician. • Prepare for possible injection of lidocaine (without epinephrine) to relieve spasm. • Document.	• Tape the catheter securely and splint the arm or leg.

Review Questions

1. It is the responsibility of the staff nurse to make sure I.V. flow rates are maintained. True or false?

2. Which of the following factors affect flow rates of I.V. solutions?
   1. Height of container
   2. Viscosity of fluid
   3. Type of administration set
   4. Size of I.V. cannula
   A. 1 only
   B. 1 and 2
   C. 1, 2, and 3
   D. 1, 2, 3, and 4

3. I.V. flow rates are checked at least once a day. True or false?

4. & 5. If you are using a microdrip set, an order for 100 ml/hour would mean running the infusion at _____ drops/minute or _____ drops every 15 seconds.

6. Name four things you might check when an I.V. infusion has stopped running.

7. to 16. Match the following complications of I.V. therapy with a cause.
Complication
7. Infiltration
8. Clotting
9. Pulmonary overload
10. Air embolism
11. Catheter embolism
12. Pyrogenic reaction
13. Phlebitis
14. Nerve damage
15. I.V. site infection
16. Hematoma
Cause
A. Armboard "unpadded"
B. Buretrol ran dry
C. Contaminated I.V. needle
D. Vein irritation
E. Rate too slow to maintain patency of device
F. Infusion at 10 times ordered rate
G. Dislodgment of needle
H. "Blown" vein on insertion
I. Sheared-off catheter
J. Unsterile I.V. solution

17. The risk of air emboli is greater when a catheter is passed into the great veins, where negative pressure may actively pull in fluid and air. True or false?

18. Check those medications that may cause extravasation injury if they infiltrate during I.V. infusion.
methotrexate
dopamine
vincristine
ampicillin
vancomycin
dactinomycin
hyalouronidase

19. Lowering the extremity and applying warm wet compresses to the site constitute treatment for an infiltrated vesicant. True or false?

20. If a peripheral, central, or arterial I.V. line is clotted, it should be removed, or treatment with a thrombolytic agent should be instituted. True or false?

21. Prevention is the best way to avoid complications of I.V. therapy. True or false?

22. Before a patient can be discharged to perform I.V. therapy at home, he must give a successful return demonstration and satisfactorily answer questions about the procedure. True or false?

Selected References

"Administering Drugs: What Are Your Legal Risks," *Nursing86*, March 1986.
Brown, A., et al. "Skin Necrosis from Extravasation of Intravenous Fluids in Children," *Plastic Reconstructive Surgery* 64, August 1979.
Burman, R., and Berkowitz, H. "I.V. Bolus: Effective, But Potentially Hazardous," *Critical Care Nurse* 6(1):22-28, January/February 1986.
Crudi, C., and Larkin, M. *Core Curriculum for Intravenous Nursing*. Philadelphia: J.B. Lippincott Co., 1984.
Gaze, N.R. "Tissue Necrosis Caused by Commonly Used Intravenous Infusions," *Lancet* 2, August 1978.

Gong, H., and King, C. "Inadequate Drug Mixing: A Potential Hazard in Continuous Intravenous Administration," *Heart and Lung* 12(5):528-32, September 1983.

Gong, H., et al. "Nursing Techniques in Preparing and Administering Intravenous Admixtures," *Journal of the National Intravenous Therapy Association*, 5:132-33, March-April, 1982.

Huey, F. "Setting Up and Troubleshooting," *American Journal of Nursing* 83(7):1026-28, July 1983.

Huey, F. "What's on the Market? A Nurse's Guide," *American Journal of Nursing* 83(6):902-10, June 1983.

Intravenous Nursing Standards of Practice, NITA, Cambridge, Mass., November 1981.

League of Intravenous Therapy Education (LITE). *Standards of Practice and Guidelines to Achieving the Standard.* Park Ridge, Ill., January 1984.

MacCara, M. "Extravasation: A Hazard of Intravenous Therapy," *Drug Intelligence and Clinical Pharmacy* 17, October 1983.

Managing I.V. Therapy. Nursing Photobook Series. Springhouse, Pa.: Springhouse Corp., 1983.

Mascaro, J. "Managing I.V. Therapy in the Home," *Nursing86* 16, May 1986.

May, C. "Antibiotic Therapy at Home," *American Journal of Nursing*, March 1984.

Piercy, S. *Extravasation.* New Orleans: Presented at the National Intravenous Therapy Association conference, May 1986.

Plumer, A. *Principles and Practice of Intravenous Therapy,* 3rd ed. Boston: Little, Brown & Co., 1982.

Schaffner, A. "Safety Precautions in Home Chemotherapy," *American Journal of Nursing*, March 1984.

Seymour, F. "Parenteral Chemotherapeutic Agents," *Journal of the National Intravenous Therapy Association* 8, May/June 1985.

Steel, J. "Too Fast or Too Slow—The Erratic I.V.," *American Journal of Nursing* 83, June 1983.

Tilden, S., et al. "Cutaneous Necrosis Associated With Intravenous Nafcillin Therapy," *American Journal of Diseases of Children* 134, November 1980.

Turco, S., ed. *The Sourcebook for I.V. Therapy.* San Diego: IVAC Corp., 1985.

Upton, J., et al. "Major Intravenous Extravasation Injuries," *American Journal of Surgery* 127, April 1979.

Weinstein, S. "Intravenous Therapy Within the Scope of Home Health Service," *Journal of the National Intravenous Therapy Association* 7, January/February 1984.

Wiseman, M. "Setting Standards for Home I.V. Therapy," *American Journal of Nursing*, April 1985.

Woodland, C. "How to Make Infusion Control Devices Work for You (Instead of Vice Versa)," *RN* 44, November 1981.

Yosowitz, P., et al. "Peripheral Intravenous Infiltration Necrosis," *Annals of Surgery* 182, November 1975.

Zenk, K., et al. "Nafcillin Extravasation Injury," *American Journal of Diseases of Children* 135, December 1981.

15

Parenteral Nutrition

Parenteral nutrition therapy has significantly decreased the morbidity and mortality of serious illnesses that preclude normal nutrition and metabolism. This chapter covers nutritional assessment, types of parenteral nutrition, indications for usage, components of solutions, and complications of total parenteral nutrition (TPN) therapy. Procedures discussed include equipment preparation and site care for TPN, patient monitoring during TPN therapy, administering peripheral vein nutrition, and preparation for home parenteral nutrition. See *NITA Standards for Hyperalimentation Therapy*, p. 23, for information on parenteral nutrition policies.

Nutritional assessment

No single test or measurement can identify and classify malnutrition, but a comprehensive profile of pertinent subjective and objective data allows prevention and early recognition of nutritional depletion. Parenteral nutrition therapy and repletion of body stores minimize the harmful effects of poor nutrition, such as indolent wound healing, increased incidence of infection and complications, and prolonged hospitalization.

During initial evaluation of the patient, obtain a dietary history to determine recent changes in appetite, food intake, and body weight. Note medical conditions that impair nutrient intake and absorption. Thorough and complete physical assessment—including inspection, palpation, percussion, and auscultation of each body system—reveals other signs and symptoms of malnutrition.

Additional objective data commonly gathered for nutritional assessment include anthropometric measurements (height, weight, triceps skinfold, midarm circumference) and biochemical determinations (serum concentrations of albumin, transferrin, prealbumin, and retinol-binding protein; total lymphocyte count; and 24-hour urinary excretion of urea and creatinine). (See *How to Take Anthropometric Measurements.*)

Fat, skeletal muscle protein, and visceral protein are the three major energy reserves of the patient with a catabolic disorder. Adipose (fat) tissue—the body's primary calorie reserve—is assessed by measuring the triceps skinfold, which includes the subcutaneous fat layer. Skeletal muscle mass can be estimated by determining midarm muscle circumference as well as the creatinine-height index. Visceral protein depletion is quantified by serum albumin and serum transferrin concentrations, and the status of the cellular immune response is shown by total lymphocyte count and recall antigen skin testing.

Critical analysis of these energy reserves is essential to determine the severity and type of malnutrition. *Marasmus*—the severe depletion of both protein and calories—results in growth retardation in children, weight loss without edema, muscular atrophy, and decreased subcutaneous tissue. The acute protein loss or deprivation known as *kwashiorkor* produces generalized edema, skin lesions, hair changes, and fatty infiltration of the liver. In many hospitalized patients, marasmus and kwashiorkor are present concurrently, resulting in depletion of fat and of skeletal and visceral protein.

HOW TO TAKE ANTHROPOMETRIC MEASUREMENTS

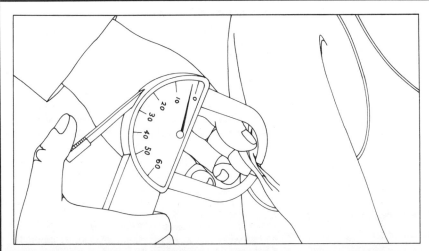

Anthropometric measurements help you assess your patient's nutritional status. Body height and weight, skinfold thickness, and midarm muscle circumference measurements allow you to identify body fat, muscle mass, and protein and caloric adequacy.

Follow these techniques for accurate anthropometric measurements:
- Weigh the patient around the same time every day and after he empties his bladder. Use the same scale, and have him wear the same amount of clothing. It's the easiest and least expensive way to assess nutritional status quickly.
- Record the patient's height and weight. Compare actual weight to ideal body weight. For some patients, you may need to determine the basal energy requirement. This will give an approximation of the number of calories needed daily to maintain the body at rest. An easy method of doing this is to multiply 10 times the ideal body weight in pounds. For example, if ideal body weight for your patient is 120 lb, then 120 × 10 equals 1,200 calories, the amount needed to maintain basal metabolism.
- Measure, record, and compare with standard values the *triceps skinfold thickness,* measured by skinfold calipers like the ones shown here.

You can also compare with standard values the *subscapular and abdominal skinfold thickness,* although these measurements are not routinely done.
- Measure, record, and compare with standard values the *midarm circumference* to estimate the size of the triceps muscles. This represents the muscle mass.
- Make sure the following laboratory values are recorded, since such data may indicate potential nutritional problems before clinical signs develop.

Laboratory Values	Purpose
Serum albumin and serum transferrin	To measure visceral protein stores
Total lymphocyte counts	To measure immune competence
24-hour urine specimens	The creatinine-height index provides an estimate of skeletal muscle mass. The urine urea nitrogen test is a measure of nitrogen balance.

TYPES OF PARENTERAL NUTRITION

Type	Solution Components/Liter
Total parenteral nutrition (TPN) via central venous line	• Dextrose 20% to 25% (1 liter dextrose 25% = 850 non-protein calories) • Crystalline amino acids 2.5% to 8.5% • Electrolytes, vitamins, trace elements, insulin, and heparin as ordered • Fat emulsion 10% to 20% (usually infused as a separate solution; can be given peripherally or centrally) • A new infusion system is available in which dextrose, protein, and fat are mixed together in the same container.
Peripheral vein nutrition	• Dextrose 5% to 10% • Crystalline amino acids 2.75% to 4.25% • Electrolytes, trace elements, and vitamins as ordered • Fat emulsion 10% or 20% (1 liter dextrose 10% and amino acids 3.5% infused at same time with liter fat emulsion = 1,440 nonprotein calories: 340 from dextrose and 1,100 from fat emulsion) • Heparin or hydrocortisone as ordered
Protein-sparing therapy	• Crystalline amino acids in same amounts as TPN • Electrolytes, vitamins, and minerals as ordered
Standard I.V. therapy	• Dextrose, water, and electrolytes in varying amounts *Examples of frequently used parenteral fluids:* D_5W = 170 calories/liter $D_{10}W$ = 340 calories/liter 0.9% NaCl (normal saline solution) = 0 calories • Vitamins as ordered

Uses	Special Considerations
• 3 weeks or more (long term) • For patients with large caloric and nutrient needs • Provides needed calories; restores nitrogen balance; replaces essential vitamins, electrolytes, minerals, and trace elements • Promotes tissue synthesis, wound healing, normal metabolic function • Allows bowel rest and healing; reduces activity in the gallbladder, pancreas, and small intestine • Improves tolerance to surgery	**Basic solution** • Nutritionally complete • Requires minor surgical procedure for central line insertion (can be done at bedside by physician) • Delivers hypertonic solutions • May cause metabolic complications (glucose intolerance, electrolyte imbalances, essential fatty acid deficiency) **I.V. fat emulsion** • May not be utilized effectively in severely stressed patients (especially burn patients) • May interfere with immune mechanisms • Irritates peripheral vein in long-term use
• 3 weeks or less • Maintains nutritional state in patients who can tolerate relatively high fluid volume; those who usually resume bowel function and oral feedings in a few days; and those who are susceptible to catheter-related infections of central venous TPN	**Basic solution** • Nutritionally complete for a short term • Cannot be used in nutritionally depleted patients • Cannot be used in volume-restricted patients since higher volumes of solution needed than with central venous TPN • Does not cause patient to gain weight • Avoids insertion and maintenance of central catheter, but patient must have good veins; I.V. site should be changed every 48 hours • Delivers less hypertonic solutions than central venous TPN • May cause phlebitis • Less chance of metabolic complications than central venous TPN **I.V. fat emulsion** • As effective as dextrose for caloric source • Diminishes phlebitis if infused at same time as basic nutrient solution • Irritates vein in long-term use
• 2 weeks or less • May preserve body protein in a stable patient • Augments oral or tube feedings	• Nutritionally incomplete • Requires little mixing • May be initiated or stopped at any point in a patient's hospital stay • Other I.V. fluids, medications, and blood byproducts may be given through same I.V. line • Not as likely to cause phlebitis as peripheral vein nutrition • Adds a major expense, with limited benefits
• Less than 1 week as nutrition source • Maintains hydration (main function) • Facilitates and maintains normal metabolic function	• Nutritionally incomplete; does not administer sufficient calories to maintain adequate nutritional status

Types of parenteral nutrition

Parenteral nutrition—the administration of nutrients by the I.V. route—can be classified according to the concentration and the extent of nutrients delivered.

Total parenteral nutrition (TPN), also known as intravenous hyperalimentation, provides the patient's total energy and nutrient requirements (proteins, carbohydrates, water, electrolytes, vitamins, trace elements, and fats) exclusively by vein. Because peripheral veins cannot tolerate the concentrated hypertonic amino acid–glucose solutions used in TPN, these solutions must be infused through a central vein. Fat emulsion, however, may be infused centrally or peripherally. The average adult patient who receives TPN for longer than several months will develop essential fatty acid deficiency unless I.V. fat emulsion is added to the regimen.

Peripheral vein nutrition is a more limited form of nutritional therapy. It provides fewer nonprotein calories but greater volume than TPN. Because concentrated hypertonic glucose solutions cannot be administered peripherally, significant weight gain rarely occurs in patients receiving this type of treatment. Therefore, it is used only for periods of less than 3 weeks in patients who do not need to gain weight yet need to maintain optimal nutritional status. (See "Administering peripheral vein nutrition," p. 249, for information on how to perform the procedure.)

Other forms of parenteral nutrition include protein-sparing therapy and standard I.V. therapy. (See *Types of Parenteral Nutrition*, pp. 234 and 235, for more information and a comparison of the four types of parenteral nutrition.)

Indications

TPN is indicated when use of the GI tract for nutritional replenishment is inadequate, ill advised, or impossible. TPN promotes normal growth and development in infants with congenital anomalies such as tracheoesophageal fistula, gastroschisis, small-bowel atresia, cystic fibrosis, meconium ileus, diaphragmatic hernia, volvulus, malrotation of the gut, and annular pancreas. (See Chapter 17, Pediatric Drug and I.V. Therapy.)

Other candidates for TPN include patients with fistulas of the alimentary tract, inflammatory bowel disease, short-bowel syndrome, burns, severe trauma, cancer, pancreatitis, and other disorders that adversely affect nutritional status. Specially prepared formulas have been devised for patients with renal and hepatic failure.

Solution components

TPN solutions are quite hypertonic, with an osmolarity of 1,800 to 2,400 mOsm/liter. These solutions are admixed in the pharmacy under laminar flow, filtered-air hoods. Usually, 500 ml of dextrose 50% are mixed with 500 ml of 8.5% crystalline amino acid solution. Rarely, 350 ml of dextrose 50% are mixed with 750 ml of 5% to 10% protein hydrolysate solution. Electrolytes, vitamins, minerals, and trace elements must be added to the base solution in sufficient amounts to satisfy daily requirements.

Dextrose

The number of nonprotein calories needed to maintain the patient's nitrogen balance depends on the severity of his illness. Maximum energy expenditure occurs in multiple trauma, severe sepsis, long-bone fractures, and burns. A patient who weighs 60 kg (132 lb) requires 1,800 to 3,000 nonprotein calories/day (usually 30 to 50 calories/kg/day).

In the absence of adequate exogenous calories, energy is generated primarily by lipolysis and gluconeogenesis. Research has confirmed that approximately 50 grams/day of dextrose can have a significant nitrogen-sparing effect; infusions of greater quantities result in only minor increases in nitrogen sparing. In fact, if the amount of dextrose provided greatly exceeds the energy expended, excess glycogen and fat can be deposited in the liver, with subsequent hepatomegaly, right upper quadrant tenderness or pain, and disordered hepatic function. For the average patient, a ratio of 150 to 200 calories per gram of nitrogen administered seems best.

Protein

The recommended dietary allowance of protein for a healthy adult is approximately 0.9 grams/kg of body weight. Protein requirements in patients with malnutrition are substantially higher. Determination of nitrogen balance is probably the best way to accurately assess individual protein requirements. The typical patient on TPN receives approximately 18 grams of nitrogen daily in the form of amino acids, the building blocks of new muscles and protein.

Protein hydrolysate solutions, the earliest form of parenteral nitrogen, are rarely used anymore. They contain peptides of minimal biological value, they do not have ideal amino acid patterns, and occasionally they may cause sensitivity reactions. These disadvantages have been overcome by the more recently developed crystalline amino acid solutions.

Electrolytes

Electrolytes are added exogenously to the TPN solution. Apparently, potassium, phosphorus, and magnesium depletion parallel the protein depletion in patients with catabolic conditions. Additions to the base solution include sodium (acetate, lactate, chloride, or bicarbonate), potassium (acetate, lactate, chloride, acid phosphate), magnesium (sulfate), phosphate (potassium acid salt), and calcium (gluconate).

Vitamins

Vitamins must be administered daily to ensure normal body functions and optimal utilization of the nutrient substrates. A mixture of fat- and water-soluble vitamins, biotin, and folic acid (MVI-12 or MVI 9+3®) is added to any single unit of a daily regimen. Because the vitamins in MVI-12 and MVC 9+3® are usually in the therapeutic dosage range, administering more than one ampule daily is neither necessary nor advisable for the adult patient, as hypervitaminosis A or D can occur within several days or weeks. In addition, the patient should receive vitamin K supplementation to maintain normal blood coagulation. Vitamin K may be given intramuscularly or intravenously, but not as a bolus.

Trace elements

Trace elements are found as contaminants in nutrient solutions. If parenteral nutrition therapy lasts longer than 2 weeks, additional trace elements may be needed. Commercial solutions contain zinc, copper, chromium, iodide, selenium, and manganese; however, many institutions compound their own solutions.

Zinc is an essential component of approximately 70 enzymes in humans. It functions in the metabolism of DNA, protein, and mucopolysaccharides. Zinc deficiency is characterized by anorexia, alopecia, impaired wound healing, hypogeusia (diminished sense of taste), hypogonadism, intractable diarrhea, and vesicular dermatitis.

Copper, together with albumin, is transported to the liver, where it is incorporated into ceruloplasmin. Copper deficiency results in anemia that does not respond to treatment with iron.

Chromium deficiency may result in glucose intolerance, since this element is important in the action of insulin.

Insulin

Most patients receiving TPN do not require exogenous insulin unless glucose intolerance is secondary to diabetes mellitus, pancreatitis, or sepsis. Crystalline insulin, preferably, is added to the I.V. bag or bottle in initial doses of 5 to 10 units/liter of TPN solution when urine and serum glucose levels exceed 200 mg/100 ml. Thereafter, the insulin dosage can be increased gradually until the desired serum glucose level is achieved. Although some of the crystalline insulin will adhere to the sides of an infusion bag or bottle, only a negligible quantity of insulin is lost. Moreover, I.V. insulin administration is preferable to subcutaneous injection, because rebound insulin shock is less likely to result if the infusion is stopped abruptly due to mechanical problems.

Fat emulsions

Ordinarily, two or three 500-ml infusions of a 10% or 20% fat emulsion are administered twice weekly to prevent essential fatty acid deficiency in adults. Signs of essential fatty acid deficiency include desquamating dermatitis, alopecia, poor wound healing, and growth retardation in children.

The fat emulsions currently available in the United States are:
- Intralipid 10% and Intralipid 20% (Kabivitrum), soybean oil emulsions
- Liposyn 10% and Liposyn 20% (Abbott), safflower oil emulsions
- Travemulsion 10% and Travemulsion 20% (Travenol), soybean oil emulsions
- Soyacal 10% and Soyacal 20% (Alphatherapeutic), soybean oil emulsions

Ten percent fat emulsions provide 1.1 calories/ml, and 20% emulsions provide 2 calories/ml. To minimize the possibility of fat overload or fat embolism, no more than 3 grams/kg/day should be administered to an adult.

The isotonicity of fat emulsions permits peripheral administration. Occasionally, piggybacking the emulsion into the TPN tubing is preferable. Note: A 0.22-micron cellulose membrane filter cannot be used during a piggyback infusion of fat emulsion because the fat particles are larger than the pores of the filter.

Ensuring the stability and sterility of a lipid emulsion before and during administration is an important nursing priority. Since lipid emulsions support the growth of bacteria, aseptic technique must be followed. Never shake the lipid container excessively or use the emulsion if there is any inconsistency in texture or color. During the initial infusion of fat, monitor the patient's vital signs as baseline indices. The flow rate should not exceed 1 ml/minute for the first 30 minutes. During this time, observe for fever, chills, flushing, diaphoresis, dyspnea, and allergic reactions.

The patient's fat tolerance can be monitored biochemically by routine measurement of serum triglyceride levels and by liver function studies. Fat overload may be accompanied by headache, irritability, low-grade fever, abdominal pain, nausea, coagulopathy, hepatomegaly, and splenomegaly. The drug of choice to help clear lipids from the patient's plasma is I.V. heparin solution.

Administration

Because TPN fluid has approximately six times the solute concentration of blood, peripheral administration results in sclerosis and thrombosis. To ensure optimal dilution, the superior vena cava—a wide-bore, high-flow vein—is catheterized. In central venous access, the catheter tip is not usually advanced into the right atrium because of the risk of cardiac perforation and dysrhythmias.

In adults and in children who weigh more than 4.5 kg (10 lb), subclavian venipuncture has been the most commonly used technique for catheterization of the superior vena cava (see "Assisting with insertion of a central venous line" in Chapter 13, p. 203).

Occasionally, the catheter is inserted into the brachial vein in the antecubital fossa or into one of the internal or external jugular veins. However, the catheter tip is always positioned in the superior vena cava.

Subclavian catheters typically remain in place 30 days or longer. When cannulation is necessary for longer than 2 months, implantation of a silicone rubber, Dacron-cuffed catheter may be preferred. The catheter is inserted into the jugular, subclavian, cephalic, thyroid, or facial vein and is then tunneled so the catheter exit site is lateral to the xiphoid process. Firm tissue ingrowth into the Dacron cuff, with secondary catheter fixation, occurs in 2 to 3 weeks; the cuff then serves as a mechanical barrier against bacterial and fungal in-

---

USE OF THE T.P.N. INFUSION LINE

When a central venous line is being used for TPN infusion, the following procedures are contraindicated:
- Infusion of blood or blood products
- Bolus injection of drugs
- Simultaneous administration of I.V. solutions
- Measurement of central venous pressure
- Aspiration of blood for routine laboratory tests
- Addition of medication to an intravenous hyperalimentation solution container
- Use of three-way stopcocks.

vasion. Many implanted catheters have remained in place 5 to 10 years. The location of the catheter exit site enables the knowledgeable and capable patient to care for his own catheter.

The medical care of patients receiving TPN is often very involved. (See *Use of the TPN Infusion Line.*)

Complications of TPN therapy

Major complications of TPN therapy may be insertion-related, septic, metabolic, or mechanical (see *TPN Complications,* pp. 240 and 241).

Catheter insertion complications

To minimize or obviate complications of central venous catheterization:
- Ensure that skin preparation before insertion is adequate.
- Serve as a quality control assistant to maintain strict sterile technique during the insertion procedure.
- Advise the patient to remain very still during the procedure, to reduce the risk of pneumothorax. Tell him to perform Valsalva's maneuver when the I.V. line is attached to the catheter hub. This increases intrathoracic pressure and central venous pressure, and prevents air from entering the vein (air embolus).
- Hang a container of dextrose 5% in water until a chest X-ray is taken to check catheter tip position. Proper catheter tip positioning in the middle superior vena cava is necessary before TPN solution can be infused.
- Assess the patient for complications associated with insertion of a central line into the subclavian vein, and report signs and symptoms to the physician immediately.

Sepsis

The most feared and serious complication of TPN is sepsis. Defects in normal defense mechanisms make the patient with malnutrition prone to infections. Furthermore, hyperglycemia, administration of steroids or immunosuppressives, chemotherapy, and radiation therapy increase the likelihood of infection caused by common skin bacteria, such as *Staphylococcus epidermidis* and *Staphylococcus aureus.* Increased incidence

---

T.P.N. DRUG COMPATIBILITY

Compatible
- Antibiotics (carbenicillin, cephalothin, cefazolin, chloramphenicol, clindamycin, erythromycin, gentamicin, tobramycin)
- insulin
- iron dextran
- aminophylline
- cimetidine
- 5-fluorouracil
- heparin
- low-dose glucocorticoids
- ranitidine
- metoclopramide
- morphine
- meperidine
- hydromorphone
- levorphanol

Incompatible
- amphotericin B
- ampicillin
- phenytoin

---

of candidiasis has been reported in patients receiving antibiotics and those with hypophosphatemia.

Sepsis is a potentially lethal complication; prevention depends on meticulous and consistent catheter care. (See "Equipment preparation and site care for TPN," p. 243.) Follow these guidelines to prevent sepsis:
- Provide catheter care at least three times weekly (once weekly for transparent dressings) and whenever the sterile occlusive dressing becomes wet, nonocclusive, or soiled.
- If possible, the same nurse should routinely change the catheter dressing to report comparative changes in skin appearance.
- Refrigerate 1-liter containers of TPN solution until 30 minutes before infusion, and 2-liter and 3-liter bags until 6 to 8 hours before infusion.
- Never incorporate a three-way stopcock into the infusion line or mix additives with the TPN solution after pharmacy preparation. The risk of contamination is too great.
- Do not manipulate the catheter unnecessarily or use it for measuring central venous pressure or infusing medication. This

T.P.N. COMPLICATIONS

COMPLICATIONS	SYMPTOMS	TREATMENT
Catheter-related		
Pneumothorax and hydrothorax	Dyspnea, chest pain, cyanosis, decreased breath sounds	Suction; insert chest tube.
Brachial plexus injury	Tingling and numbness along arm in peripheral TPN catheters	Remove catheter.
Air embolism	Apprehension, chest pain, tachycardia, hypotension, cyanosis, seizure, loss of consciousness, cardiopulmonary arrest	Clamp catheter. Place patient in Trendelenburg position on left side. Give oxygen as ordered. If cardiac arrest occurs, do CPR with patient on his left side. Keep patient in this position until asymptomatic.
Sepsis	Fever, chills, leukocytosis, erythema or pus at insertion site	Remove catheter and culture tip. Start appropriate antibiotics.
Metabolic		
Hyperglycemia	Polyuria, dehydration, elevated blood and urine glucose levels	Start insulin therapy or adjust flow rate.
Hyperosmolar hyperglycemic nonketotic coma	Confusion, lethargy, seizures, coma, hyperglycemia, dehydration, glycosuria	Stop dextrose. Give insulin and 0.45% NaCl to rehydrate.
Hypokalemia	Muscle weakness, paralysis, paresthesias, dysrhythmias	Increase potassium supplementation.
Hypomagnesemia	Tingling around mouth, paresthesias in fingers, mental changes, hyperreflexia	Increase magnesium supplementation.
Hypophosphatemia	Irritability, weakness, paresthesias, coma, respiratory arrest	Increase phosphate supplementation.
Hypocalcemia	Paresthesias, twitching, positive Chvostek's sign	Increase calcium supplementation.
Metabolic acidosis	Increased serum chloride level, decreased serum bicarbonate level	Use acetate or lactate salts of Na^+ or H^+.
Hepatic dysfunction	Increased serum transaminases, LDH, and bilirubin levels	Use special hepatic formulations. Decrease carbohydrate, and add I.V. fats.
Hypoglycemia	Sweating, shaking, irritability when infusion is stopped	Infuse with dextrose 10%.
Mechanical		
Obliteration of catheter lumen	Interrupted flow rate, hypoglycemia	Reposition catheter. Attempt to aspirate clot. If unsuccessful, instill urokinase as a fibrinolytic agent to declot catheter.
Air embolism	Apprehension, chest pain, tachycardia, hypotension, cyanosis, seizure, loss of consciousness, cardiopulmonary arrest	Clamp catheter. Place patient in Trendelenburg position on left side. Give oxygen as ordered. If cardiac arrest occurs, do CPR with patient on his left side. Keep patient in this position until asymptomatic.

(continued)

T.P.N. COMPLICATIONS (continued)

COMPLICATIONS	SYMPTOMS	TREATMENT
Mechanical (continued)		
Thrombosis	Erythema and edema at puncture site; ipsilateral swelling of arm, neck, or face; pain along vein; malaise; fever; tachycardia	Remove catheter promptly. Administer anticoagulant doses of heparin, if ordered. Venous flow studies may be done.
Fluid extravasation	Swelling of neck and shoulder area on affected side; pain	Stop I.V. infusion. Observe patient for cardiopulmonary abnormalities by assessment and chest X-ray.

may increase the risk of sepsis. Discourage the use of the central venous line catheter and delivery mechanism for any purpose other than supplying parenteral nutrients.
• Unless an emergency arises, do not use the catheter for obtaining aliquot portions of venous blood.

New double- and triple-lumen catheters are available for simultaneous infusion of medications that are incompatible with TPN solutions. (See *TPN Drug Compatibility*, p. 239, for information on which drugs are compatible with TPN.) A peripheral venous route is recommended for infusion of blood or blood products, for bolus injection of medication, and for administration of additional solutions during TPN therapy.

Do not automatically stop nutritional therapy if the patient suddenly develops a fever. Temporarily replace the TPN solution with dextrose 10% in water. Change the catheter dressing and tubing, and culture the TPN solution container, the administration tubing, and a sample of peripheral blood.

If the patient becomes afebrile 4 to 6 hours later, a culture may identify the source of the fever. (Negative cultures indicate a nonspecific pyrogenic response.) However, if the patient's temperature remains elevated or his condition deteriorates, peripheral blood is cultured a second time. Blood from the catheter is withdrawn for fungal culture and aerobic and anaerobic bacterial culture, and a sepsis workup is completed. Whenever the catheter must be removed, it is cultured for bacteria and fungi.

If the catheter is the source of the fever, the patient's adverse reaction usually subsides in 12 to 24 hours. Systemic antibiotic or antifungal medication is not required unless the patient fails to respond to catheter removal and develops septic shock.

In most cases, a new feeding catheter is not inserted until all blood cultures are negative; however, if interruption of nutrient delivery is life-threatening, a new catheter can be inserted immediately and changed every 48 to 72 hours using a modified Seldinger technique (over-the-wire procedure).

Metabolic abnormalities
The most common and serious metabolic complications are glucose intolerance and imbalances of potassium, phosphate, and magnesium.

Glucose intolerance and hyperglycemia
Endogenous insulin output increases gradually after the start of TPN therapy. The average adult tolerates 1 liter of TPN solution during the first 24 hours, then progresses to 1 liter every 12 hours for at least 2 consecutive days. Within the first 3 to 5 days, the typical adult can accommodate a daily ration of 3 liters of TPN solution or 500 mg/kg/hour of glucose without suffering adverse effects. This infusion schedule

allows pancreatic islet cells to adapt to the continuous dextrose load by increasing insulin output.

Hyperglycemia can occur when the total dextrose load is excessive, the delivery rate is too rapid, or glucose tolerance is lowered. In a patient with normal renal function, desirable glucose tolerance is verified by routinely measuring fractional urine and ketone concentrations every 6 hours. (Note: If your patient is receiving cephalosporins, methyldopa, aspirin, or vitamin C, do not use reagent tablets to analyze the urine since they produce false-positive readings.) Glycosuria is one of the first signs of sepsis when the infusion rate has not been altered.

A high serum glucose level also increases serum osmolality, causing a fluid shift from the intracellular space to the extracellular space. The expanded plasma volume dilutes serum sodium and bicarbonate concentrations, producing hyponatremia with hypertonic metabolic acidosis. This results in osmotic diuresis with both intracellular and extracellular dehydration.

Other symptoms of hyperglycemia include nausea, vomiting, diarrhea, confusion, headache, and lethargy. Untreated hyperosmolar hyperglycemic dehydration can lead to convulsions, coma, and death.

Hypokalemia
Severe hypokalemia can develop quickly since, during TPN-induced anabolism, potassium is transported into the cells. The hypertonicity of the glucose-insulin solution augments this flow.

Hypokalemia is suggested by muscle cramps and weakness, nausea, vomiting, paresthesias, and elecrocardiographic aberrations. Catastrophic myocardial dysfunction and dysrhythmias with ventricular asystole or fibrillation occur when serum potassium levels fall below 2 mEq/liter. A patient with severe cachexia may require as much as 60 to 100 mEq of potassium to reach equilibrium. As anabolism progresses and metabolism stabilizes, protein turnover slows, and potassium requirements are reduced.

Hypophosphatemia
Phosphorus depletion parallels potassium and protein depletion in the patient with malnutrition. Although high phosphate concentrations are found in bone, phosphate is not sufficiently labile or available for rapid redistribution throughout the body. If exogenous phosphorus is not provided in the TPN solution (usually 10 to 15 mEq/liter), blood levels may fall below 0.5 mg/dl. Neurologic and hematologic dysfunctions occur, exhibited by paresthesias, weakness, lethargy, and respiratory difficulty. Low serum phosphate levels are associated with impaired platelet function and decreased phagocytic and bactericidal activity of granulocytes.

Hypocalcemia
Calcium levels must be monitored closely because of the relationship between calcium and phosphorus. Calcium deficiency increases neuronal membrane permeability and allows sodium to enter cells more easily than usual, thus facilitating spontaneous depolarization. The central and the peripheral nervous systems can be affected, resulting in nausea, vomiting, diarrhea, hyperactive reflexes, muscular irritability, dysrhythmias, diminished cardiac contractility, and bleeding due to abnormal clotting. Usually, 4.8 to 9.6 mEq/day of calcium gluconate prevents hypocalcemia in the patient receiving TPN therapy.

Hypomagnesemia
Magnesium concentrations are much higher in the intracellular compartment than in the extracellular compartment, and loss of body cell mass probably results in relative magnesium deficiency. This may be manifested by muscle weakness, tremors, spasms, confusion, delirium, and seizures. Diuretics and cisplatin administered concurrently with TPN solution make the patient even more prone to hypomagnesemia. Usually, 10 to 15 mEq of magnesium sulfate/liter of TPN solution is sufficient to maintain normal blood levels.

Mechanical complications
The most common mechanical complications of the feeding catheter are obliteration of the catheter lumen, air embolism, thrombosis, and fluid extravasation.

Obliteration of the catheter lumen
This mechanical difficulty may be caused by kinking of the catheter. Repositioning it

and replacing the suture can resolve the problem. Unless the catheter is heparinized, any interruption in the continuous infusion of I.V. solution, such as catheter kinking, can precipitate clot formation as well as occlusion of the catheter.

To restore catheter patency, attempt to aspirate the clot by applying slightly negative pressure to the barrel of a sterile syringe fixed snugly into the hub of the catheter. *Never* push a clot or precipitate into the patient's venous system, since either could become a fatal embolus.

If aspiration is ineffective, notify the physician. Urokinase, a fibrinolytic agent, may be ordered to lyse the clot, and the following procedure may be used:
- Instill a volume of urokinase (5,000 IU/ml) equal to that of the catheter lumen.
- Wait 5 minutes and attempt to aspirate the clot; if unsuccessful, repeat every 5 minutes for 1 hour.
- Waste 3 to 5 ml of blood after the clot has been lysed.

Air embolism
To prevent this potentially lethal complication, use only Luer-Lok connections or secure any I.V. tubing junctions with tape. Replace tubing if a hairline crack develops. Before disconnecting the catheter from the infusion line and exposing its open hub to the atmosphere, make sure the patient is in the supine or Trendelenburg position. An additional precaution is to instruct the patient to perform Valsalva's maneuver or to hold his breath after deep inspiration.

A significant air embolism with sudden vascular collapse may be accompanied by apprehension, chest pain, tachycardia, hypotension, cyanosis, seizure, loss of consciousness, and cardiopulmonary arrest. Emergency nursing intervention includes immediate action to stop air infiltration into the bloodstream. The patient is then positioned on his left side, with his head down. Air can thus be dissipated slowly by way of the pulmonary outflow tract as normal circulation returns. Several minutes can elapse before the patient becomes asymptomatic.

Thrombosis
Thromboses of the subclavian or jugular vein or of the superior vena cava—although rare—are often associated with sepsis or a malpositioned catheter. The risk of this complication is lessened by optimal nursing care of the catheter exit site, by X-ray confirmation of proper catheter position, and by securing the catheter to the skin.

Evidence of thrombosis includes erythema and edema of the catheter insertion site; ipsilateral swelling of the arm, neck, or face; pain along the course of the vein; inability to obtain venous backflow of blood and sluggish flow rate; and systemic manifestations such as malaise, fever, and tachycardia. When thrombosis or thrombophlebitis occurs, the catheter must be removed promptly and the patient given anticoagulant doses of heparin to prevent thrombus propagation. With prompt action, signs and symptoms of venous obstruction usually subside within several days.

Fluid extravasation
If the feeding catheter ruptures or comes out of the vein, close observation for pulmonary and cardiac abnormalities, in conjunction with X-ray studies, is critical. Because of the proximity of the catheter tract to the thoracic cavity, this complication is serious. Furthermore, infusion of TPN solution into subcutaneous tissue can produce tissue necrosis, with sequential sloughing of the epidermal and dermal layers.

Equipment preparation and site care for TPN

Because TPN solution is a good medium for bacterial growth and the central venous line gives systemic access, contamination and sepsis are always a risk. Strict surgical asepsis is required during equipment preparation and dressing, and during tubing, solution, and filter changes. Site care and dressing changes should be performed at least three times weekly (once weekly for transparent dressings) and whenever the dressing becomes wet, nonocclusive, or soiled.

Tubing and filter changes are performed every 24 hours (according to NITA policy standards).

Equipment and materials
You will need an infusion pump, sterile tubing, two pairs of sterile gloves, an organic solvent (such as 10% acetone or 70% alcohol), an antimicrobial solution (such as

povidone-iodine), povidone-iodine ointment or a substitute, sterile 4"x4" gauze sponges, precut drainage gauze sponge, antiseptic adhesive balsam, and nonallergenic tape. You may need two face masks, sterile scissors, and a 0.22-micron cellulose membrane filter.

Newer administration sets include single tubing with an in-line filter incorporated into the tubing. Prepackaged dressing kits are available commercially.

Preparation
• Remove 1-liter bags or bottles of TPN solution from the refrigerator 30 minutes before use, and 2- or 3-liter bags 6 to 8 hours before use. Infusion of a chilled solution can cause pain, hypothermia, venous spasm, and venous constriction.
• Compare the contents of the solution with the physician's order. Then, observe the solution for cloudiness, turbidity, and particles, and inspect the container for cracks. If any of these are present, return the solution to the pharmacy.
• Wash your hands.
• Connect, in sequence, the pump tubing, filter (if applicable), and extension tubing. Tubing connections should be secured with Luer-Loks or tape to prevent accidental separation, which can lead to air embolism, exsanguination, and sepsis.
• Using strict aseptic technique, insert the pump tubing spike into the port of the TPN container, and start the flow of solution to prime the tubing and remove air. Gently tap the tubing to dislodge air bubbles trapped in the Y-sites.
• Attach a time tape to the TPN container to allow approximate measurement of fluid intake.

Steps
• Explain the procedure and clean the patient's overbed table with isopropyl alcohol (if you are not using a cart).
• If required, put on a mask, and position the patient so he is supine, with his head turned away from the catheter insertion site. If institutional policy dictates and the patient can tolerate it, place a mask over his nose and mouth. Place a sterile drape over the patient who is connected to a ventilator.
• Remove the dressing carefully, pulling the tape gently from the skin to minimize trauma. Then, inspect the skin for signs of infection and the catheter for leakage or other mechanical problems. (See *TPN Complications*, pp. 240 and 241.) Check that the sutures are intact.
• Put on sterile gloves, and cleanse the catheter insertion site with sterile sponges or swabs soaked in an organic solvent (such as 10% acetone or 70% alcohol). Work in a circular motion, moving from the insertion site 4" to 5" (10 to 14 cm) outward to the edge of the adhesive border to avoid introducing contaminants from the uncleansed area. To prevent damage, do not allow the organic solvent to touch the tubing.
• Working in a circular motion, as before, cleanse the insertion site and the catheter for 2 minutes with the povidone-iodine solution.
• Instruct the patient to perform Valsalva's maneuver or to hold his breath after inspiration as you change the I.V. tubing. If the patient is connected to a ventilator, change the tubing immediately after the machine delivers a breath. These measures increase intrathoracic pressure and prevent air embolism.
• Ensure that the junction of the catheter tubing is secure, remove the contaminated gloves, and put on a sterile pair.
• Continue to cleanse the skin with povidone-iodine solution for 3 minutes. Avoid removing this solution from the skin because its antimicrobial effects are long-lasting and continue after drying.
• Using a sterile swab or sponge, apply povidone-iodine ointment to the skin at the insertion site and to the hub of the catheter at the catheter-tubing junction, being careful not to loosen the connections.
• Arrange the sterile dressing sponges to shield the catheter and skin from airborne contaminants. A precut drainage sponge may be used around the catheter.
• Apply adhesive balsam to the skin at the perimeter of the dressing sponges.
• With the patient's arm abducted, tape the dressing securely and occlusively to the skin.
• Write the catheter insertion date, the date of the dressing change, and your initials on a strip of tape and apply this to the dressing.

- Using the chevron method, loop and tape the tubing (but not the filter) over the intact dressing to prevent tension on the catheter and its inadvertent removal if the tubing is pulled.
- Record the times of dressing, filter, and solution change, the condition of the catheter insertion site, your observations on the patient's condition, and any complications and resulting treatments.

Nursing considerations
- If the patient is allergic to iodine, use 70% alcohol for the antimicrobial treatment, increase skin preparation time to 10 minutes, and substitute a combination of antimicrobial and antifungal ointments for the povidone-iodine ointment.
- When using a filter, position it between the pump tubing and the extension tubing to avoid disturbing the underlying dressing.
- Observe the patient for signs of thrombosis or thrombophlebitis, such as erythema and edema at the catheter insertion site; ipsilateral swelling of the arm, neck, or face; pain along the course of the vein; and other systemic manifestations. If such signs occur, notify the physician immediately; he will remove the catheter and start heparin infusion at a peripheral site.
- Be alert for swelling at the catheter insertion site. This indicates extravasation of the TPN solution, which can cause necrosis. Check the catheter tubing for leaks from mechanical or chemical disruption.

Monitoring TPN

Because the patient receiving TPN is frequently in a protein-wasting state, the therapy causes marked changes in fluid and electrolyte status and in glucose, amino acid, mineral, and vitamin levels. Careful patient monitoring is necessary to assess his response to the nutrient solution and to detect early signs of complications. The TPN regimen can then be changed to preclude or alleviate complications.

Assessment of the patient's nutritional status includes physical examination, anthropometric measurements, biochemical determinations, and occasionally tests of cell-mediated immunity. Assessment of the patient's condition to detect complications requires recognition of the signs and symptoms of possible complications, understanding of laboratory test results, and careful record keeping.

Because the TPN solution is high in glucose content, the infusion must start slowly to allow the patient's pancreatic beta cells to adapt to it by increasing insulin output. Usually, if the adult patient tolerates the solution well the first day, the physician increases the intake to 1 liter every 12 hours for at least 2 days. After the first 3 to 5 days of TPN, the typical adult patient can usually tolerate 3 liters of solution per day without adverse effects.

Equipment and materials
You will need a test kit for urine glucose and ketone, a stethoscope, a sphygmomanometer, a watch with second hand, a scale, intake and output chart, a time tape, and additional equipment for nutritional assessment, as ordered.

If the patient is receiving cephalosporins, methyldopa, aspirin, or large doses of ascorbic acid, Tes-Tape should be used in place of Clinitest reagent tablets to avoid false-positive results in urine glucose and ketone determinations.

Steps
- Explain the procedure to the patient to diminish his anxiety and ensure cooperation. Instruct him to inform you if he experiences any unusual sensations during the infusion.
- Begin the infusion at a slow rate (usually 40 ml/hour), as ordered, to reduce the risk of hyperglycemia. Then, as ordered, increase the infusion rate (usually in 40 ml/hour increments) in adults to allow the pancreatic beta cells to increase endogenous insulin production, and to establish carbohydrate and water tolerance.
- Check the infusion pump's volume meter and the time tape every 30 minutes, or more often if necessary, to avoid an irregular flow rate, which can cause disturbances in glucose metabolism.
- Record vital signs every 4 to 8 hours, or more often if necessary, because increased temperature is one of the earliest signs of catheter-related sepsis.
- Collect a double-voided urine specimen every 6 hours and test for glucose and acetone. Notify the physician if observed glycosuria equals or exceeds ¼% (+ +).

CYCLIC T.P.N.: AN ALTERNATIVE TO CONTINUOUS T.P.N.

Cyclic TPN is a scheduled parenteral nutrition plan whereby a patient receives 1,000 to 2,000 calories parenterally overnight and the rest of his nutritional requirements orally during the day.

Cyclic TPN allows your patient freedom while receiving parenteral therapy. Instead of continuous feedings, he receives parenteral feedings of I.V. dextrose and amino acids for 12 to 16 hours. Then, during the remaining 8 to 12 hours, depending on the patient's particular regimen, he may receive I.V. fluids without glucose,* no I.V. fluids, and/or restricted enteral feedings.

Who receives cyclic TPN?
- A patient who is being weaned from TPN to enteral feedings.
- A patient on home TPN. Parenteral feedings overnight allow your patient to follow a routine life-style during the day.

Tips for stopping the TPN solution
When your patient stops continuous TPN and starts cyclic TPN, his blood glucose level must adjust to the new therapy. Stopping the TPN solution should not cause a hypoglycemic episode in a patient with normal endocrine function if you follow this procedure:
- Reduce the flow rate to one-half its normal rate for 1 hour before TPN is discontinued.
- Stop the infusion after 1 hour at this slower rate.
- Observe the patient closely for hypoglycemic symptoms (tachycardia, sweating, tremors, weakness, and hunger) for the first 2 hours after the infusion is stopped.
- Draw a blood sample 1 hour after the infusion is stopped, to measure blood glucose level. Rarely will patients develop symptoms or have blood glucose levels below 60 to 70 mg/dl.
- To maintain patency, flush the I.V. line after TPN infusion is discontinued. Follow institutional policy. Heparin (100 units/ml) in an amount equal to the volume of the catheter is recommended.

*When no parenteral glucose is given, insulin levels fall, allowing the normal process of lipolysis of essential fatty acids and transport of nonessential fats from the liver to occur.

- Accurately record daily fluid intake and output. Specify the volume and type of each fluid, and calculate the daily caloric intake. This record is a diagnostic tool for prompt, precise replacement of fluid and electrolyte deficits.
- Physically assess the patient daily. Weigh him at the same time each morning (after voiding), in similar clothing, using the same scale. Suspect fluid imbalance if the patient gains more than 1.1 lb (0.5 kg) per day. If ordered, measure arm circumference, triceps, and skinfold thickness.
- Monitor the results of routine laboratory tests, and report abnormal findings to the physician to allow appropriate changes in the TPN solution. Laboratory tests usually include serum electrolytes, BUN, and blood glucose at least three times a week and liver function studies, complete blood count and differential, serum albumin, phosphorus, calcium, magnesium, and creatinine every week. Less frequently ordered studies include serum transferrin, creatinine-height index, nitrogen balance, and total lymphocyte count.
- Monitor the patient for signs and symptoms of disturbances of glucose metabolism, fluid and electrolyte imbalances, and nutritional aberrations. Remember that some patients may require supplementary insulin for the duration of TPN; the pharmacy usually adds this directly to the TPN solution.
- Record serial monitoring indices on the appropriate flowchart to determine the patient's progress and response. Note any abnormal, adverse, or altered responses.
- Document signs and symptoms of complications and nursing interventions in the nurses' notes.

Nursing considerations
- When discontinuing TPN therapy, decrease the infusion rate slowly, depending on the patient's current glucose intake.

HOME PARENTERAL NUTRITION: A CHECKLIST

The home care patient receiving TPN may need instructions about some or all of the procedures and special topics listed below. Assess him carefully for possible knowledge deficits in these areas.

Basic Procedures	Special Topics
• Catheter heparinization	• Detection of complications
• Destruction of needles and syringes	• Financial support, home referral, medical alert, and networking services
• Dressing changes	• Follow-up appointments
• Drug administration	
• Handwashing	• Performance of necessary procedures when traveling
• I.V. fat emulsion administration	• Procurement and storage of supplies
• I.V. tubing changes	• Schedule for infusion and free time
• Pump operation	• Troubleshooting (air embolism; infection; thrombosis; clotted catheter; catheter fracture; pump malfunction; metabolic complications, such as deficiency and excess symptoms; broken I.V. container; contaminated solution or fat emulsion bottle)
• Self-monitoring (intake and output, daily weight, urine testing, temperature, diet record if patient is allowed partial oral intake)	
• Solution preparation	
• Use of sterile equipment (packages, gloves, syringes)	• Weaning

• Although most patients receiving between 2,000 and 3,000 calories/day tolerate sudden termination of the TPN infusion without incident, others experience profound reactive hypoglycemia. Therefore, taper the TPN solution dosage gradually over 24 to 48 hours. More rapid weaning is safe when the patient is ingesting sufficient carbohydrates or when peripheral I.V. infusion of dextrose 10% in water is begun.

• Cyclic TPN administration can also be used if a patient is being weaned from TPN to enteral feedings (see *Cyclic TPN: An Alternative to Continuous TPN*).

Preparing the patient for home parenteral nutrition

Home parenteral nutrition (HPN) enables prolonged or indefinite I.V. hyperalimentation. This technique has dramatically improved the health of patients with such chronic conditions as Crohn's disease and malabsorption syndrome, and with such acute conditions as incomplete bowel obstruction and antineoplastic therapy. It has also decreased the duration of hospitalization. Preparation for HPN usually requires 10 days to 2 weeks of extensive patient teaching and, when possible, of instructing the patient's family or others involved in his care.

To prepare for parenteral nutrition, a barium-impregnated silicone rubber catheter with a Dacron cuff is implanted in the superior vena cava. About 2 to 3 weeks after implantation, firm tissue covers the catheter cuff to provide a physical barrier to microbial contamination.

Usually, HPN patients can ingest part of their caloric requirements, requiring 10 to 14 hours of infusion nightly to supply the remaining nutrients. For both cyclic and continuous infusion, patient teaching must include all techniques for proper care (see *Home Parenteral Nutrition: A Checklist*).

Equipment and materials

You will need teaching aids, as available, I.V. infusion apparatus, dressings, TPN solution, a volumetric infusion pump, and a portable I.V. pole.

TPN solution is available in either premixed or component form. Not every patient is trained to mix the solution, because it requires precision and absolute aseptic technique to prevent contamination and subsequent sepsis.

Steps

- Assess the patient's ability to perform the care routines necessary for HPN, and determine if family members or friends can assist with or perform them, as needed. Consider the patient's motivation, mental aptitude, job or other daily activities, home environment, and the accessibility of hospitals, home nursing services, and other health care support systems.
- Formulate a teaching plan based on this assessment and on the patient's expectations. Be sure the plan incorporates goals, specifies criteria for meeting them, and proceeds from simple to complex tasks to allow the patient to develop confidence. Avoid placing time limits on goals, because learning ability and mastery of tasks requiring manual dexterity vary from patient to patient.
- If desired, develop a written contract between you and the patient that specifies the goals of HPN and the means to achieve them. Revise the contract as necessary to reflect changes in the patient's needs and performance. Use of the contractual relationship enhances the patient's independence, minimizes conflict and frustration between patient and nurse, encourages open communication, and promotes a cooperative patient-nurse relationship.
- Implement teaching sessions based on the goals specified in the contract. Conduct these sessions in a quiet area, and if possible arrange to have a family member present. When the family member understands the patient's pathophysiology, medical management, and progress, he tends to be less anxious, more satisfied with the quality of health care, and able to acknowledge the limitations and constraints of HPN.
- Use a variety of teaching-learning materials to accommodate differences in the ability of the learner. Some patients will benefit from the use of an extensively illustrated manual that includes the goals, equipment, procedures (with rationales), suggested learning activities, and evaluation of equipment for HPN. Procedures should be demonstrated with mannequins and real equipment to involve the patient actively and reduce anxiety about performing them. The patient's interest can be stimulated with audiovisual teaching aids.
- Offer positive feedback during all teaching phases.
- Before discharge, critically evaluate the patient's ability to perform HPN procedures, and ensure that all essential learning goals have been met.
- Remind the patient to change the catheter site dressing according to the recommended procedure, or whenever it becomes soiled or nonocclusive, and to change administration tubing as scheduled. Tell the patient that after the implanted catheter has been in place for 1 month or longer, his physician may allow him to remove his dressing and bathe or shower.
- Instruct the patient about the complications of home parenteral nutrition and how to handle them. (See *Troubleshooting Home Total Parenteral Nutrition*, pp. 250 and 251.)
- Remind the patient to prevent contact of the catheter with granular or lint-producing surfaces to avoid local tissue reaction from airborne particles and surface contaminants.
- Confirm a suitable HPN schedule with the patient, considering his nutritional needs as well as his life-style. Emphasize his adherence to the prescribed schedule and volume to prevent glucose imbalance.
- As ordered, arrange for a home referral service to help the patient adjust to HPN and resolve any difficulties.
- At discharge, provide the patient with supplies such as dressings, tubing, and TPN solution, and tell him how and where to obtain these supplies.
- Arrange for a follow-up physical examination and for obtaining specimens for laboratory analysis to detect fluid, electrolyte, and nutrient imbalances.
- Record the patient's learning progress in the nurses' notes.

Nursing considerations

- During teaching and treatment, recognize that conflicts can arise between you and the patient unless lines of authority and expectations are clear. Arrange nursing conferences to evaluate the patient's adaptation, to discuss counseling techniques for use during periods of maladaptation or crisis, and to provide management of expected stress in the patient.
- Suggest that the patient wear a Medic-Alert bracelet or subscribe to another medical alert service. Ensure that at least one nurse from the home health care team is always available to the patient in case of emergency.
- Because the financial burden of long-term or permanent HPN can be devastating—even with health insurance—provide the patient with the names of hospitals and philanthropies that provide services or financial support. Inform the elderly patient that Medicare may assume the cost of supplies and pharmaceuticals if he meets eligibility requirements.

Administering peripheral vein nutrition

Using a combination of an amino acid–dextrose (5% to 10%) solution and a fat emulsion, peripheral vein nutrition (PVN) can supply full caloric needs without the risks associated with use of a central venous catheter. Because this combined solution has a lower tonicity than a TPN solution, the success of PVN depends on the patient's tolerance of the large volumes of fluid necessary to supply full nutritional needs. PVN that includes a fat emulsion is associated with a lower incidence of phlebitis than an amino acid–dextrose solution infused alone. PVN is used only for periods of less than 3 weeks in patients who do not need to gain weight yet need to maintain optimal nutritional status. PVN is contraindicated in patients with malnutrition or disorders of fat metabolism, such as pathologic hyperlipemia, lipid nephrosis, and acute pancreatitis accompanied by hyperlipemia. It should be used cautiously in patients with severe hepatic damage, coagulation disorders, anemia, and pulmonary disease and in those who are at increased risk of fat embolism. In the premature or low-birth-weight infant, PVN with fat emulsion may cause lipid accumulation in the lungs.

Equipment and materials

You will need amino acid–dextrose solution, fat emulsion, two controllers, a Y-type nonphthalate administration set, alcohol sponges, and an I.V. pole. You may need venipuncture equipment.

A nonphthalate administration set, designed especially for simultaneous infusion of fat emulsion and amino acid–dextrose solution, consists of two lines in a Y configuration. This special tubing is necessary because lipids can extract small amounts of phthalates from phthalate-plasticized polyvinylchloride tubing. The vented line is used for the fat emulsion; the nonvented line, containing a filter, for the amino acid–dextrose solution.

Controllers that can accommodate the special tubing are needed to ensure the correct infusion rate, because the risk of phlebitis is decreased when two components are administered at approximately the same rate.

Preparation

- Inspect the fat emulsion for opacity and consistency of color and texture. If the emulsion looks frothy or oily, or if it contains particles or its stability or sterility is questionable, return the bottle to the pharmacy. Avoid excessive shaking of the bottle to prevent aggregation of fat globules. Similarly, inspect the amino acid–dextrose solution for cloudiness, turbidity, and particles and the bottle for cracks; if any of these are present, return the bottle to the pharmacy.
- Wash your hands and, using aseptic technique, take the nonphthalate tubing from its package.
- Remove the protective cap from the fat emulsion bottle, and wipe the rubber stopper with an alcohol sponge. Hold the bottle upright, and insert the vented spike through the inner circle of the rubber stopper. Hang the bottle, and squeeze the drip chamber until it fills to the level indicated in the tubing package instructions. Open the flow clamp, allow fat emulsion to flow through to the Y-connector, and then close the clamp. (See *Y-Connector Administration Set*, p. 252.)

TROUBLESHOOTING HOME TOTAL PARENTERAL NUTRITION

Complications, although rare, may develop while the patient is undergoing home total parenteral nutrition. Here are signs and symptoms he should watch for, and what he can do about them.

Problem	What to watch for	What to do
Infiltration	Swelling of tissues around catheter insertion site (shoulder, neck, or arm), discomfort, pain in shoulder or arm on catheter side; swollen tissues cooler than rest of body tissues	• Call the physician immediately if you think the catheter has come out of the vein or has ruptured. • Slow the flow rate if you cannot reach the physician immediately.
Cloudy solution or sediment in solution	Solution cloudy or showing undissolved particles	• Do not use. Solution may be contaminated. Return solution container to pharmacy at once for exchange. • If you are mixing your own solution, take extra care with preparation, and do not prepare more than 24 hours' worth of solution at a time.
Too rapid infusion	Nausea, headache, lassitude	• Check to be sure solution is flowing at the rate ordered by your physician. If you are using an infusion pump, check for mechanical problems. • If the flow rate is correct and symptoms persist, contact your physician.
Catheter dislodged	Catheter pulled out of vein	• Place a sterile gauze pad on insertion site, and apply pressure. • Notify your physician.
Crack or break in catheter tubing	Fluid leaking out through crack or break in tubing	• Apply padded hemostat above break, to prevent entry of air. • Call your physician at once.
Clotted catheter	Solution flow stops and does not enter the vein	• Notify physician. He may instill streptokinase or heparin into the catheter to try to dissolve clot.

(continued)

TROUBLESHOOTING HOME TOTAL PARENTERAL NUTRITION *(continued)*

Problem	What to watch for	What to do
Hyperglycemia (high blood glucose)	Fatigue, restlessness, confusion, anxiety, weakness, urine tests positive for sugar, and (in severe cases) possibly delirium and/or coma	• Notify physician at once.
Phlebitis	Pain, tenderness, skin redness, and warmth	• Rest, and apply gentle heat to the site. Elevate your arm if the catheter is inserted in your arm. • Relief should occur within 24 to 72 hours, and condition should subside within 3 to 5 days. • Notify your physician immediately. He may want to examine you or give you additional care instructions.
Infection	Fever (body temperature above 100° F. [37.8° C.]), redness and/or pus at insertion site	• Notify your physician so he can determine the fever's source. • If infection is present, the physician will remove the catheter to have the tip cultured.
Thrombosis	Redness and swelling around catheter entrance site; swelling of catheterized arm and of neck or face on same side of body; pain at insertion site and along vein; rapid heartbeat; fever	• Notify your physician at once. He will evaluate the catheter for removal. • These symptoms usually indicate blood clot formation around the catheter, a problem that requires prompt medical and nursing treatment.
Air embolism	Apprehension, chest pain, rapid heartbeat, low blood pressure resulting in dizziness and fainting, bluish appearance; problem caused by air entering catheter, usually during bottle changes	• Lie on your left side, with your head slightly lower than the rest of your body. • Stop the air leak. • Call 911 (emergency).

Note: Complications from home total parenteral nutrition are uncommon *if* proper technique is maintained. Despite the possibility of these problems, home total parenteral nutrition results in decreased hospitalization and significant cost savings for the patient. In addition, this therapy lets him maintain a more normal life-style.

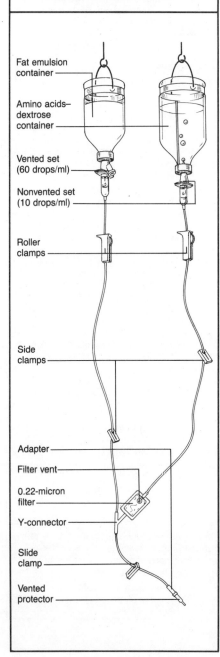

Y-CONNECTOR ADMINISTRATION SET

Labels: Fat emulsion container; Amino acids–dextrose container; Vented set (60 drops/ml); Nonvented set (10 drops/ml); Roller clamps; Side clamps; Adapter; Filter vent; 0.22-micron filter; Y-connector; Slide clamp; Vented protector

- Remove the protective cap from the container of amino acid–dextrose solution, and wipe the rubber stopper with an alcohol sponge. Hold the bottle upright, and insert the nonvented spike. Hang the bottle, and squeeze the drip chamber until the fluid reaches the desired level. Hold the filter with the Y-connector facing upward and the air vent downward. Open the clamp and let the solution flow until the filter and line are free of air. Close the clamp.
- Then, attach the controllers to the I.V. pole, and prepare them according to manufacturer's instructions.

Steps
- Explain the procedure to the patient.
- Obtain baseline vital signs, as ordered. If necessary, perform venipuncture. Select a relatively large, straight, unused peripheral vein. Use an over-the-needle catheter rather than a metal or winged device. (See "Inserting a peripheral line," p. 195.)

Starting the infusion
- Connect the administration set to the I.V. needle or catheter hub. Then, turn on the controllers and set them to the desired flow rate. Next, completely open the flow clamps to allow the controllers to regulate the flow rate.
- Monitor vital signs every 10 minutes for the first 30 minutes and every hour thereafter.

Changing solutions
- Remove the protective caps, and wipe the stoppers of the solution bottles with alcohol sponges.
- Turn off the controllers, and close the flow clamps. Using strict aseptic technique, remove each spike and insert it in the new bottle.
- Hang the bottles, turn on the controllers, and set the flow rate. Completely open the flow clamps.

Changing solutions and tubing
- Hang the new solution bottle and tubing alongside the old ones.
- Examine the skin above the insertion site for signs of phlebitis: redness, warmth, and pain. If such signs are present, remove the existing I.V. line and start a line in a different vein.

- Turn off the controllers, and close the flow clamps on the old tubing. Disconnect the tubing from the needle or catheter hub, and connect the new tubing.
- Open the flow clamps on the new bottles to equal, slow flow rates to prevent clot formation in the needle or catheter while inserting the tubing into the controllers.
- Remove the old tubing from the controllers, and insert new tubing according to the manufacturer's instructions.
- Turn on the controllers, set them to the desired flow rate, and completely open the flow clamps.
- Remove the old equipment and dispose of it properly.

Changing a dressing and needle or catheter
- Change the dressing at intervals specified by institutional policy, and inspect the insertion site for signs of phlebitis. Change the needle or catheter after 48 hours or at the onset of signs of phlebitis. Loop and tape the tubing over the dressing or use the chevron method so it will not be dislodged from the needle or catheter hub.
- Record the dates and times of all dressing and needle or catheter changes, the duration and amount of each infusion, and the patient's condition and response to therapy.

Nursing considerations
- Always use strict aseptic technique when handling equipment, and never reuse a partially empty bottle of fat emulsion, because it is an excellent medium for bacterial growth. Be alert for signs of sepsis: elevated temperature, glycosuria, chills, malaise, leukocytosis, and altered level of consciousness.
- Observe the patient's reaction to the fat emulsion. Usually, it is a feeling of satiety, but occasionally it is an unpleasant metallic taste.
- Fat emulsion may clear from the blood at an accelerated rate in a patient with full-thickness burns, multiple trauma, and metabolic imbalance, because catecholamines, adrenocortical hormones, thyroxine, and growth hormone enhance lipolysis and mobilization of fatty acids.
- Check serum triglyceride levels; these should return to normal within 18 hours after infusion of a bottle of fat emulsion. Typically, SGOT, SGPT, alkaline phosphatase, cholesterol, triglyceride, plasma free fatty acid, and coagulation tests are performed weekly to monitor the patient's response to therapy.
- Because lipase synthesis increases insulin requirements, increase the insulin dosage of the patient with diabetes, as ordered. For the patient with hypothyroidism, administer thyroid-stimulating hormone—which affects lipase activity—as ordered, to prevent intravascular accumulations of triglycerides.
- Immediate or early adverse reactions to fat emulsion therapy, which reportedly occur in fewer than 1% of patients, include fever, dyspnea, cyanosis, nausea, vomiting, headache, flushing, diaphoresis, lethargy, syncope, chest and back pain, slight pressure over the eyes, irritation at the infusion site, hyperlipemia, hypercoagulability, and thrombocytopenia. Thrombocytopenia has been reported in infants receiving 20% I.V. fat emulsion.
- Delayed but common complications associated with prolonged administration of fat emulsion include hepatomegaly, splenomegaly, jaundice secondary to central lobular cholestasis, and blood dyscrasias (thrombocytopenia, leukopenia, and transient increases in results of liver function studies). For unknown reasons, a few patients receiving 20% I.V. fat emulsion have developed brown pigmentation (I.V. fat pigment) in the reticuloendothelial system.

Review Questions

1. What is the most nutritionally complete form of parental nutrition?
    A. Total parenteral nutrition (TPN)
    B. Peripheral vein nutrition (PVN)
    C. Protein-sparing therapy
    D. Standard I.V. therapy

2. Which of the following is/are true regarding TPN?
    1. It must be administered through a central line
    2. It is a hypertonic solution
    3. It is for short-term use
    4. It may cause minor metabolic complications
        A. 1 only
        B. 1 and 2
        C. 1, 2, and 3
        D. 1, 2, 3, and 4

3. What is the *most* important nursing consideration in fat emulsion administration?
A. Not shaking the lipid container
B. Monitoring laboratory results
C. Administering I.V. heparin solution
D. Adhering to aseptic technique

4. An infusion control device is necessary for TPN administration. True or false?

5. Complications of TPN therapy include:
1. Catheter-insertion complications
2. Sepsis
3. Metabolic complications
4. Mechanical complications
A. 1 only
B. 1 and 2
C. 1, 2, and 3
D. 1, 2, 3, and 4

6. The most feared and serious complication of TPN therapy is sepsis. True or false?

7. The following symptoms indicate which TPN complication: apprehension, chest pain, tachycardia, hypotension, cyanosis, seizure, loss of consciousness, and cardiopulmonary arrest.
A. Sepsis
B. Hyperglycemia
C. Air embolism
D. Thrombosis

8. Which of the following is *not* a nursing action to clear a blocked catheter?
A. Reposition the catheter
B. Flush the catheter
C. Aspirate the clot
D. Instill a fibrinolytic agent

9. State four symptoms of hypokalemia.

10. What actions can you take to prevent air embolism?
1. Assist the patient to a supine or Trendelenburg position before disconnecting the infusion line
2. Ask the patient to perform Valsalva's maneuver or hold his breath after deep inspiration when tubing is changed
3. Use Luer-Lok connections, or tape all I.V. junctions
4. Replace tubing if a hairline crack develops
5. Purge all air from the tubing before attaching it to the catheter
A. 1 and 2
B. 1, 2, and 3
C. 1, 2, 3, and 4
D. All of the above

11. How often should site care for TPN be performed?

12. State three contraindicated uses for a central venous line being used for TPN.

13. TPN solutions should remain refrigerated until immediately before they are to be administered. True or false?

14. After the first 3 to 5 days of TPN the typical adult patient can usually tolerate 3 liters of solution per day without adverse reactions. True or false?

15. State two nursing actions for monitoring a patient during TPN therapy.

16. TPN infusions must be discontinued slowly to prevent hyperinsulinemia and resulting hypoglycemia. True or false?

17. Preparation for home parenteral nutrition usually necessitates 10 days to 2 weeks of extensive patient teaching. True or false?

18. What are two of the benefits of home parenteral nutrition?

19. PVN is used for long-term therapy. True or false?

20. For PVN a large, straight, unused peripheral vein should be selected for venipuncture and an over-the-needle catheter should be used. True or false?

Selected References

Drugs, 2nd ed. Nurse's Reference Library. Springhouse, Pa.: Springhouse Corp., 1984.

Elwyn, D.H. "Nutritional Requirements of Adult Surgical Patients," *Critical Care Medicine* 8:9, January 1980.

Englert, D.M. "The Role of the Nurse in Intravenous Hyperalimentation in the United States," in *Symposia: Second European Congress of Parenteral and Enteral Nutrition.* Edited by Wright, P. Stockholm: Almovist and Wiksell Periodical Co., 1981.

Grant, J.P. *Handbook of Total Parenteral Nutrition.* Philadelphia: W.B. Saunders Co., 1980.

"Hyperalimentation Standards of Practice of the National Intravenous Therapy Association (NITA)," *Journal of the National Intravenous Therapy Association* 3(6):234, 1981.

Lawson, M., et al. "The Use of Urokinase to Restore the Patency of Occluded Central Venous Catheters," *American Journal of Intravenous Therapy and Clinical Nutrition,* October 1982.

Plummer, A. *Principles and Practices of Intravenous Therapy.* Boston: Little, Brown and Co., 1982.

Procedures. Nurse's Reference Library. Springhouse, Pa.: Springhouse Corp., 1985.

Wilhelm, L. "Helping Your Patient 'Settle-in' with TPN," *Nursing85* 15(4):60, April 1985.

Blood and Blood Component Therapy

Blood and blood component therapy has become an increasingly common part of nursing care. It is the nurse's responsibility to provide safe transfusions; the patient's health depends in large part on your knowledge and ability to peform this complex procedure. This chapter discusses blood composition and physiology, nursing responsibilities in transfusion therapy, and specific transfusion procedures.

Blood composition and physiology

Blood plays a fundamental role in maintaining life. It carries everything the tissues require for metabolism and removes all cellular waste products.
• It supplies oxygen and nutrients for energy production and for tissue maintenance, growth, and repair.
• It transports cellular waste, including carbon dioxide, to the organs of elimination.
• It provides a defense against infection by transporting antibodies.
• It regulates and equalizes body temperature.
• It helps to maintain acid-base balance.
• It regulates fluid and electrolyte balance.

Because blood has so many important functions, any deficiency in its components requires correction. The objectives of transfusion therapy are to maintain blood volume, oxygen-carrying capacity, and coagulation. Transfusion therapy is also necessary in blood exchange (see the discussion of neonatal exchange transfusion in Chapter 17) and in cardiac surgery to prime the bypass machine and maintain circulation.

Blood components

Blood is made up of two basic components: cellular or formed elements and plasma. The cellular component, composed of erythrocytes (red cells), leukocytes (white cells), and thrombocytes (platelets), makes up approximately 45% of blood volume. Plasma, the liquid component, makes up approximately 55%. Plasma is composed of water (serum) and protein (albumin, globulin, and fibrinogen), as well as lipids, electrolytes, vitamins, carbohydrates, non-protein nitrogen compounds, bilirubin, and gases. (See *Blood Composition in the Average Adult.*)

Current techniques allow separation of freshly donated whole blood into its component fractions: red cells, plasma, platelets, granulocytes, $Rh_o(D)$ immune globulin, albumin, and plasma protein. Because each component can correct a particular hematologic deficiency, use of whole blood is seldom necessary. Whole blood is indicated only when a patient has lost considerable quantities of blood within a short time.

Component transfusion—the technique of administering specific components rather than whole blood to a patient—has several advantages. In addition to providing deficiency-specific therapy, it increases the potential uses of a single blood donation and helps ease the chronic shortage of blood. The risks of viral hepatitis and exposure to sensitizing agents or drugs in blood are also reduced. For a summary of the uses of each component, see *Blood Component Therapy,* pp. 270 and 271.

Immunohematology

Immunohematology is the study of antigen-antibody reactions and their effect on blood. An *antigen* is a substance that can initiate an immune response and induce the formation of a corresponding antibody. The estab-

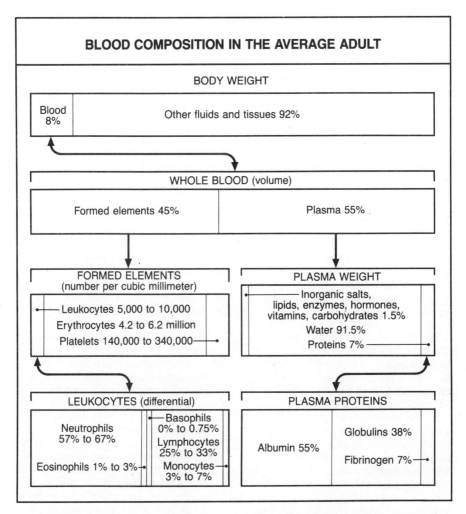

lished major antigens found in blood are inherited, such as those in the ABO system and the Rh-Hr system; others can be introduced into the body from exogenous sources, such as blood transfusions or drugs. An *antibody* can be defined as an immunoglobulin molecule synthesized in response to a specific antigen. Successful blood transfusions require tests that identify these naturally occurring or acquired antigens and antibodies to enable correct matching of donor and recipient blood. Among the most important of these tests are ABO blood typing, Rh typing, cross matching, the direct antiglobulin test, and the antibody screening test. If a transfusion reaction occurs despite correct transfusion of compatible blood, tests for other antibodies (such as leukoagglutinins) help identify the cause and prevent further reactions.

ABO blood group

All blood group classifications are based on the types of antigens present or absent on the surfaces of red blood cells (RBCs). Karl Landsteiner, Austrian immunologist and winner of a Nobel Prize in 1930 for his work in physiology, created the most important of these classifications—the ABO blood group system. Landsteiner classified human

RBCs as A, B, AB, or O, depending on the presence or absence of these surface antigens. Persons with group A blood have RBCs with A antigens. Those with group B blood have B antigens. AB blood contains both A and B antigens. Group O blood contains neither.

The ABO system also classifies two naturally occurring antibodies, anti-A and anti-B; one, both, or neither of these are found in the serum. Group A blood has anti-B antibodies, rather than anti-A antibodies, which would destroy the RBCs. Similarly, group B blood has anti-A antibodies. Group O blood has both anti-A and anti-B antibodies. And AB blood has neither type of antibody.

Because group O blood lacks both A and B antigens, it can be transfused in limited amounts to any recipient in an emergency, regardless of the recipient's blood type, with little risk of agglutination. For this reason, a person with group O blood is called a *universal donor*. (However, the transfusion should be given as packed RBCs, from which the plasma has been removed.) Because a person with AB blood has neither anti-A nor anti-B antibodies, he can receive A, B, or O blood (packed cells) and is called a *universal recipient*.

Typing and cross matching of donor and recipient blood are required before transfusion, to establish compatibility. (See *Transfusions: Blood Type Compatibility*.) These tests minimize the risk of a hemolytic reaction—the greatest danger with blood transfusions. A hemolytic reaction is the immune reaction that occurs when the donor's and recipient's blood types are mismatched—that is, when blood containing anti-A antibodies is mixed with blood containing A antigens or when blood containing anti-B antibodies is mixed with blood containing B antigens. When mismatching happens, the antibodies attach to the surfaces of the recipient's RBCs and cause the cells to clump together. The clumped cells can eventually plug small blood vessels and arterioles.

This antibody-antigen reaction activates the body's complement system—a group of enzymatic proteins—which promotes and accelerates RBC hemolysis and phagocytosis by the reticuloendothelial cells. RBC hemolysis releases free hemoglobin into the bloodstream, which can damage the renal tubules and lead to renal failure and death.

Rh blood group

In 1940, Landsteiner and immunoserologist Alexander S. Wiener developed the Rh blood group system after discovering a certain antigen on the surface of RBCs in virtually all rhesus monkeys. Among humans, about 85% of whites and an even higher percentage of blacks, Native Americans, and Asians carry this Rh antigen, $Rh_o(D)$ factor, on their RBCs. Such blood is therefore classified Rh-positive. The blood of the remaining portion of the population lacks this factor and is typed Rh-negative.

The Rh antigen is highly immunogenic—that is, it is more likely to stimulate formation of an antibody than are other known antigens.

Consequently, a person with Rh-positive blood does not carry anti-Rh antibodies in his serum, because they would destroy his RBCs. However, a person with Rh-negative blood develops anti-Rh antibodies following exposure to Rh-positive blood (by transfusion or pregnancy). A transfusion reaction usually does not occur after the initial exposure to Rh-positive blood, however. Anti-Rh antibodies generally develop slowly, over several months, causing the transfusion recipient to become sensitized to the Rh antigen. Subsequent exposure to Rh-positive blood then provokes a transfusion reaction and hemolysis, as in hemolytic disease of the newborn (HDN).

An important variant in the Rh system is the D^u antigen, which is somewhat less immunogenic than $Rh_o(D)$. The D^u antigen may not provoke antibody production in persons lacking it. However, all prospective donors must be screened for this antigen, which is more commonly found in blacks than in whites. Persons whose blood contains it are considered Rh-positive donors but are generally considered Rh-negative recipients. This precaution is taken to protect persons with a D^u variant whose blood may not be distinguished serologically from that of D^u blood.

Other clinically significant Rh antigens have been discovered since Landsteiner's and Wiener's work; these additional anti-

TRANSFUSIONS: BLOOD TYPE COMPATIBILITY

Precise blood-typing and cross matching are essential—if the donor's blood is incompatible with the recipient's, the transfusion can be fatal. In most instances, determining the recipient's blood type and cross matching it with available donor blood takes less than 1 hour.

The four blood groups are distinguished by their agglutinogen (antigen in RBCs) and their agglutinin (antibody in serum or plasma).

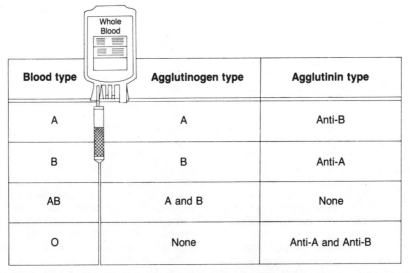

Blood type	Agglutinogen type	Agglutinin type
A	A	Anti-B
B	B	Anti-A
AB	A and B	None
O	None	Anti-A and Anti-B

After determination of the recipient's blood type, it can be cross matched with a donor's. The following chart shows the groups that are compatible:

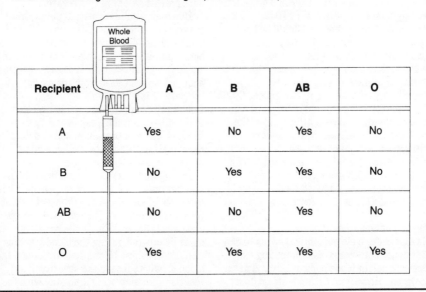

Recipient	A	B	AB	O
A	Yes	No	Yes	No
B	No	Yes	Yes	No
AB	No	No	Yes	No
O	Yes	Yes	Yes	Yes

gens, such as rh′ (C), rh″ (E), rh′ (c), and hr″ (e), are much less immunogenic and not so likely to provoke an antibody reaction. Tests for these antigens are done only in special cases, such as establishing paternity, studying families, or distinguishing between heterozygous and homozygous Rh-positive factors.

Selection and screening of blood donors
To qualify for selection, prospective blood donors must meet strict criteria established by the Scientific Committee of the Joint Blood Council and the Standards Committee of the American Association of Blood Banks. The purpose of these guidelines is to protect the donor and the recipient and to ensure safe, therapeutic blood transfusions.

Before donation, a detailed medical history must be obtained from the prospective donor, to detect conditions that may exclude or defer the donation. These include exposure to diseases that can be transmitted by blood transfusion (such as viral hepatitis, malaria, or acquired immune deficiency syndrome [AIDS]), active tuberculosis, alcoholism, drug addiction or drug therapy, pregnancy, and recent immunizations or dental surgery.

A physical examination and laboratory tests must then be done to determine if the prospective donor meets the following minimum health standards.
- Age: should be between 17 and 65 years.
- Weight: should be at least 110 lbs (50 kg).
- Systolic blood pressure should be between 90 and 180 mm Hg; diastolic, between 50 and 100 mm Hg.
- Pulse rate should be between 50 and 100 beats per minute and regular.
- Oral temperature should not exceed 99.6° F. (37.5° C.).
- Skin should be free of all lesions at the venipuncture site and show no evidence of intravenous drug abuse.
- Hemoglobin should be 12.5 grams/dl for females and 13.5 grams/dl for males.
- Hematocrit should be 38% or more for females and 41% or more for males.

Testing of donor blood
Except in the case of identical twins or of a self-donor (autotransfusion), testing for donor-recipient blood compatibility is never foolproof. However, certain tests on donor blood ensure the best possible blood selection for the recipient. These include:
- determining ABO and Rh blood groups
- detecting unexpected antibodies that can coat, hemolyze, or agglutinate RBCs
- cross matching of donor blood and recipient blood (usually done while testing for unexpected antibodies)
- determining white cell antigens through HLA (human leukocytic antigens) testing necessary for organ donation
- screening for hepatitis B, syphilis, and AIDS.

Nursing responsibilities

The most important nursing responsibility in transfusion therapy is to make sure you match the *right* blood with the *right* patient. Hemolytic reactions are most often caused by giving blood to the wrong person. Double-check the patient's name, medical record number, and ABO and Rh status, preferably with another nurse or a physician. If there is a discrepancy—no matter how slight—*do not* administer the blood. Instead, notify the blood bank immediately, so a substitution can be made without delay. Preventing potentially fatal hemolytic reactions from mismatched blood transfusions ranks among the most critical of nursing responsibilities. Uncompromising thoroughness and strict adherence to protocol ensure patient safety in this regard.

Depending on institutional policy, transfusion may require identification of the patient and blood product by two nurses before administration, to prevent errors and a possibly fatal reaction. It always requires a signed consent form from the patient. If the patient is a Jehovah's Witness, transfusion requires special written permission.

It is also a nursing responsibility to inspect blood prior to transfusion to detect abnormalities, and to be well versed in proper transfusion procedures.

During and after blood administration, another important nursing responsibility is to watch for signs and symptoms of a transfusion reaction. (See *Transfusion Reactions and Complications.*) Check the patient's vital signs before and during the blood transfusion. For the first 15 minutes, transfuse the blood slowly to lessen the severity of any reaction that may occur, and stay with the

TRANSFUSION REACTIONS AND COMPLICATIONS

Reaction	Cause	Signs and Symptoms
Acute intravascular hemolysis	ABO donor-recipient incompatibility (rare)	Rapid onset of hemolysis with chills, fever, low back or chest pain, hypotension, nausea, vomiting, and bleeding disorders
Delayed extravascular hemolysis	Immunogenicity (as in Rh incompatibility); previous immunization through pregnancy	Slow onset of hemolysis with symptoms listed above
Allergy	Sensitivity to foreign plasma protein very common in transfused blood	Onset of pruritus and urticaria, possibly with facial swelling, dyspnea, and wheezing
Circulatory overload	Rapid or excessive blood infusion over a short time	Onset of dyspnea and enlarged neck veins, leading to congestive heart failure or pulmonary edema
Febrile nonhemolytic	Sensitization to leukocyte, platelet, or protein antigens (very common); bacterial contamination (rare)	Onset of chills and fever; later symptoms resemble a hemolytic reaction

Complication	Cause	Signs and Symptoms
Hepatitis	Blood transfusion containing hepatitis surface antigen or core antibody	Delayed onset of hepatitis B with fatigue, nausea, and yellow scleras
Potassium toxicity	Potassium leakage (out of RBCs into plasma) during blood storage (rare)	Immediate onset of hyperkalemia with tachycardia and later bradycardia, nausea, and muscle weakness
Citrate toxicity	Massive transfusion of citrated blood; citrate binds with plasma calcium because the liver cannot metabolize it (rare)	Onset of hypocalcemia after several hours, with tingling in fingers, cramps, and convulsions
Syphilis	Blood contaminated with *Treponema pallidum* (rare)	Onset of syphilis after 4 to 6 weeks with painless genital chancres, rash, and headache
AIDS	Transfusion of blood contaminated with AIDS virus (rare)	Insidious onset of AIDS with fever, adenopathy, and skin nodules

patient. If a reaction occurs, stop the transfusion and begin an infusion of 0.9% NaCl at a keep-vein-open rate. Then notify the physician.

Many state laws require that only certified registered nurses administer blood and blood component therapy. However, in some places, a licensed practical nurse is allowed to regulate the transfusion flow rate, observe the patient for reactions, discontinue the transfusion, and document the procedure. Be aware of your state and institutional policies.

Transfusing whole blood, packed cells (RBCs), washed cells, and WBCs

Whole blood transfusion replenishes both the volume and the oxygen-carrying capacity of the blood. Transfusion of packed cells, in which 80% of the plasma is removed, restores only the oxygen-carrying capacity. Both types of transfusion treat decreased hemoglobin and hematocrit levels. Whole blood is usually transfused only when the decreased levels result from hemorrhage. Packed cells are transfused when the levels are decreased but blood volume is normal, to avoid possible fluid and circulatory overload.

Washed cells are similar to packed red cells in that 80% of the plasma has been removed, but they have been treated so that fewer white blood cells (WBCs) and platelets are present. Washed cells are used to replenish oxygen-carrying capacity in patients who have been previously sensitized by transfusions.

WBCs, primarily granulocytes, are sometimes used in the treatment of septicemia and other life-threatening infections unresponsive to routine therapies, and in severely granulocytopenic patients. Because some RBCs are normally found in WBC concentrates, compatibility testing (ABO, Rh type, and HLA, when possible) is recommended. Administration of WBCs must be repeated daily for 4 to 5 days or longer to be effective.

For a summary of blood component therapy, see *Blood Component Therapy,* pp. 270 and 271.

Equipment and materials
You will need a blood recipient set (filter and tubing with drip chamber for blood, or combined set); whole blood, packed red cells, washed cells, or WBC concentrates; 250 ml of normal saline solution; an I.V. pole; and a plasma transfer set (for transfusing packed cells with a straight set). You may need venipuncture equipment.

Both straight and Y-type blood administration sets are commonly used. Although both mesh and microaggregate filters are available, the latter type is preferred, especially when transfusing multiple units of blood. The microaggregate filter should not be used to transfuse WBC concentrates, however, because it will trap the granulocytes.

Preparation
• Prepare the normal saline solution for infusion. Insert the tubing spike, and prime the filter and tubing according to the manufacturer's instructions.
• Avoid obtaining whole blood or packed cells until you are ready to begin the transfusion because red cells deteriorate after 2 hours when stored at room temperature.
• If multiple units of blood are to be transfused, use a blood warmer, as ordered, to prevent hypothermia. (See *Using Blood-Warming Devices.*)

Steps
• Confirm the identity of the patient by checking the name, room number, and bed number on his wristband.
• Explain the procedure to him, and *make sure he has signed a consent form.*
• Take vital signs to serve as baseline values.
• If the patient does not have an I.V. line in place, perform venipuncture, preferably using an 18G catheter or 19G needle (see "Inserting a peripheral line," p. 195). Avoid using an existing line if the needle or catheter lumen is smaller than 20G.
• Attach the saline solution to the catheter or needle hub, and start the infusion at a keep-vein-open rate (about 10 drops/minute).
• Obtain whole blood, packed red cells, washed cells, or WBC concentrates from the blood bank. Check the expiration date on the bag, and observe for abnormal color, red cell clumping, gas bubbles, and extraneous material. Return outdated or abnormal blood to the blood bank.

USING BLOOD-WARMING DEVICES

Use the blood-warming devices shown below for massive, rapid blood transfusions and for exchange transfusions in the newborn, according to hospital policy, because rapid transfusion of cold blood can lead to hypothermia. You can also use these devices for transfusions in the patient with cold agglutinins. Both devices maintain a constant temperature of 98.6° F. (37° C.).

To use either blood warmer, first plug in the device. Then, prepare the patient and equipment as you would if using a straight-line set (for the blood-warming coil) or a Y-set (for the dry-heat warmer). After the administration set is free of air, close the flow-control clamp.

• Close the blood warmer's door and secure the latch. Turn the machine on, and allow it to operate for at least 2 minutes to warm the blood to 98.6° F. Avoid opening the door until completion of the transfusion to prevent loss of vacuum and mandatory replacement of the warming bag.
• While the blood is warming, connect the blood line's adapter to the female adapter on the bottom lead. When the desired temperature is reached, open the saline line clamp and the main flow clamp to fill the blood-warming bag with saline solution. Squeeze the outlet chamber on the top lead until it is flat, and continue to hold the chamber. When saline solution ap-

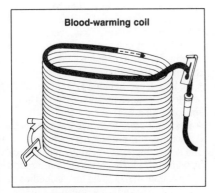

Blood-warming coil

To use a blood-warming coil
• Turn on the machine.
• Using aseptic technique, remove the coil from its sterile wrapper and close the clamps. Attach the blood line's male adapter to the coil's female adapter. Then, attach the needle to the opposite end of the coil.
• Immerse the coil in a basin of water warmed to 98.6° F. Keep the adapters dry to prevent water from entering the tubing and contaminating the entire setup.
• When the administration set and coil are fully flushed with blood, proceed as you would for straight-line administration. When the blood bag empties, flush the coil with normal saline solution to remove blood from the line. Replace the coil after 24 hours.

To use a dry-heat warmer
• Insert the warming bag into the blood warmer. Match the bottom lead (for the blood line) and the top lead (for the patient) to the corresponding openings in the blood warmer. *Note:* The top lead has a special outlet chamber attached to it. Mount the warming bag on the support pins, keeping the bag flat against the back panel. Then, secure the pins.

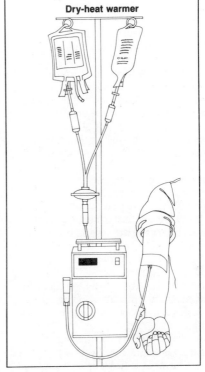

Dry-heat warmer

pears in the top lead chamber, close the main flow clamp and release the chamber. The chamber then automatically fills halfway with saline solution.
• Remove the adapter cover on the top lead and open the clamp. Expel residual air from the line. Then, close the clamp and recap the line. Next, proceed as you would when administering blood with a Y-set.

- Compare the name and number on the patient's wristband with that on the blood bag label. Check the blood bag identification number and ABO and Rh compatibility. Also, compare the patient's blood bank identification number, if present, with the number on the blood bag. Ask another nurse to verify all information to prevent transfusion error and a possibly fatal reaction.
- If you are administering *packed cells* with a *straight set,* use a plasma transfer set to add 50 ml of saline solution to the bag. With the flow clamp closed, insert one spike into the blood bag and the second spike into the saline container. Lower the packed cells, open the flow clamp, and allow 50 ml of saline solution to flow into the packed cells. Close the flow clamp, and gently rotate the bag to mix the saline solution and the cells. Then, insert the straight set spike into the other port on the blood bag. Leave the plasma transfer set in place during the transfusion.
- If you are administering *packed cells* with a *Y-type set,* add saline solution to the bag to dilute the cells by closing the clamp between the patient and the drip chamber and opening the clamp on the blood line. Then, lower the blood bag below the saline container and let 30 to 50 ml of saline flow into the packed cells. Finally, close the clamp on the blood line, rehang the bag, rotate it gently to mix the cells and saline solution, and close the clamp on the saline line.
- If you are administering *whole blood,* gently invert the bag several times to mix the cells.
- Open all clamps between the blood bag and the patient, and adjust the flow clamp closest to the patient to deliver 25 to 30 drops/minute. This rate will minimize any transfusion reaction, which usually occurs within this period.
- Remain with the patient, monitor vital signs according to institutional policy, and watch for signs of transfusion reaction. If signs develop, take and record vital signs, and proceed accordingly. (See "Managing transfusion reactions," p. 273.) If no signs of a reaction appear within 30 minutes, adjust the flow clamp to the ordered infusion rate. Raising and lowering the blood bag to adjust the rate reduces the risk of hemolysis from pressure on the tubing.
- After completion of the transfusion, flush the filter and tubing with saline solution, if recommended by the manufacturer. Then, reconnect the original I.V. fluid or remove the I.V. line.
- Return the empty blood bag to the blood bank, and discard the tubing and filter.
- Take and record the patient's vital signs.
- Record the date and time of transfusion, the type and amount of transfused blood, the patient's vital signs, and your check of all identifying data. Document any transfusion reaction and treatment.

Nursing considerations
- Although some microaggregate filters can be used for up to 10 units of blood, always replace the filter if more than 1 hour elapses between transfusions.
- Avoid piggybacking blood, because the secondary set can become dislodged from the injection site, causing contamination of the transfused blood.
- Adding drugs to blood is contraindicated because it complicates identifying the source of an adverse reaction.
- Despite increasingly accurate compatibility testing, transfusion reactions can occur, and despite donor screening, hepatitis can be transmitted. However, current practices of screening donor blood for antibodies to the AIDS virus will prevent transmission of AIDS via transfusion because blood banks will not accept blood in which the antibodies are found.
- Circulatory overload and hemolytic, allergic, febrile, and pyrogenic reactions can result from any transfusion.
- Coagulation disturbances, citrate intoxication, hyperkalemia, acid-base imbalance, loss of 2,3-diphosphoglycerate, ammonia intoxication, and hypothermia can result from massive transfusion.
- Blood may be transfused under pressure when rapid replacement is necessary. (See *Transfusing Blood Under Pressure.*)
- If a hematoma develops at the needle site, stop the infusion immediately. Remove the needle or catheter, and cap the tubing with a new needle and guard. Notify the physician. He will probably want you to place ice on the site for 24 hours, and after that warm compresses. Promote reabsorption of

TRANSFUSING BLOOD UNDER PRESSURE

Transfuse blood under pressure only when rapid replacement is necessary. Begin this procedure by selecting the proper equipment—a pressure cuff or a positive-pressure set. The *pressure cuff*, which resembles a sleeve, is placed over the blood bag and inflated; a pressure gauge, attached to the cuff, is calibrated in millimeters of mercury. The *positive-pressure set* is a gravity administration set containing a built-in pressure chamber that increases the flow rate when manual pressure is applied externally to the chamber.

Prepare the patient and set up equipment in the same way as with a standard administration set. Prime the filter and tubing to remove all air from the administration set. Connect the tubing to the needle or catheter hub. Throughout transfusion, watch the patient closely for complications, such as infiltration or extravasation, which can occur quite rapidly.

• To set the flow rate, turn the screw clamp on the pressure cuff counterclockwise. Compress the pressure bulb of the cuff to inflate the bag until you achieve the desired flow rate. Then, turn the screw clamp clockwise to maintain this constant flow rate. *Note*: As the blood bag empties, the pressure decreases, so check the flow rate regularly and adjust the pressure in the pressure cuff as necessary to maintain a consistent flow rate. But do not allow the cuff needle to exceed 300 mm Hg, because excessively high pressure may cause hemolysis of red blood cells.

To use a positive-pressure set
• Open the upper and lower flow clamps on the administration set. Manually compress and release the pump chamber to force blood down the tubing and into the patient. Allow the pump chamber to refill completely before compress-

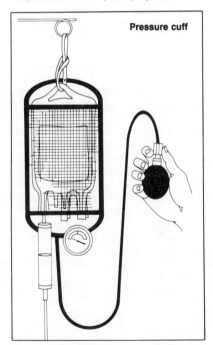

Pressure cuff

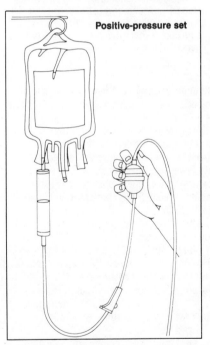

Positive-pressure set

To use a pressure cuff
• Insert your hand into the pressure cuff sleeve and pull the blood bag upward through the center opening. Then, grasp one loop of the sleeve, slip it through the blood bag loop, and pull the other sleeve loop through it.
• Hang the blood bag on the I.V. pole. Open the flow clamp on the tubing.

ing it again. Continue to compress and release the chamber until the blood bag empties or until rapid administration is no longer necessary. To discontinue transfusion under pressure, stop compressing the chamber and adjust the flow rate as for standard administration.

ENCOURAGING VOLUNTARY BLOOD DONATIONS

If your patient needs a blood transfusion, he can expect it to be expensive. But you can suggest ways to help him cut that cost. If time permits, he should be advised that he can donate his own blood and have it held for his own use when his surgery is performed. Or, family and friends can be encouraged to become volunteer blood donors. Then, the blood your patient receives will be free, even though the administration fees will remain the same.

Start your explanation of the volunteer blood donor program by asking if the potential donors are already enrolled in a program at either their place of employment or a religious institution. If they are not, suggest they contact a Red Cross center. Explain how a trained staff member draws each donor's blood. Remind them that it is simple, almost painless, and relatively hazard-free. Reassure donors that AIDS is not transmitted through donation.

As you may know, almost anyone between ages 17 and 65 can donate blood. But a person is ineligible if he is receiving medication, has an infectious disease, or has traveled in a malarial area within the past 3 years. A healthy, eligible adult can donate a pint of blood once every 2 months. However, only about 3% of the eligible donors in the United States give blood annually.

Because of this, blood banks frequently replenish their supplies with purchased blood. And when they do, they risk collecting blood that is unhealthy. With purchased blood the chances of transmitting disease are up to 10 times greater than with donated blood.

Encourage eligible donors to give blood whenever possible. Make sure you know the location of local blood collection centers, and keep printed material about them handy.

---

the hematoma by gently exercising the involved limb. Restart the line in another site as ordered.
• If the transfusion stops running, check the distance between the blood bag and the insertion site. Make sure it is at least 3' (1 m) above the site. Check the flow clamp to make sure it is open. Observe the filter to see if it is completely immersed in blood. Rock the bag back and forth gently to agitate blood cells that may have settled to the bottom. Squeeze the tubing and flashbulb to get the fluid moving again. Untape the dressing over the insertion site, and make sure the needle or catheter is still correctly placed in the vein. Reposition it, if necessary. If you are using a Y-set, open the saline solution line to dilute the blood and facilitate its flow.
• If the blood bag is empty and a new unit has not arrived from the blood bank, hang a container of normal saline solution (if not hung already), and administer it slowly until the new unit arrives. If you are using a Y-set, close the blood line clamp, open the saline solution line clamp, and let the saline solution run slowly until the new unit arrives. Decrease the flow rate or clamp the line before you attach the new unit of blood.
• Provide emotional support to the patient and family. Remember that they will probably be anxious and frightened. Many people associate blood transfusions with serious illness. Do what you can to ease their stress. Encourage questions and answer them honestly. Correct misconceptions, but do not mislead your patient or his family by minimizing the importance of the therapy. Explain the procedure in simple terms so they understand what is happening.
• When appropriate, explain to the patient and family about voluntary blood donation. (See *Encouraging Voluntary Blood Donations.*)
• At some institutions, transfusion of hemoglobin solutions may be done to treat patients who have suffered massive hemorrhage. (See *Learning About Hemoglobin Solutions.*)
• For nursing considerations relevant to each blood component, see *Blood Component Therapy,* pp. 270 and 271.

LEARNING ABOUT HEMOGLOBIN SOLUTIONS

Soon, you may find yourself giving a hemoglobin solution to a patient who has suffered massive hemorrhage. Although not yet in clinical use in the United States, this oxygen-carrying blood substitute may soon be a standard treatment for short-term restoration of circulating oxygen levels.

Hemoglobin solutions are prepared from outdated red blood cells (RBCs). By crystallizing hemoglobin molecules, researchers have developed a simple, rapid method for preparing a hemoglobin solution that is free of toxic substances released by RBC membranes during processing.

Advantages. Why give a hemoglobin solution rather than whole blood? One reason is that hemoglobin solution is less viscous. And, unlike whole blood, it has no microaggregates to clump together in the microcirculatory system. For both these reasons, hemoglobin solution is especially useful when the patient's microcirculation is compromised.

Hemoglobin solution has other advantages, too. For example, it:
- requires no blood-typing or cross matching.
- is compatible with I.V. solutions and blood, for easy administration.
- will not cause an antigen reaction.
- can be stored for long periods.
- has an osmotic effect, so it tends to hold fluid in blood vessels.

Disadvantages. Crystalloid hemoglobin solutions under study have a very high oxygen affinity; in other words, they resist releasing oxygen to tissues. When arterial oxygen levels are already low, as in hypovolemic shock, the oxygen affinity is even greater. These solutions also tend to increase the oxygen affinity of free hemoglobin.

Transfusing plasma and plasma fractions

Transfusion of plasma and its fractions serves a variety of therapeutic purposes. For example, transfusion of platelets, which are suspended in 30 to 50 ml of plasma, is ordered to correct an extremely low platelet count (below 10,000/mm³), which can occur in patients with hematologic diseases, such as aplastic anemia and leukemia, and in those receiving antineoplastic chemotherapy. Platelet transfusion is not indicated in disseminated intravascular coagulation and in disorders causing rapid platelet destruction, such as idiopathic thrombocytopenic purpura. Usually, a large quantity of platelets—typically four or more units for an adult—are required to prevent or control bleeding.

Transfusion of fresh or fresh frozen plasma (FFP), which contains most clotting factors but no platelets, is ordered to treat an undetermined clotting factor deficiency, a specific factor deficiency when that factor alone is not available, and factor deficiencies resulting from hepatic disease or blood dilution. Transfusion of FFP is the only treatment for Factor V deficiency.

Although plasma functions as a blood volume expander, the blood products used more commonly for this function are plasma protein fraction (PPF), which is a 5% solution of selected proteins (albumin and some globulins) from pooled plasma in a buffered, stabilized saline diluent, and albumin, which is extracted from plasma, heat-treated, chemically processed, and available in 5% (isotonic) and 25% (hypertonic) preparations. Both preparations are also used to treat hypoproteinemia and hypoalbuminemia. Hypertonic albumin also reduces cerebral edema by drawing large amounts of extravascular fluid into the vascular system. Albumin transfusion is contraindicated in severe anemia because of the risk of cellular dehydration, and should be administered cautiously in cardiac and pulmonary disease because of the risk of congestive heart failure caused by circulatory overload.

Transfusion of cryoprecipitate, which forms when FFP thaws slowly, replaces missing clotting factors in hemophilia A, von Willebrand's disease, and fibrinogen and Factor XIII deficiencies. However, transfusion of Factor VIII (antihemophilia factor) concentrate is the long-term treatment of choice for hemophilia A because the amount of Factor VIII per vial varies less than with cryoprecipitate. Prothrombin complex (Factors II, VII, IX, and X), obtained through chemical fractionation of pooled plasma, can be used to treat hemophilia B, severe liver disease, and acquired deficiencies of Factors II, VII, IX, and X. However, it is used infrequently because of the associated high risk of transmitting hepatitis and AIDS.

Equipment and materials
You will need plasma or plasma fraction, an administration set (see *Transfusion Sets*), normal saline solution, an alcohol sponge, an 18G to 20G 1" needle, and adhesive tape. You may need venipuncture equipment.

Preparation
- Obtain the necessary unit of plasma or plasma fraction from the blood bank just before transfusion. Check the expiration date, and carefully inspect the plasma for cloudiness and turbidity, and the plastic bag for leaks.
- Use FFP within 4 hours, because it does not contain preservatives.
- When transfusing a *Factor VIII* or *prothrombin preparation,* carefully reconstitute it according to the manufacturer's directions, if you did not receive it already prepared by the pharmacy.
- For administration of *Factor VIII concentrate,* avoid using a glass syringe, to prevent binding to ground glass surfaces.

Steps
- Positively identify the patient by carefully comparing the name and number on his wristband with the information on the laboratory slip.
- Explain the procedure to him to ease his anxiety and promote cooperation.
- *Make sure he has signed a consent form.*
- Obtain baseline vital signs.
- Wash your hands.
- If an I.V. line is already in place, check the insertion site for inflammation and the line for patency. If the primary solution cannot be interrupted or if no I.V. line is in place, perform a venipuncture and start the saline infusion at a keep-vein-open (KVO) rate.
- If you are using an existing I.V. line, replace the infusing solution with saline, and adjust the flow to a KVO rate. Insert a sterile plug in the original solution container to prevent contamination.

Administering plasma, FFP, albumin, Factor VIII concentrate, or prothrombin complex
- Attach the administration set to the plasma or plasma product and the needle to the tubing. Then, prime the system.
- Using an alcohol sponge, wipe the Y-injection port of the primary administration set. Then, insert the needle from the plasma product administration set into the

ADMINISTRATION OF GAMMA GLOBULIN

Gamma globulin, the antibody-containing portion of plasma that is obtained by chemical fractionation of pooled plasma, is used to prevent infectious hepatitis (Type A), rubeola, mumps, pertussis, and tetanus (if given before clinical symptoms develop) and to treat hypogammaglobulinemia and agammaglobulinemia. Administration of gamma globulin is contraindicated in patients with known hypersensitivity to it or an anti-immunoglobulin (anti-IgA) antibody.

Gamma globulin is administered intramuscularly. Follow the manufacturer's instructions. If you are injecting more than a 5-ml dose, divide it into two doses, and administer them at different sites. Discard equipment after use or return it to the blood bank, according to institutional policy.

TRANSFUSION SETS

The component syringe set contains two side clamps: one located slightly below the bag spike, the other slightly below the Y-connector (as shown at right). After you have primed the tubing and connected the set to the patient, draw the platelets into the syringe and depress the plunger. Control the administration rate by depressing the plunger at various speeds.

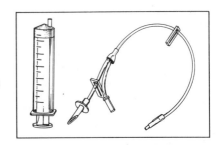

The component drip set contains tubing, a drip chamber, and filter (as shown at right). Prepare for transfusion by compressing the drip chamber until the filter is completely covered. Then, close the flow rate clamp, hang the set, and connect the I.V. line to it. Control the administration rate by adjusting the flow clamp. This set also comes in a Y type; saline is connected on one side to prime and flush the system, and the blood product is connected on the other side.

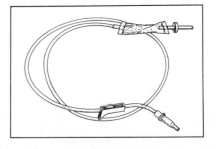

injection port, stop the saline infusion, and adjust the flow rate of the plasma or plasma product, as ordered. (See *Blood Component Therapy*, pp. 270 and 271.)

Administering platelets or cryoprecipitate with a component drip set

- Open the port of the platelet or cryoprecipitate bag by pulling back the tabs. Then, remove the protective cover of the administration set spike.
- Close the flow clamp and, using a twisting motion, insert the administration set spike into the port. Hang the bag, compress the drip chamber until fluid fully covers the filter, and open the clamp. Then, prime the tubing and close the clamp.
- Using an alcohol sponge, wipe the Y-injection port of the primary administration set. Then, insert the needle from the component drip set into the injection port and stop the saline infusion.
- Completely open the flow clamp on the component drip set to administer the platelets or cryoprecipitate rapidly, preventing clumping or loss of activity.
- Administer additional bags of platelets by removing the administration set spike and inserting it in a new bag. Close the clamp and attach the new bag before the drip chamber empties, to keep air from entering the line.
- After completion of the infusion, flush the line with 20 to 30 ml of saline solution. Then, disconnect the I.V. line, or if therapy is scheduled to continue, hang the original I.V. solution and adjust the flow rate, as ordered.
- Record the type and amount of plasma or plasma fraction administered, duration of transfusion, baseline vital signs, and any adverse reactions.

Administering platelets or cryoprecipitate with a component syringe set

- Close both clamps on the syringe set. Then, open the port of the platelet or cryoprecipitate bag by pulling back the tabs. Next, remove the protective cover of the administration set spike.
- Using a twisting motion, insert the administration set spike into the port. Then, attach the syringe to the Luer-tip port.

BLOOD COMPONENT THERAPY

All blood component products are extracted from whole blood, but because each has different characteristics some components treat certain hematologic disorders better than others. The physician will choose a blood component product based on how well it will treat your patient's condition. For example, if your patient needs volume replenishment quickly, he will receive a volume expander. If his blood is not clotting properly, he will receive a product with clotting factors.

Here is a table to help you learn more about blood component products and their uses.

Type	Contents	Uses	Nursing Considerations
Whole blood	• Red blood cells (RBCs), white blood cells (WBCs), platelets, plasma, and plasma clotting factors	• To restore blood volume and to replenish oxygen-carrying capacity in a patient with massive hemorrhage	• Administer through a large-gauge needle or angiocath over 2 to 4 hours, or as ordered.
Packed cells	• RBCs and 20% plasma • Less sodium and potassium than whole blood	• To replenish blood's oxygen-carrying capacity while minimizing risk of fluid overload in patients with severe anemia, slow blood loss, or congestive heart failure	• Administer more slowly than whole blood (unless diluted with saline solution).
Washed cells	• RBCs and 20% plasma • Fewer WBCs and platelets than packed cells	• To replenish blood's oxygen-carrying capacity in patients previously sensitized by transfusions	• Administer at a slower rate than whole blood (unless diluted with saline solution).
Granulo-cytes	• WBCs and 20% plasma	• To treat life-threatening granulocytopenia (<500/mm^3)	• Administer rapidly. • Expect the patient to develop fever, chills, hypertension, or disorientation during transfusion; these are considered to be transfusion reactions.

(continued)

BLOOD COMPONENT THERAPY (continued)

Type	Contents	Uses	Nursing Considerations
Plasma (fresh frozen)	• Clotting Factors II, III, V, VII, IX, X, and XIII; fibrinogen; prothrombin; albumin; and globulins	• To treat patients with clotting factor deficiencies (the only treatment for Factor V deficiency) • To expand volume	• Fresh frozen plasma takes 20 minutes to thaw, so call the blood bank ahead of time. • Administer one unit over 1 hour.
Platelets	• Platelets, WBCs, and plasma	• To correct low platelet counts ($<10,000/mm^3$)	• Administer one unit over 10 minutes.
Cryoprecipitate	• Factors VIII and XIII and fibrinogen	• To replace clotting factors in patients with disseminated intravascular coagulation, hemophilia A, von Willebrand's disease, fibrinogen deficiency, or Factor XIII deficiency	• Administer rapidly immediately after thawing to ensure factor activation.
Albumin (5% and 25%)	• 5% and 25% albumin from plasma	• To replace volume in patients suffering from shock, burns, hypoproteinemia, or hypoalbuminemia	• Administer 1 ml/min or, *if the patient is in shock,* administer rapidly. • May administer with dextrose 5% in water.
Plasma protein fraction	• 5% albumin and globulin solution in saline solution	• To expand volume in patients with burns, hemorrhage, or hypoproteinemia	• Administer 1 ml/min. • Risk of hepatitis or sensitization is low.
Prothrombin	• Factors II, VII, IX, and X	• To replace clotting factors in patients with hemophilia B or bleeding secondary to severe liver disease	• Prothrombin is used infrequently because of increased hepatitis risk.

- Open the clamp above the Y-connection, aspirate the contents of the bag into the syringe, and close the clamp. Then, open the clamp below the Y-connection, hold the syringe upright, prime the tubing, and close the clamp.
- Using an alcohol sponge, wipe the Y-injection port of the primary administration set.
- Insert the needle from the syringe set into the injection port, and stop the saline infusion. Depress the syringe plunger and rapidly administer the platelets or cryoprecipitate to prevent clumping or loss of activity.
- Administer additional bags of platelets by removing the administration set spike and inserting it in a new bag. Close the clamp closest to the patient before aspiration.
- After completion of the infusion, flush the line with 20 to 30 ml of saline solution. Then, disconnect the I.V. line, or if therapy is scheduled to continue, hang the original I.V. solution and adjust the flow rate, as ordered.
- Record the type and amount of plasma or plasma fraction administered, duration of transfusion, baseline vital signs, and any adverse reactions.

Nursing considerations
- Because platelet transfusion can be time-consuming, schedule your daily patient care duties around it.
- During transfusion therapy, check frequently for signs of bleeding, and instruct the patient to report even slight bleeding.
- If the patient requires whole blood or packed cells after plasma transfusion, first administer the plasma with a blood set. Then, maintain the I.V. line with saline solution at a KVO rate until you are ready to transfuse blood.
- If you have difficulty establishing the flow of an albumin infusion, suspect an air lock in the vent on the tubing spike. To correct this, wipe the container's rubber stopper with an alcohol sponge and insert a 20G 1" needle. If unsuccessful, change the tubing. If still unsuccessful, obtain a new container of albumin and a new administration set, and return the defective set.
- If albumin has been diluted or added to another solution, use it as soon as possible to prevent bacterial growth.

- Always use an administration set supplied by the manufacturer, because it contains a small concealed filter that removes particles and other contaminants.
- For other nursing considerations, see *Blood Component Therapy*, pp. 270 and 271.

Managing transfusion reactions

Transfusion reactions can result from a single or massive transfusion of blood or blood products. Most transfusion reactions occur during or shortly after transfusion and require immediate recognition and prompt nursing intervention to prevent further complications and, possibly, death. Recognition and intervention are particularly important if the patient is unconscious or so heavily sedated that he cannot report the common signs and symptoms.

Equipment and materials
You will need normal saline solution, an I.V. administration set, a sterile urine specimen container, a needle and syringe and tubes for blood samples, and a transfusion reaction report form. You may need emergency equipment.

Steps
- As soon as you suspect an adverse reaction, stop the transfusion, change the I.V. tubing, and start the saline infusion at a keep-vein-open rate to maintain venous access. *Do not discard the blood bag or administration set.*
- Notify the physician.
- Place the patient in a supine position, with legs elevated, and monitor vital signs every 15 minutes as indicated by the severity and type of reaction. (See *Recognizing Transfusion Reactions* to determine the type of reaction.)
- Compare the labels on all blood containers to corresponding patient identification forms to ensure that the correct blood or blood product was used.
- Notify the blood bank of a possible transfusion reaction and collect blood samples, as ordered. Immediately send these samples, all transfusion containers (even if empty), and the administration set to the blood bank. The blood bank will test these materials to further evaluate the reaction.

RECOGNIZING TRANSFUSION REACTIONS

During a blood transfusion, your patient is at risk for developing any of five types of reactions. To learn to recognize them and to intervene appropriately, study this table.

If your patient develops any sign or symptom of a reaction, immediately follow this procedure:
- Stop the infusion.
- Change the I.V. tubing to prevent infusing any more blood. Save the tubing and blood bag for analysis.
- Administer saline solution I.V. to keep the vein open.
- Take the patient's vital signs.
- Notify the physician.
- Obtain urine and blood samples from the patient and send them to the laboratory.
- Prepare for further treatment.

Reaction	Signs and Symptoms	Nursing Considerations
Hemolytic	Include chills, fever, low back pain, headache, chest pain, tachycardia, dyspnea, hypotension, nausea and vomiting, restlessness, anxiety, shock	• Expect to place the patient in a supine position, with his legs elevated 20 to 30 degrees, and to administer oxygen, fluids, and epinephrine to correct shock. • Expect to administer mannitol to maintain the patient's renal circulation. • Expect to insert an indwelling (Foley) catheter to monitor the patient's urinary output (should be about 100 ml/hr). • Expect to administer antipyretics to lower the patient's fever. If his fever persists, expect to apply a hypothermia blanket or to give tepid sponge or alcohol baths.
Plasma protein incompatibility	Include chills, fever, flushing, abdominal pain, diarrhea, dyspnea, hypotension	• Expect to place the patient in a supine position, with his legs elevated 20 to 30 degrees, and to administer oxygen, fluids, and epinephrine to correct shock. • Expect to administer corticosteroids.
Blood contamination	Include chills, fever, abdominal pain, nausea and vomiting, bloody diarrhea, hypotension	• Expect to administer fluids, antibiotics, corticosteroids, vasopressors, and a fresh transfusion.
Febrile	Range from mild chills, flushing, and fever to extreme signs and symptoms resembling a hemolytic reaction	• Expect to administer an antipyretic and an antihistamine for a mild reaction. • Expect to treat a severe reaction the same as a hemolytic reaction.
Allergic	Range from pruritus, urticaria, hives, facial swelling, chills, fever, nausea and vomiting, headache, and wheezing to laryngeal edema, respiratory distress, and shock	• Expect to administer parenteral antihistamines or, for a severe reaction, epinephrine or corticosteroids. • If the patient's only sign of reaction is hives, expect to restart the infusion, as ordered, at a slower rate.

COMPLICATIONS OF MASSIVE TRANSFUSION

If refrigerated properly, whole blood preserved with citrate-phosphate-dextrose (CPD) is suitable for transfusion within 21 days of collection. Blood preserved with CPD-adenine is usable for 35 days. During storage, whole blood undergoes changes that can cause complications in the patient receiving blood volume replacement (8 to 10 units for an adult) within 24 hours. These complications include the following:
- **Coagulation disturbances.** These may result from poor survival of platelets, Factor V, and Factor VIII.
- **Citrate intoxication.** This rare reaction may result from the binding of citrate (present in the anticoagulant preservative solution) to serum calcium, causing hypocalcemia. It occurs with too-rapid, massive transfusion of citrated blood and, most frequently, in the patient with existing hepatic or renal dysfunction, because citrate is metabolized in the liver and excreted by the kidneys.
- **Hyperkalemia.** This complication may result from the release of potassium into the plasma during red cell lysis, thereby elevating potassium levels. It is rare except in patients with conditions causing potassium retention, such as renal failure.
- **Acid-base imbalance.** Gradual acidification of stored blood occurs and may result in metabolic acidosis. Particularly at risk is the patient with existing acidosis associated with decreased tissue perfusion. Such an imbalance precedes delayed metabolic alkalosis, caused by rapid citrate metabolism and the resulting bicarbonate excess.
- **Loss of 2,3-diphosphoglycerate.** This can lead to tighter binding of oxygen to hemoglobin, resulting in a shift of the oxygen dissociation curve to the left. The seriously ill patient may then experience inadequate tissue oxygenation.
- **Ammonia intoxication.** This complication results from increased levels of ammonia in stored blood and primarily affects the patient with hepatic impairment.
- **Hypothermia.** Rapid infusion of large amounts of cold blood can cause hypothermia, which may decrease cardiac output and rate and reduce blood pH.
- **Circulatory overload.** This complication results when transfusion volume exceeds circulatory system capacity, particularly in the debilitated or elderly patient.
- **Bacterial or viral infection.** Although this complication can occur with single or multiple blood transfusions, its risk increases with each transfused unit because various donors are involved. Viral hepatitis, the most common infection transmitted by transfusion, occurs despite screening for hepatitis antigens.

- Collect the first posttransfusion urine specimen, mark the collection slip "Possible Transfusion Reaction," and send it to the laboratory immediately. The laboratory will test this specimen for the presence of hemoglobin, which indicates a hemolytic reaction.
- Closely monitor intake and output. Note evidence of oliguria or anuria, because hemoglobin deposition in the renal tubules can cause renal damage.
- If ordered, administer oxygen, epinephrine, or other drugs. If ordered, give a tepid bath or apply a hypothermia blanket to reduce fever. (See *Recognizing Transfusion Reactions*, p. 273.)
- Make the patient as comfortable as possible, and provide reassurance as necessary.
- Record the time and date of the transfusion reaction, the type and amount of infused blood or blood products, the clinical signs of the reaction in order of occurrence, the patient's vital signs, any specimens sent to the laboratory for analysis, any treatment, and the patient's response to treatment. If required by institutional policy, complete the transfusion reaction form.

Nursing considerations
- Treat all transfusion reactions seriously until they are proven otherwise.
- If the physician anticipates a transfusion reaction, as in leukemia patients, he may order prophylactic treatment with antihis-

tamines, corticosteroids, or antipyretics to precede blood administration.
- For more information on specific nursing considerations for each type of reaction, see *Recognizing Transfusion Reactions*, p. 273.
- For information on complications of massive blood transfusion, see *Complications of Massive Transfusion*.

Performing therapeutic plasma exchange (plasmapheresis)

In therapeutic plasma exchange (TPE), or plasmapheresis, blood withdrawn from a patient's vein (usually in the antecubital fossa) flows to a cell separator and is separated into plasma and formed elements (red cells, white cells, platelets) by centrifugation. The plasma is then collected in a container for disposal, and the formed elements are mixed with a plasma replacement fluid (proteins, fluid, and electrolytes) and returned to the patient through another vein. Because the extracorporeal circuit contains 150 to 400 ml of blood during plasma exchange, the patient must tolerate decreased blood volume.

TPE may benefit patients with immune-related disorders, such as multiple myeloma, rapidly progressive glomerulonephritis, and systemic lupus erythematosus, and neuromuscular disorders, such as multiple sclerosis. It is usually combined with steroid immunosuppressant therapy to suppress pathologic immune responses, thereby preventing further organ or system destruction. The procedure can be performed at bedside or in a special unit and requires a specially trained technician or nurse to operate the cell separator, another nurse to monitor and maintain the patient, and the presence of a specialized physician in the institution.

Equipment and materials
You will need vascular access needles, if not in place; gloves; sterile gauze pads; aids to help maintain blood flow, such as a rolled gauze pad, blood pressure cuff, or heating pad; and a bedpan. You may need heparin.

The technician or specially trained nurse usually provides all equipment necessary to operate the cell separator.

Preparation
Using sterile technique, the technician or specially trained nurse assembles all necessary equipment and primes the extracorporeal circuit with normal saline solution to remove air bubbles, preventing formation of an air embolus. Then, an anticoagulant, usually anticoagulant-citrate-dextrose (ACD) is added, which prevents clotting by citrate binding to the blood's ionized (free) calcium; ACD works only in the extracorporeal circuit and is neutralized on return to the patient. The physician may order the addition of calcium gluconate to the plasma replacement solution to prevent hypocalcemic reactions, because albumin in this solution can also bind the returned blood's ionized calcium.

Steps
- Confirm the identity of the patient by checking the name, room number, and bed number on his wristband.
- Explain the procedure to the patient, and verify that he has signed a consent form. Tell him the procedure usually takes 1 to 2 hours but may take longer, depending on the volume of plasma exchanged. Advise him to eat lightly before this procedure.
- Instruct the patient to urinate before the procedure and during the procedure, as necessary. A full bladder may cause mild hypotension because of fluid shift or vasovagal reaction.
- Tell the patient to report any symptoms of hypocalcemic paresthesias—tingling of mouth, chin, or fingers—during treatment.
- Take vital signs to serve as baseline values. Put on gloves to prevent transmission of hepatitis or other diseases from contaminated plasma.
- If an I.V. line is not in place, perform venipunctures to establish vascular access routes. Use large-bore needles to minimize resistance and prevent damage to blood cells. Obtain blood samples, as ordered. If ordered, administer 2,000 to 3,000 units of heparin I.V. just before TPE to prevent clot formation in the vascular access sites.
- The technician or specially trained nurse then connects the patient to the cell separator and starts it. While the machine is operating, observe all solutions to avoid an air embolus from an empty container.

- Monitor the patient for signs of hypotension, hypocalcemia, or allergic reaction, which may result from the replacement solution. Temporary reduction of blood flow rate relieves paresthesias from hypocalcemia.
- Take one or more of the following measures to ensure optimal blood flow, as necessary: Place the patient in an elevated, semi-Fowler position to promote gravity drainage, and hyperextend the arm on a firm surface, with the wrist supported to bring large veins to the skin surface. Instruct the patient to squeeze a small, rolled gauze pad to promote venous blood flow and prevent vessel collapse. Apply a tourniquet or blood pressure cuff above the vascular sites to provide pressure and increase blood pooling. Place heating pads over the access sites to dilate the vessels, but observe for reddening skin, especially in the elderly patient with diminished heat sensitivity. Slightly withdraw or shift the needle to augment blood flow.
- After plasma exchange is completed, remove the needles (while wearing gloves) and elevate the affected arm slightly.
- Firmly hold sterile gauze pads over the puncture sites until bleeding stops. Then, apply sterile pressure dressings. Avoid bending the extremities to prevent vessel scarring and to allow use of the veins for further treatment. If necessary, note on the patient's chart that the veins should not be used for other purposes between TPE treatments.
- Mark all disposable equipment and plasma bags as contaminated, and discard according to institutional policy.
- Record the time of the procedure, the patient's vital signs, the vascular access sites, the volume of exchanged plasma, the replacement solution, any adverse reactions, and any administration of drugs. Determine the patient's fluid balance from the following formula, and note it on the intake and output sheet:

$$\frac{\text{Replacement solutions} + \text{ACD solution}}{\text{Volume removed}} \times 100 = \% \text{ return}$$

Nursing considerations
- Advise the patient of TPE aftercare (see *Therapeutic Plasma Exchange Aftercare*).

THERAPEUTIC PLASMA EXCHANGE AFTERCARE

After therapeutic plasma exchange (TPE), the patient may experience fatigue for 1 or 2 days as a result of decreased plasma protein levels. Advise him to rest frequently during this period and to reschedule strenuous activities, if possible. Unless contraindicated, tell him to maintain a high-protein diet to replace lost proteins and to take multivitamins with iron daily. If the patient is receiving steroids and requires a low-sodium diet, emphasize the importance of observing the diet.

Because TPE and concurrent therapy can cause immunosuppression, advise the patient to avoid persons with colds and other illnesses. Tell him to notify the doctor if any symptoms of an infection develop—even a scratchy throat—so the schedule for TPE and other therapy can be altered, if necessary. Also, advise the patient to notify the physician of any muscle weakness or cramping.

- If possible, withhold drugs until completion of the procedure to prevent their removal from the blood.
- If an unstable patient with myasthenia gravis is undergoing TPE, have emergency equipment available. Monitor the patient's blood pressure and pulse rate at least every 30 minutes. As ordered, give pyridostigmine bromide only if the patient experiences dysphagia or respiratory difficulty.
- If a patient is receiving TPE treatments frequently, he may require transfusions of fresh frozen plasma to replace the normal clotting factors removed from his plasma.
- As ordered, give deep intramuscular injections of gamma globulin in divided doses for 3 days after the procedure, to replace normal immunoglobulins removed in the plasma. If permitted by institutional policy, mix 2 ml of 2% lidocaine with 10 ml of gamma globulin to promote patient comfort during injection.
- If the patient is receiving immunosuppressant or steroid therapy, watch for signs of infection and an abnormally low WBC count.

- Hypotension can result from fluid shifts without protein replacement or from decreased blood volume.
- In the elderly patient, diminished cardiac output may cause hypotension after the procedure.
- Hypocalcemia can result from the binding of ionized calcium by citrate; hypomagnesemia can follow repeated TPE, producing severe, prolonged muscle cramping and tetany.
- Any allergic reaction can result from the protein replacement solution, particularly from the plasma protein fraction.
- In a patient with myasthenia gravis, cholinergic crisis is possible.
- In a patient connected to a respirator, increased respiratory secretions can occur for 1 to 2 days after treatment.

Performing autotransfusion

Autotransfusion is the collection, filtration, and reinfusion of the patient's own blood. Autotransfusion techniques are used after traumatic injury and before, during, and after surgery. *The trauma technique,* most commonly used for hemothorax, can also be used in primary injuries of the lungs, liver, chest wall, heart, pulmonary vessels, spleen, kidneys, inferior vena cava, and iliac, portal, and subclavian veins. In this technique, the collection system uses citrate-phosphate-dextrose (CPD) to prevent clotting of the collected blood. *The preoperative technique* is used when patients know they are going to have surgery and wish to have their own blood transfused. It is used primarily for patients with rare blood types, patients afraid of acquiring AIDS through a blood transfusion, and patients in whom isoimmunization may complicate future transfusion needs. This technique follows standard blood bank donation and transfusion procedures. *The intraoperative technique,* used most often for thoracic and cardiovascular surgery, can also be used in hip resection, spinal fusion, liver resection, and ruptured ectopic pregnancy. In this technique, a commercial cell washer-processor reduces anticoagulated collected whole blood to washed cells for later reinfusion. *The postoperative technique* is used solely to collect shed mediastinal blood after cardiac surgery.

Autotransfusion has several advantages over transfusion of banked blood. Most important, because autotransfused blood is autologous, it eliminates disease transmission, transfusion reactions, and exposure to incompatible blood antigens. Autotransfusion can overcome the objections of certain religious groups who oppose transfusion of donor blood.

Unlike banked blood, autologous blood contains normal levels of 2,3-diphosphoglycerate (2,3-DPG)—advantageous for tissue oxygenation—potassium, ammonia, and clotting factors (except for fibrinogen); has normal pH; and appears to have viable platelets. Occasionally, it causes transient hemoglobinuria, due to RBC trauma during collection.

Autotransfusion is contraindicated in patients with malignant neoplasms, intrathoracic or systemic infections and infestations, coagulopathies, enteric contamination, or excessive hemolysis, and use of an antibiotic at the venipuncture site that is not suitable for I.V. administration.

Equipment and materials
- For the *trauma* technique, you will need an I.V. pole or floor stand, a 500-ml bottle of CPD, chest tubes for hemothorax, a trauma drainage tubing set, a volume-control set (usually 150 ml), a Receptal canister, a 1,900-ml sterile disposable trauma blood liner with 170-micron filter, and a microemboli filter with recipient set.
- For the *intraoperative* technique, you will need an I.V. pole or floor stand, two connected Receptal canisters, a 1,900-ml sterile disposable autotransfusion liner with 170-micron filter, a 1,900-ml sterile disposable overflow liner, double-lumen aspiration tubing with autotransfusion liner connector, an administration set with macrodrip chamber, a suction wand, anticoagulant solution (CPD or heparin), and a cell washer. You may need an overflow shutoff valve.

Liners and double-lumen tubing with administration set are available as kits.
- For the *postoperative* technique, you will need a Receptal canister, a sterile disposable mediastinal liner, a recipient set with microemboli filter, and a mediastinal drainage tubing set.

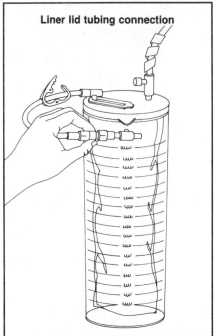

Liner lid tubing connection

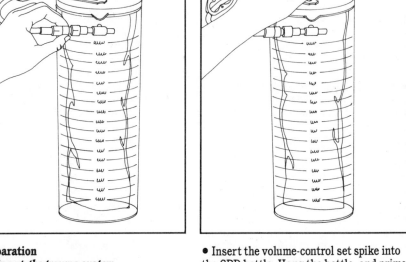

Anticoagulant line attachment

Preparation
Setting up the trauma system
• Remove the sterile liner from the package and extend it to its full length, so it expands in the canister when the vacuum is applied. Avoid contaminating the sterile spacer that caps the drainage port.
• Insert the liner in the canister and snap the lid securely in place, with the thumb tab directly over the canister tee to facilitate connection to suction.
• With the sterile spacer, connect the liner lid tubing to the canister tee (illustration above). The sterile spacer prevents contamination of the port by the nonsterile canister tee. Attach the vacuum tubing to the opposite end of the canister tee.
• Temporarily occlude the tubing between the vacuum regulator and canister to set the vacuum pressure between 10 and 30 mm Hg. A higher setting increases hemolysis.
• Remove the protective cap from the patient port, and attach the yellow sterile (proximal) end of the drainage tubing with the anticoagulant connector to the patient port of the liner.

• Insert the volume-control set spike into the CPD bottle. Hang the bottle, and prime the administration set.
• Remove the yellow cap from the anticoagulant connector, and attach the anticoagulant administration line (illustration above).
• Run 100 ml of CPD into the liner to prevent clotting of any blood.

Setting up the intraoperative system
• Open the outer sterile wrap of the equipment, and gently drop the inner package onto the sterile field. Using sterile technique, remove the inner wrap.
• Remove the overflow liner (orange lid) from the sterile field and extend it to its full length, so it expands in the canister when vacuum is applied.
• Insert the orange-lidded liner in the left canister and connect its tubing to the canister's tee or shutoff valve. The shutoff valve prevents aspiration of overflow blood into the vacuum line. Snap the orange lid in place, with the thumb tab directly over the tee.
• Remove the red-lidded liner from the sterile field, extend it to its full length, insert it in the right canister, and snap it securely in

Blood and Blood Component Therapy 279

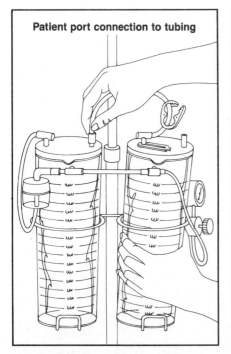

Patient port connection to tubing

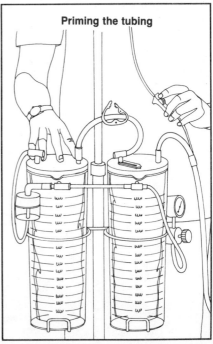

Priming the tubing

place, with the thumb tab placed directly over the canister tee.
- Remove the white protective cap from the orange-lidded patient port, and connect this port to the tubing with the orange connector, which originates at the red lid (illustration above).
- Connect the vacuum tubing to the canister tee on the canister with the red-lidded liner. Temporarily occlude the tubing between the regulator and the canister to set the vacuum pressure between 30 and 60 mm Hg.
- Label the red lid with pertinent patient information to prevent misidentification when the patient's blood is removed to the cell processor.
- Remove the red connector end of the aspiration tubing from the sterile field, and attach it to the patient port on the red lid. The clear end of the aspiration tubing remains within the sterile field for connection to the suction wand.
- Close the roller clamp on the administration set (illustration above, right), insert the spike into the anticoagulant container, and prime the tubing.

- Check that all components are securely in place, because any break in the system interferes with vacuum suction.

Setting up the postoperative system
- Remove the sterile liner from the package and extend it to its full length, so it expands in the canister when the vacuum is applied.
- Insert the liner in the canister, and snap the lid securely in place, with the thumb tab placed directly over the canister tee.
- With the sterile spacer, connect the liner lid tubing to the canister tee. Attach the vacuum tubing to the opposite end of the canister tee.
- Temporarily occlude the tubing between the vacuum regulator and canister to set the vacuum pressure between 25 and 30 mm Hg.
- Remove the protective cap on the patient port, and connect the drainage tubing to the port.

Steps
Confirm the patient's identity.

Liner removal	Air removal from liner bag
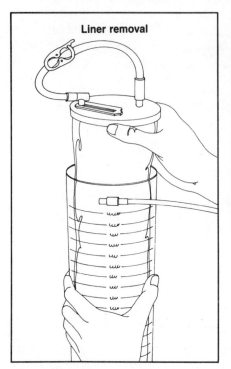	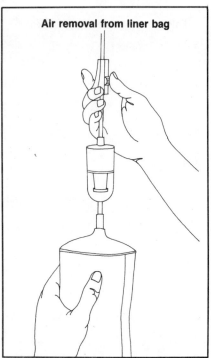

Trauma technique
- To collect blood, attach the proximal end of the drainage tubing to the chest drainage catheter. During drainage, add one part CPD to seven parts blood.
- To transfuse collected blood, clamp the patient's line to prevent pneumothorax when the vacuum is lost. Then, disconnect the patient and anticoagulant lines from the liner lid.
- Disconnect the liner lid tubing and sterile spacer from the canister tee, and remove and discard the sterile spacer.
- Attach the liner lid tubing to the patient port, close the white cricket clamp, push up on the thumb tab to unsnap the liner lid, and remove the liner from the canister (illustration above).
- Invert the liner and raise the recessed stem at the bottom of the liner. Remove the yellow cap. Using a twisting motion, insert the microemboli filter set into the liner port.
- Hold the filter and recipient set upright, open the clamp, and gently compress the bag to remove all air (illustration above, right). Close the clamp.

- Then, hang the liner, open the clamp, partly fill the drip chamber, and prime the tubing.
- Transfuse blood in the usual way. If you are using a pressure cuff, avoid exceeding pressure of 150 mm Hg.

Intraoperative technique
- When collecting blood, ensure that the anticoagulant flow rate is sufficient to prevent clotting.
- To transfuse collected blood, disconnect the aspiration tubing from the red-lidded patient port. Then, disconnect the tubing from the orange connector on the orange lid, and connect it to the red-lidded patient port. Close the white cricket clamp, and remove and discard the orange adapter from the orange lid.
- Push upward on the red-lidded thumb tab to unsnap it, and remove the liner from the canister (illustration, next page).
- To collect additional blood, insert a new red-lidded liner into the canister and make the connections to the orange lid and aspiration tubing.

Blood and Blood Component Therapy

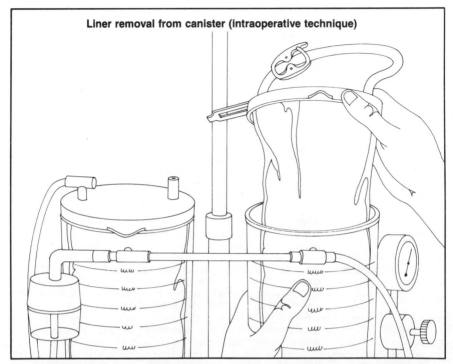

Liner removal from canister (intraoperative technique)

• Place the blood collected in the red-lidded liner in the blood processor, and follow the manufacturer's instruction for operation. The processor washes the blood and the saline solution and packs red cells to a hematocrit of 60% to 75%.
• Transfuse the washed, packed cells, using proper equipment and technique.

Postoperative technique
• To collect blood, attach the sterile drainage tubing to the thoracic catheters, release the chest tube clamp with the vacuum on, and collect up to 800 ml of blood.
• To transfuse collected blood, clamp the chest drainage tube, disconnect the liner lid tubing and sterile spacer from the canister lid, and remove and discard the spacer.
• Attach the liner lid tubing to the patient port. Push upward on the thumb tab to unsnap the liner lid, and remove the liner from the canister. (To collect additional blood, insert a new liner and secure all connections.)
• Place your thumb under or behind the liner's white port to facilitate valve closure as you separate the liner's sections. If blood remains in the upper section of the liner, alternately compress upper and lower sections to transfer it to the lower one.
• Clamp the recipient set line. Using a twisting motion, insert the microemboli filter in the bottom port of the liner.
• As recommended in "Trauma technique," compress the liner to remove all air, prime the line, and transfuse the blood.

Documentation
Record the duration of collection, suction pressure, and the type and amount of anticoagulant. Also note the duration of transfusion and the use of a blood filter or washed cells. Record the amount and characteristics of drainage and any complications.

Nursing considerations
• Cover canisters and avoid unwrapping sterile components until ready to use.
• Secure all connections and clamp the chest drainage system before stopping suction, to prevent pneumothorax.

COMPLICATIONS OF AUTOTRANSFUSION

Complication	Cause
Blood clotting	Insufficient anticoagulant added to collected blood in trauma and intraoperative systems (postoperative system does not use anticoagulant)
Hemolysis	Blood trauma from turbulence, possibly caused by excess vacuum pressure
Coagulopathies	Same as those associated with banked blood
Thrombocytopenia	Insufficient platelets in the transfused blood; less common than with banked blood, because autotransfused blood contains some viable platelets. If patient receives more than 4,000 ml of blood, he may require transfusion of fresh frozen plasma or platelet concentrate.
Particulate and air emboli	Microaggregate debris causes particulate emboli. When microemboli filters remove this debris, adult respiratory distress syndrome occurs less frequently than with banked blood. Air emboli can occur with a roller pump or pressure system.
Sepsis	Breakdown in aseptic technique or use of blood with known enteric contamination or pulmonary infection
Citrate toxicity	Rare and unpredictable complication; occurs as frequently in the trauma system as in banked blood transfusion. Citrate-phosphate-dextrose is removed during cell washing in the intraoperative system; none is used in postoperative system.

- If suction fails, place a Heimlich valve between the canister tee and the vacuum.
- Avoid excessively high suction pressure, which can collapse the tubing.
- If the liner fails to expand after you turn on the vacuum, check for leaks at the canister tee, liner lid, and suction connections. If the liner still fails to expand, remove it from the canister, extend it fully, and return it to the canister.
- In the trauma and intraoperative systems, periodically agitate the liner to mix the blood and anticoagulant thoroughly.
- Avoid storing blood in a liner; transfuse it within 4 hours of the start of collection.
- Monitor the volume of collected blood to prevent overflow and estimate blood loss; precise measurement is not critical because the blood is returned to the patient.
- Do not be concerned if clots become trapped in the 170-micron liner filter, because these will not interfere with transfusion. Change the microemboli filter after collecting 1,900 ml.
- If you are using the trauma system, remember to vent the volume-control set.
- If you anticipate heavy bleeding, set up two canisters to eliminate changing liners.
- For selected patients, autotransfused blood can be washed and processed before reinfusion.
- If you are using the intraoperative system, remember that the orange-lidded liner functions only as an overflow trap. Because this liner does not contain a 170-micron filter or a spike port, overflow blood collected within it is not autotransfused. An overflow shutoff valve prevents the aspiration of blood from this liner into the vacuum system.
- For a summary of complications, see *Complications of Autotransfusion*.

Review Questions

1. What are the functions of the blood?
   1. Supplying oxygen and nutrients for tissue maintenance, growth, and repair
   2. Transporting cellular waste, including carbon dioxide
   3. Providing defense against infection by transporting antibodies
   4. Regulating and equalizing body temperature
   5. Helping maintain acid-base balance
   6. Regulating fluid and electrolyte balance

   A. 1 and 2
   B. 1, 2, 3, and 5
   C. 1, 2, 3, 4, and 5
   D. All of the above

2. What are the objectives of transfusion therapy?

3. Why is blood component transfusion performed more frequently than whole blood transfusion?

4. Define antigen.

5. Define antibody.

6. Which are genetically inherited—antigens or antibodies?

7. What determines a patient's blood group?

8. What is the blood type of a person who is called a universal donor? Define universal donor.

9. What is the blood type of a person who is called a universal recipient? Define universal recipient.

10. What is the purpose of testing donor and recipient blood for compatibility?

11. What does Rh-positive mean?

12. When transfusing blood and blood components, what are the *five* major nursing responsibilities?

13. White blood cells must be ABO- and Rh-matched. True or false?

14. Washed cells are administered to restore oxygen-carrying capacity in a patient previously sensitized to blood transfusion. True or false?

15. All blood transfusions require use of a filter. True or false?

16. Blood warming is done *routinely* to prevent hypothermia. True or false?

17. What is the purpose of beginning a blood transfusion slowly?

18. Describe, in order, the steps to take in managing a transfusion reaction.

19. What is plasmapheresis?

20. Define autotransfusion.

21. What are the advantages of autotransfusion over banked blood?

22. When is autotransfusion used?

23. Name *three* situations in which autotransfusion is contraindicated.

Selected References

Berkman, Eugene, and Umlas, Joel. *Therapeutic Hemapheresis.* Washington, D.C.: American Association of Blood Banks, 1980.

Diagnostics, 2nd ed. Nurse's Reference Library. Springhouse, Pa.: Springhouse Corp., 1986.

Emergency Care Handbook. Springhouse, Pa.: Springhouse Corp., 1986.

Plummer, A. *Principles and Practices of Intravenous Therapy.* Boston: Little, Brown & Co., 1982.

Procedures. Nurse's Reference Library. Springhouse, Pa.: Springhouse Corp., 1983.

Shock. Nursing Now Series. Springhouse, Pa.: Springhouse Corp., 1984.

Standards for Blood Banks and Transfusion Services. Arlington, Va.: American Association of Blood Banks, 1983.

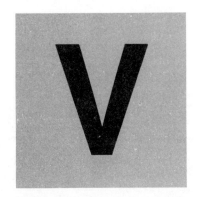

Pediatric and Geriatric Considerations

17 Pediatric Drug and I.V. Therapy 286

18 Geriatric Drug and I.V. Therapy 308

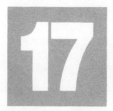

Pediatric Drug and I.V. Therapy

This chapter covers principles and procedures of drug administration and I.V. therapy in infants and children. Although the principles are essentially the same for patients of any age, caring for infants and children requires changes in approach and technique because of special anatomic, physiologic, and developmental considerations.

MEDICATION ADMINISTRATION
Physiologic considerations

Administering medications to children can be more complex than it seems. During a child's development, the child's ability to absorb, distribute, metabolize, and excrete drugs undergoes profound changes that affect drug dosage. If these variables are ignored, underestimation or overestimation of dosage may result, causing therapeutic failure, toxicity, or even death. Furthermore, dosage calculations are only the starting point of therapy. Drug regimens must be tailored to each patient's requirements to ensure optimal drug effect and minimal toxicity.

Absorption
Drug absorption in children depends on the form of the drug; its physical properties; other drugs or substances, such as food, taken simultaneously; physiologic changes; and concurrent disease. The rate and completeness of drug absorption also varies according to the route of administration.

Oral administration
Several physiologic differences affect absorption of orally administered drugs in a child. The pH of neonatal gastric fluid is neutral or slightly acidic and becomes more acidic as the infant matures. This affects drug absorption. For example, nafcillin and penicillin G, erratically absorbed or malabsorbed in an adult due to degradation by gastric acid, are *better* absorbed in an infant due to low gastric acidity.

Various infant formulas or milk products may increase gastric pH and impede absorption of acidic drugs. So, if possible, a child should be given oral medications when his stomach is empty. Gastric emptying time and transit time through the small intestine, which are greater in children than in adults, can increase absorption. Also, intestinal hypermotility (as in diarrhea) can diminish the drug's absorption.

The child's activity level also affects gastrointestinal (GI) absorption. During exercise, blood is shunted away from the GI tract to the arms and legs, decreasing GI blood supply and reducing drug absorption.

Topical administration
Unlike most drugs administered orally, topically administered drugs are absorbed faster and more completely in a child than in an adult. Absorption increases because the child's keratin and epithelial layers are much thinner than an adult's. In fact, some topically administered drugs can cause serious adverse reactions in children. Hydrocortisone ointment, for example, can suppress growth after long-term use. And antibiotic ointments, such as bacitracin, may trigger an allergic reaction, especially if applied in excessive amounts.

Intramuscular administration
Drugs administered intramuscularly (I.M.) are absorbed erratically in young children, especially newborns and infants. One reason is their relatively low muscle mass. In addition, blood flow to muscle tissue is variable, making absorption rates difficult to predict.

Distribution

Normal changes in weight and physiology during childhood can significantly influence a drug's distribution and effects. As in an adult, drug distribution is influenced by plasma protein binding, body mass, and membrane permeability.

Plasma protein binding

As the result of a decrease in either albumin concentration or intermolecular attraction between a given drug and plasma protein, a child has fewer protein-binding sites than an adult. Many drugs, therefore, are less bound to plasma proteins in children than in adults, and their effects are intensified. Furthermore, drugs that bind to plasma proteins may displace endogenous compounds, such as steroids or hormones. Conversely, an endogenous compound may displace a weakly bound drug. Since only an unbound, or free, drug has a pharmacologic effect, any alteration in ratio of protein-bound to unbound active drug can greatly influence effect. In addition, several diseases, such as malnutrition and nephrotic syndrome, can also decrease plasma protein and increase the concentration of unbound drug, intensifying the drug effect or producing toxicity.

Body mass

An infant has a much higher percentage of body fluid than an adult. In a premature infant, body fluid makes up about 85% of total body weight; in a full-term infant, 55% to 70%; and in an adult, 50% to 55%. Extracellular fluid (mostly blood) makes up 40% of a neonate's body weight, compared with 20% in an adult. (Intracellular fluid remains fairly constant throughout life and has little effect on drug dosage.) Since most drugs travel through extracellular fluid to reach their receptors, extracellular fluid volume influences a water-soluble drug's concentration and effect. Because children have a larger proportion of fluid to solid body weight, their distribution area is proportionately greater.

The proportion of fat to lean body mass increases with age, and the distribution of fat-soluble drugs is more limited in children than adults. As a result, a drug's lipid- or water-solubility affects the dosage for a child.

Note: Body-surface area correlates closely to a child's extracellular fluid volume. Because extracellular fluid volume is so important to drug distribution in an infant or child, pediatric drug dosages are commonly calculated on the basis of body-surface area rather than body weight.

Membrane permeability

The child's blood-brain barrier is immature, and certain drugs can penetrate to the central nervous system (CNS) more easily in a child than in an adult. Lipid-soluble drugs, for example, readily cross the blood-brain barrier, possibly causing CNS toxicity.

Metabolism

A newborn's ability to metabolize a drug depends on the integrity of his hepatic enzyme system, his intrauterine exposure to the drug, and the nature of the drug itself.

Certain metabolic mechanisms are underdeveloped in newborns. Glucuronidation, the mechanism that neutralizes drugs, for example, is insufficiently developed to permit full pediatric doses until the infant is 1 month old. Because of this, the use of chloramphenicol in a newborn may cause *gray syndrome*, illustrating the newborn's inability to metabolize the drug. Use of chloramphenicol in newborns, therefore, requires decreased dosage (25 mg/kg/day) and monitoring of blood levels.

However, intrauterine exposure to drugs may induce precocious development of hepatic enzyme mechanisms, increasing the infant's capacity to metabolize potentially harmful substances. Also, preparations given concurrently to a child may alter hepatic metabolism and induce release of hepatic enzymes. Phenobarbital, for example, can induce hepatic enzyme production and accelerate metabolism of drugs given concurrently.

Older children can metabolize some drugs (theophylline, for example) more rapidly than adults. This ability may be due to their increased hepatic metabolic activity. Larger doses, based on weight, than those recommended for adults may be required.

Excretion

Renal excretion of a drug is the net effect of glomerular filtration, active tubular secretion, and passive tubular reabsorption. Because so many drugs are excreted in the urine, the degree of renal development or presence of renal disease can profoundly affect a child's dosage requirements. If a child is unable to excrete a drug renally, drug accumulation and possible toxicity may result unless the dosage is reduced.

Physiologically, an infant's kidneys differ from an adult's in that they have:
• high resistance to blood flow and subsequent decreased renal fraction of cardiac output
• incomplete glomerular and tubular development and short, incomplete loops of Henle. (An infant's glomerular filtration rate reaches adult values by age 2½ to 5 months; his tubular secretion may reach adult values by age 7 to 12 months.)
• low glomerular filtration rate
• decreased ability to concentrate urine or reabsorb various filtered compounds
• reduced proximal tubular ability to secrete organic acids.

Both children and adults have diurnal variations in urine pH that correlate with sleep-wake patterns.

Developmental considerations

An adequate knowledge of child development is necessary to understand and predict the responses of most children to medication administration. Safe and effective administration of a correct dose depends upon using approaches and techniques that are appropriate to the child's age and stage of development. The theories of Erikson, Freud, and Piaget, as well as physical growth patterns, must be taken into consideration, since *all* aspects of a child's development will influence his behavior.

Calculating and monitoring pediatric dosages

When calculating pediatric dosages, do not use formulas that modify adult dosages; a child is not a scaled-down version of an adult. Pediatric dosages should be calculated on the basis of either body weight (mg/kg) or body-surface area (mg/m^2). (See *Calculating Pediatric Dosages.*) Calculations using body-surface area and body weight may be confusing, however, so another source of information should be used, if available. Drug information giving the recommended dosage per kilogram (or pound) of body weight is the most accurate source of pediatric dosage information.

Although they are useful for adults and older children, do not use dosages based on body-surface area in premature or full-term newborns. Use the body weight method instead. Also, do not exceed the maximum adult dose when calculating amounts per kilogram of body weight (except with certain drugs, such as theophylline, if indicated).

To monitor drug response, know administration times and when to draw blood to measure drug levels. (Discuss findings with the physician and pharmacist.) Dosages should also be reevaluated at regular intervals to ensure necessary adjustments as the child develops.

Obtain an accurate maternal drug history—prescription and nonprescription drugs, vitamins, and herbs or other health foods taken during pregnancy. In utero exposure may harm the newborn and hinder subsequent drug therapy.

Drugs passed through breast milk can have adverse effects on the nursing infant. Before a drug is prescribed for a breast-feeding mother, the potential effects on the infant should be investigated. For example, sulfa drugs given to a breast-feeding mother for a urinary tract infection appear in breast milk and may cause kernicterus at lower-than-normal levels of unconjugated bilirubin. High concentrations of isoniazid also appear in breast milk. Since this drug is metabolized by the liver, an infant's immature hepatic enzyme mechanisms cannot metabolize the drug, and the infant may suffer CNS toxicity.

Emergency drug administration

To treat pediatric emergencies effectively, quick dosage calculation and administration are essential. A list of appropriate emergency drug dosages should be placed in pediatric areas and on emergency equipment.

CALCULATING PEDIATRIC DOSAGES

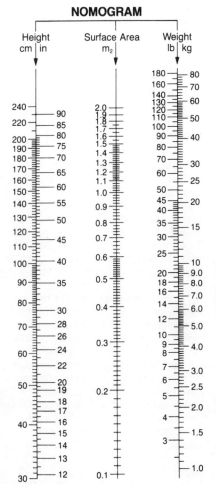

Before administering any medication to an infant or child, it is the nurse's responsibility to double-check and make sure that the prescribed dosage is appropriate for that infant or child. The two most accurate methods for calculating safe pediatric dosages are as follows:

Body-surface area
Using the nomogram at the right, lay a straightedge on the correct height and weight points for the patient, then see the intersecting point on the surface area scale. That point indicates the child's body-surface area (BSA). The dosage is then determined using the following equation:

$$\frac{BSA (m^2)}{1.7} \times \text{adult dosage} = \text{estimated child's dosage}$$

Body weight
Determine the child's body weight in kilograms (1 kg = 2.2 lb). Then, calculate the total amount of drug to be given over 24 hours (number of doses × amount in milligrams). Check a pharmacology text or hospital formulary to find the recommended safe pediatric dosage (RPD), and calculate the recommended safe dosage (RSD) for the patient:

RPD × child's weight in kg = RSD

Compare the prescribed dosage with the RSD.

Reprinted from Hayman, L., and Sparing, E. *Handbook for Pediatric Nursing*, John Wiley & Sons, Inc., New York, 1985.

Reprinted from Behrman, Richard, and Vaughan, Victor. *Nelson Textbook of Pediatrics*, 12th ed. Philadelphia: W.B. Saunders Co., 1983.

Giving oral medication

The oral route is the most acceptable route for a child. When giving an oral medication to an infant or young child, administer it in liquid form if possible. However, refrain from adding a drug to the child's bottle or other large amount of liquid, because he may not drink it all and may thus receive an inadequate dose.

Make oral medication as palatable as possible but, unless ordered, avoid mixing it with milk or milk products, which can hinder absorption, or with foods that the child may come to dislike through association. If only a tablet is available, crush it in a mortar; then mix it with a compatible syrup. Clean the mortar thoroughly to remove the complete dose and avoid incompatibilities. (Check with the pharmacist or an appropriate drug reference book to ensure that crushing the tablet does not inactivate it.)

Break only scored tablets to prepare reduced doses and do not open capsules; ask the pharmacist to prepare lower doses. Use a syringe or calibrated dropper to measure a liquid medication dose, because it is more accurate than a medication cup. If you are using a medication cup, however, place it on a flat surface at eye level to check the dose.

If the child takes medicine by spoon at home, use a spoon to administer it, but do not use the spoon to measure the dose, because it is inaccurate. To provide consistent care, check the child's records for information about how he prefers to take medication. Look for such statements as "Mix with jelly" or "Takes best for mother."

Before administering any medication, confirm the identity of the child by checking the name, room number, and bed number on his wristband. Explain the procedure to him in terms he can understand, and to his parent(s), if present. If possible, let a parent stay with the child during the administration to provide comfort. However, if the child must be restrained during administration, do not ask the parent to act as a primary restrainer; the child may then view him as your accomplice.

Every drug has its specific possible complications and adverse effects. If you must administer an unfamiliar drug, check an appropriate drug reference book for information to help you recognize a drug reaction. That is especially important in treating children, who often cannot tell you how they are feeling, but can suddenly develop severe reactions.

Carefully observe the child for any rash, itch, cough, or other sign of adverse reaction to a previously administered drug, and provide privacy, especially for the older child. If a child is receiving nothing by mouth, oral medications such as cardiac drugs and seizure control medications should be given by an alternative route. Consult the physician in that case.

Giving oral medication to an infant

Oral medications are relatively easy to give to infants because of their natural sucking instinct and, in infants under 3 to 4 months, their poorly developed sense of taste. The older the infant, however, the more difficult it may become to give oral medications as he develops anxiety toward strangers and the ability to spit medication out.

The most important consideration in giving oral medications to an infant is to position him in such a way as to prevent aspiration. Because development of trust, so important to this stage of development, is fostered by happy feeding experiences, the infant should be given oral medication while in his normal feeding position. Whenever possible, the infant should be held and cuddled when given medication. That also provides a relatively pleasant means of restraining him.

Steps
- Use a plastic syringe without a needle, or a plastic medicine dropper, to administer the medication.
- Holding the infant in a normal feeding position and restraining his limbs as needed, gently press down on his lower lip with the syringe or dropper to open his mouth.
- Place the syringe or medicine dropper alongside or across the tongue and slowly release the medication. Release only enough to be swallowed at one time to prevent choking. (See *Administering Liquid Medications to an Infant.*)

ADMINISTERING LIQUID MEDICATIONS TO AN INFANT

Holding the infant in a normal feeding position, place the syringe or dropper (as shown below), alongside or across the tongue. Slowly release the medication in small amounts to prevent choking. Cuddle the infant after all the medication has been administered, and document the procedure.

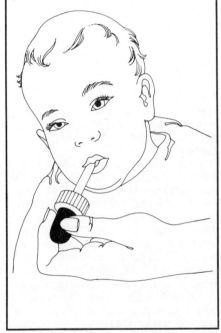

- For small infants, allow the infant to suck on the syringe as you slowly expel the medication, or allow the infant to suck the medication from a baby bottle nipple.
- After all the medication has been administered, comfort the infant and give him a fruit juice chaser.
- Then, if he is a small or inactive infant, place him on his side or abdomen to prevent aspiration. If the infant is very active, allow him to assume a comfortable position, because forcing a side-lying position may agitate him.
- Document the procedure.

Giving oral medication to a toddler

Administering oral medication to a toddler may be extremely difficult if not approached properly. The toddler's developing sense of independence and control of his body and environment, countered by his inability to make choices, his need for ritual, and his negativism, can make this experience frustrating for all involved. Ask the parents about any rituals surrounding medication administration, and try to continue them if possible. Firmly establish that the child has no choice about taking the medication. Support him in his dislike for the procedure, but remind him that the medication will help him get well. If advisable, and if time permits, allow the child to play at giving medication to a doll with a medication cup or syringe.

Steps
- Place the medication in a cup. Then pick up the toddler and have him sit on your lap or on a chair facing you, or if in bed, elevate his head and shoulders to prevent aspiration.
- If possible, enlist the toddler's cooperation by asking him to help hold the cup. If he is unable to drink by himself, hold the cup to his lips and give it to him in small amounts. If he is uncooperative or agitated, use a syringe or a spoon, and proceed as described for an infant, making sure the child drinks all the medication.
- Give the desired chaser.
- Afterward, praise the child and comfort him if he is distressed.
- Document the procedure.

Giving oral medication to an older child

Preschoolers and school-age children usually will take oral medications without much difficulty. The use of play and simple visual aids can assist them in working through concerns and fears regarding medications. The child, at this point, responds well to being given truthful explanations about the need for and taste of a medication, as well as choices in the method of administering it.

Steps
- If possible, allow the child to choose the mixer and the chaser for liquid medication.

- If feasible, let the child choose where he will take the medication, such as sitting in bed or on his parent's lap.
- Place the medication in a cup and let the child take it himself.
- If the child will not take the medication himself, use the technique described for the toddler.
- If the medication is in tablet form, and if the child is old enough (usually age 4 to 6), teach him or review with him the method for swallowing tablets or capsules.
- Have him place the pill on the back of his tongue and immediately swallow it with water or juice. Emphasize swallowing the liquid rather than calling attention to the pill.
- Make sure the child takes sufficient liquid to swallow the pill and prevent it from lodging in the esophagus. Have him open his mouth so you can check to ensure that he has swallowed the pill.
- If the child is unable to swallow the pill, crush it and place it in the proper mixer, allowing a choice of mixers if possible.
- Praise the child after he takes the medication.
- Document the procedure.

Giving oral medication to a child who refuses medication

Because of a previous bad experience or because he wants to assert his independence, a child of any age may refuse oral medication. It is important to work with the child to gain first his trust and then his cooperation.

If medication must be given before time can be spent gaining a child's trust and cooperation, try asking the parents to help, and see if the child will take it from them. If the child still will not cooperate, position him on an assistant's lap.

If the child refuses to open his mouth, apply firm, gentle downward pressure along his jaw, pressing his cheek inward. When his mouth is open wide enough for the oral syringe, place the syringe across the tongue to prevent his spitting it out (as for the infant), and instill the medication in small amounts to prevent choking.

If he refuses to swallow, stroke his throat gently in a downward motion. Comfort him afterward.

When a child spits out medication, repeat the dose if he spits out all of it, or repeat half the dose if he spits out more than half, but not all of the dose. If he spits out less than half, or if you have trouble estimating how much has been spit out, notify the physician, and readminister the dose according to his recommendations.

Giving oral medication through a nasogastric tube

Occasionally, medication must be given via nasogastric (NG) tube. The technique is the same in the child as in the adult. (See Chapter 7, Administering Oral Medications.)

Giving an injection

Because of immunization requirements, most children receive some form of injectable medication before entering school. It is not a simple task to perform, and a child may develop a fear of injections and of the health care professional who administers them.

You must be knowledgeable about anatomy and site selection, as well as about the amount of solution recommended for injection into that site. (See *Guidelines for Maximum Amounts of Solutions to be Injected into Muscle Tissues.*) Your responsibility is not only to safely administer an injection to an infant or child, but also to do so in a way that will decrease the physical and emotional trauma. If his age is appropriate, allow the child to play with syringes and other equipment associated with giving an injection, to decrease anxiety.

Prepare injections out of the child's sight to avoid frightening him. Carefully calculate the dosage and have another nurse verify the calculations, according to institutional policy. If you are giving two drugs simultaneously, check their compatibility on any up-to-date compatibility chart. Then, calculate the combined dosage volume, and check the need for divided doses by determining whether the combined volume will be too great for proper absorption from a single injection site. For I.M. injections, determine if a low platelet count, volume depletion, or other conditions prevent the use of this route, and consult the physician about any conflict.

GUIDELINES FOR MAXIMUM AMOUNTS OF SOLUTIONS TO BE INJECTED INTO MUSCLE TISSUES

Muscle group	Birth to 1½ years	1½ to 3 years	3 to 6 years	6 to 15 years	15 years to adulthood
Deltoid	Not recommended	Not recommended unless other sites are not available 0.5 ml	0.5 ml	0.5 ml	1 ml
Gluteus maximus	Not recommended	Not recommended unless other sites are not available 1 ml	1.5 ml	1.5 to 2 ml	2 to 2.5 ml
Ventrogluteal	Not recommended	Not recommended unless other sites are not available 1 ml	1.5 ml	1.5 to 2 ml	2 to 2.5 ml
Vastus lateralis	0.5 to 1 ml	1 ml	1.5 ml	1.5 to 2 ml	2 to 2.5 ml

Reprinted with permission from Howry, Linda Berner, et al. *Pediatric Medications*, Philadelphia: J.B. Lippincott Co., 1981.

For accurate measurement of small dosages for an infant, use a tuberculin syringe with a ½" (1-cm) needle. For the toddler or older child, use a syringe with a 1" (2.5-cm) needle to measure dosage.

When preparing to give the injection, make sure you have chosen a needle of appropriate size. To determine the correct size, consider the child's age, muscle mass, and nutritional status, and the drug's viscosity. As a general rule, choose a 25G to 27G ½" to 1" needle for subcutaneous injection, a 22G to 25G ⅝" (2-cm) to 1" needle for an I.M. injection, and a 26G to 27G ⅜" to ⅝" needle for an intradermal injection. Because a child may jump when the needle is inserted, causing it to come out of the skin, always have an extra needle available to replace the contaminated one.

As with administering *any* medication, confirm the identity of the child, explain the procedure to him (and to the parent[s], if present), in terms he can understand, and assess him for any adverse reaction from a previously administered medication. Make sure you rotate the site to reduce tissue irritation.

Always awaken a sleeping child before giving an injection to avoid instilling suspicion and fear of going back to sleep. Provide privacy, especially for the older child.

Giving an I.M. injection to an infant

One of the most important considerations in giving an injection to an infant is to restrain him adequately to avoid giving the injection in the wrong site or having the needle become dislodged, contaminated, or broken. An infant under 6 months can usually be restrained by one person; an older infant may require two. Always be sure to have a firm grasp on the syringe to ensure that the medication is injected at the site of aspiration, and that a second needle is readily available if necessary.

It is also important to establish a pleasant relationship with the infant before administering the injection. If he receives only pain from strangers, his natural fear of strangers at this stage will increase. Be sure to comfort the infant after giving the injection; the parents are the best source of comfort.

Steps
- Select the injection site. Usually, the vastus lateralis muscle in the anterolateral aspect of the thigh is chosen. This is the largest and most developed muscle in the child under age 2. The rectus femoris muscle on the anterior aspect of the thigh is smaller, but it may be used if care is taken to avoid the femoral artery. If necessary, you can use the ventrogluteal muscle, located between the greater trochanter of the femur and the iliac crest, but maintaining the infant's position to use this site is sometimes difficult. (Note: Avoid using the posterior gluteal muscles in an infant, because these do not develop until the child has been ambulatory for at least 1 year.)
- If an injection site is contaminated with feces, cleanse it well with soap and water before injection to avoid introducing pathogens into the site.
- Place the infant in a secure position, and have an assistant immobilize him if necessary.
- Cleanse the injection site with an alcohol sponge, moving outward from the center with a spiral motion to avoid contaminating the clean area.
- Grasp the skin between your thumb and forefinger to immobilize it and to create a muscle mass for the injection. Then, insert the needle with a quick darting motion. If injecting into the vastus lateralis or rectus femoris muscle, inject at a 45° angle toward the knee.
- Withdraw the syringe plunger slightly to ensure that the needle is not in a blood vessel. If no blood appears, inject the medication slowly so the muscle can distend to accommodate the volume.
- Withdraw the needle and rub the area with a 2" × 2" gauze pad to stimulate circulation and enhance absorption, unless contraindicated. Place a small adhesive bandage over the injection site.
- Hold and comfort the infant to reassure him or, preferably, have his parent do this.
- Document the procedure and the injection site.

Giving an I.M. injection to a toddler or older child

It is usually best to have two people available to restrain a toddler or preschooler when giving an injection. The school-age child may or may not require restraint. To reduce the stress associated with this painful experience, it is helpful to offer honest explanations in terms the child can understand, to provide time for the child to play giving the injection, and to reward the child after the injection with such things as stickers, a favorite beverage, or a colorful adhesive bandage.

Do not spend time on lengthy explanations of injections. Instead, try to divert the child's attention so his muscle will be more relaxed—unless watching increases his sense of control. If he is old enough, suggest he start counting just as you insert the needle and see if he can reach 10 before you are finished. Or have him shout "ouch" as loud as he can.

Steps
- Explain each step to the child in a way that matches his level of understanding and cooperation. Explain that the injection will hurt briefly, but will help him get better, and that it is not a punishment. Allow him to help as much as possible and as he desires.
- Have an assistant standing by to distract or immobilize the child for the injection, if necessary.
- Select the injection site. The lateral and anterior aspects of the thigh are the least threatening and safest sites for the toddler or preschooler. The ventrogluteal site may be used. The upper outer quadrant of the dorsogluteal muscle may be used for the older school-age child, but accuracy is crucial because of the danger of damaging the sciatic nerve. The deltoid muscle may be used for injecting small volumes to older, larger children.
- Cleanse the injection site with an alcohol sponge, working with a spiral motion outward from the center to avoid contaminating the clean area.

- Grasp the skin between your thumb and forefinger to immobilize it and to create a muscle mass for the injection. Then, insert the needle. For anterior and lateral thigh sites, insert the needle at a 45° angle directed toward the child's knee. For posterior and ventrogluteal sites, insert the needle at an angle perpendicular to the surface the child is lying on, rather than to the skin surface.
- Withdraw the plunger slightly. If no blood appears, slowly inject the medication. Then withdraw the needle, rub the site (unless contraindicated), and cover it with a small adhesive bandage.
- Hold the child for a few minutes or, preferably, ask his parent to hold him, to calm and comfort him.
- Document the procedure and the injection site.

Giving a subcutaneous injection

Usually, adult sites and techniques can be used (see "Giving a subcutaneous injection," p. 93). Although some subcutaneous medications, such as heparin and insulin, are given abdominally in adults, abdominal sites are not used for infants or small children.

Giving an intradermal injection

Generally, adult techniques may be used to give an intradermal injection (see "Giving an intradermal injection," p. 92). Intradermal injections are most commonly given to children in the tine test, the tuberculin test, and allergy tests. The dorsal forearm is the preferred site.

Instilling nasal medications

Although the procedure is basically the same for all age-groups, consider the child's stage of development when instilling nose drops. Warm nose drops to body temperature for an infant by running warm water over the container for several minutes or by carrying the container in your pocket for 30 minutes.

Steps
- Place a pillow under the child's shoulders and allow his head to drop back over the edge; have him lie on the bed so his head hangs over the edge; or hold him with your arm under his neck and his head tilted back.
- Draw the warmed medication into the dropper.
- Instill the prescribed number of drops or amount of medication without touching the dropper to the nasal mucosa, to avoid contaminating the remaining nose drops with bacteria. For the infant who is an obligate nose breather, open his nostrils for instillation by gently pushing up on the tip of his nose.
- Repeat the procedure in the other nostril, if ordered.
- After instillation, keep the child's head tilted back for 3 to 5 minutes to achieve full drug absorption. If the child coughs or shows signs of aspiration, place him upright and pat his back to clear the lungs.
- When administering decongestant (saline) drops, give them 20 minutes before mealtime, to make eating easier. If you are giving them to an infant, gently suction the nostrils with an infant bulb syringe before administration to remove excess mucus, and suction again approximately 20 minutes after administration.
- Document the procedure.

Instilling ear medications

Eardrops must be warmed for a child of any age. Warm them to body temperature by running warm water over the container for several minutes or by carrying the container in your pocket for 30 minutes. *Cold eardrops can cause pain and vertigo.* Test the temperature of the drops before administering them.

Steps
- Have the child lie on his side with the affected ear up. The young child may need to be restrained.
- Draw the warmed medication into the dropper.
- If the child is under age 3, gently pull the pinna *down* and straight back before instillation, because the auditory canal of infants and toddlers differs from that of older children and adults. For the child over age 3, pull the pinna *upward* and back.
- Instill the prescribed number of drops. Then, gently massage the area immediately

RESTRAINING A CHILD

To help a parent easily administer eye drops or eye ointment to a struggling 2-year-old, try teaching the restraining position shown here. The steps are as follows:
   First, place a pad on the floor and sit on it, or sit in the middle of a bed. Then, place the child between your legs, and put your thighs over the child's arms, as shown. The child's head and body are then secured between your thighs, and he cannot use his arms to struggle.
   Now you can freely administer the medication without help.

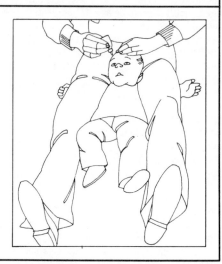

behind the ear, if this does not cause the child discomfort, to facilitate entry of the drops.
• Maintain the child's position for 5 minutes to ensure absorption of medication. Place a piece of loosely packed cotton in the external canal, if ordered, to keep the drops from running out.
• Repeat the instillation in the other ear, if ordered.
• Document the procedure.

Administering eye medications

Children fear having anything placed in their eyes. They are quick to close their eyes tightly, preventing administration of the medication. If the child is old enough, explain the procedure and demonstrate how you will retract the eyelid to administer the medication in the lower conjunctival sac. Also suggest that he close his eyes while you retract his eyelid, to keep him from looking at the dropper or applicator as it comes toward his eye.
   Adequate restraint is necessary to prevent injury to the eye. Otherwise, use the same technique as for an adult. (See "Administering eye medications," p. 128.) If necessary, obtain assistance to restrain the child. If therapy must be continued at home, show the parent(s) how to adequately restrain the child and administer the medication. (See *Restraining a Child.*) Document the procedure carefully.

Administering rectal suppositories

Rectal administration is not the best route of administration in children because of unpredictable absorption from the colon. However, it may be the route of choice when the child is vomiting.
   Most children do not like having a rectal suppository inserted, so restraint is necessary. The preschooler may become extremely upset at receiving medication this way because of his fear of body entry. For the child over age 2, explanations and developmental approaches are important to decrease anxiety.

Steps
• Explain the procedure to the child and the reasons for giving the medication this way.
• Take the suppository from the refrigerator and open the suppository package immediately before use to keep it from melting.

- Put on a clean examination glove or a finger cot. Then, lubricate the suppository with a water-soluble lubricant.
- Insert the suppository beyond the anal sphincter, using your fifth digit in infants and toddlers, and, usually, your index finger in older children. Withdraw your finger, and hold the child's buttocks together until he no longer feels the urge to defecate.
- If the child defecates within 10 to 30 minutes after insertion, check the stool for the suppository. If it was not given as a laxative and it is expelled, notify the physician.
- Document the procedure. Note expulsion of a suppository as well as any nursing actions taken.

Applying topical medications

Use the same techniques for applying topical medications in children and adults. (See Chapter 10, Topical Application of Medication.) If applying a medication for dermatitis, you can apply mitten or elbow restraints to prevent scratching.

Administering inhalants

If possible, avoid using inhalants in very young children. Obtaining their cooperation is difficult because they are frightened by the equipment. Some inhalant medications are given via cool vapor in a mist tent. The mist tent should be sealed around the child for maximum absorption. Toys may be placed in the mist tent with the child to keep him occupied. A face mask is used for a young child, and he will respond more positively if he is held during the procedure. An older child may feel he will be unable to breathe during the treatment.

Before attempting to administer medication through a metered-dose nebulizer to an older child, explain the nebulizer to him. After explaining the procedure, have him hold the nebulizer upside down, close his lips around the mouthpiece, and exhale. Then, pinch his nostrils shut, and when he starts to inhale, release one dose of medication into his mouth. Tell the patient to continue inhaling until his lungs feel full. Make sure you always clean the inhaler after use to minimize bacterial contamination.

I.V. THERAPY

I.V. therapy allows administration of drugs, replacement of electrolytes, delivery of parenteral nutrition, and maintenance of fluid balance. As with administering medications, providing I.V. therapy for infants and children requires consideration of special anatomic, physiologic, and developmental needs.

Anatomic considerations

Anatomic differences, mainly those of size and vein availability, affect the selection of cannulas and other equipment used to deliver I.V. therapy, as well as the selection of an appropriate venipuncture site. Because a child's veins are so small, he has fewer easily available I.V. sites than an adult. You must choose a site wisely and take special care to preserve the vein. The site chosen should involve minimum risk and allow maximum efficiency and safety.

In an infant, a scalp vein may be the preferred infusion site, because it is more accessible and often larger than a peripheral vein. However, the head must be shaved around the site and additional disfigurement may result from needle insertion and infiltrated fluids. For these reasons, scalp veins are not used as frequently as they have been in the past. Check your institution's policy on using scalp veins.

In an older infant, a toddler, or a child, a peripheral vein in the hand, wrist, or foot is the usual site, because it is easy to stabilize. Also consider how long the child will be receiving I.V. therapy. If he is scheduled for long-term therapy, plan venipuncture sites in advance, and rotate them every 72 hours, or according to institutional policy. Regular rotation reduces the risk of infection, thrombophlebitis, and other complications. (*Note:* Avoid a site over a joint, since the joint would have to be immobilized.)

When selecting equipment, use a small-gauge (21G to 27G) needle or catheter for a child. A winged-tip or butterfly needle is frequently used. A small needle is less likely to irritate the vein wall. It will also look less frightening to the child than a larger needle. For long-term therapy, a flexible catheter is used instead of a needle, to minimize the risk of vein injury. In an emergency, if venipuncture is difficult, a surgical cutdown may be performed.

You will administer most pediatric I.V. medications with a volume-control set and microdrip tubing (although you may use the I.V. push method under some circumstances). The volume-control set delivers small amounts of medication or fluid over an extended period of time. For greatest accuracy, however, use an infusion pump with the volume-control set. Remember, a child's size and metabolism make him especially susceptible to overdose, fluid overload, or dehydration.

Physiologic considerations

Maintaining fluid and electrolyte balance is an extremely important factor in administering I.V. therapy to an infant or child. A child's size increases the risk of both fluid overload and medication overdoses and decreases his ability to overcome them if they occur. His metabolic rate, which determines his body's water requirements, is about three times greater than an adult's, and his insensible water losses are greater because he has a larger surface area in relation to weight. Thus, a child needs more water per kilogram of body weight than an adult and can easily become dehydrated. An immature renal system may also cause more water to be excreted in the urine. To administer I.V. infusions safely and prevent fluid and electrolyte imbalance, you should know about solution compatibilities, dilution requirements, maximum administration times, maximum infusion rates, and maintenance of flow rate and fluid balance.

Solution compatibilities
If a medication is routine and compatible with the main I.V. solution, it may be diluted in enough fluid to run over 30 to 60 minutes regardless of the resulting concentration. (Administering a drug over 30 to 60 minutes can offset most concentration problems.) Usually, medications are diluted in a volume-control set in a volume of fluid at least equal to that of the reconstituted medication itself.

Occasionally, a medication must be administered using a solution that is unfavorable to the child's condition or course of treatment. In such a case, use the minimum amount of solution and infuse it over 30 to 60 minutes regardless of the resulting concentration.

If a second drug is to be run through the same I.V. tubing, first flush the tubing with a small amount of solution that is compatible with the second drug.

Dilution requirements
Some drugs are hyperosmolar; in infants, these drugs must be diluted to prevent radical changes in fluid that might induce CNS hemorrhage. Sodium bicarbonate, for example, must be diluted to half strength to lower osmolality and lessen the risk of CNS bleeding.

In general, however, use the minimum amount of compatible fluid over the shortest recommended period of time. Remember also to check the total daily fluid intake and the amount allotted to medication.

Maximum administration time and infusion rate
Whether you are infusing a *stat* or regularly scheduled medication, you should know both the maximum total administration time and the maximum infusion rate per minute. Phenytoin, for example, should be infused at no more than 50 mg/minute. If the medication has no maximum infusion rate or special concentration requirements, it may possibly be given by I.V. push. Check with the physician or pharmacist. If it has a maximum rate, follow the recommendation.

Flow rate and fluid balance
While administering a continuous I.V. infusion to a child, monitor flow rate and check the patient's condition and insertion site at least hourly—more frequently when giving medication intermittently. Flow should be adequate because some drugs (calcium, for example) can be very irritating at low flow rates. Adjust the flow rate only while the patient is composed; crying and emotional upset can constrict blood vessels.

An infusion pump should be used for accurate administration. Remember, though, the pump is not foolproof; it will continue to

FLUID AND NUTRITIONAL BALANCE: MEETING INFANTS' AND CHILDREN'S NEEDS

Maintaining proper fluid and electrolyte levels in infants is critical. An infant's body is 70% to 75% water, whereas an adult's is only 50% to 60%. Therefore, gastrointestinal upset in an infant may lead to severe dehydration and dangerous disturbance of acid-base and electrolyte balance. Also, administering I.V. fluids too fast can lead to dangerous fluid overload. To help guard against severe dehydration or fluid overload, watch closely for these signs of fluid imbalance:

Fluid overload

- Rapid pulse rate
- Hypertension
- Increased urinary output
- Decreased urine specific gravity
- Edema
- Fine crackles

Dehydration

- Rapid pulse rate
- Hypotension
- Decreased urinary output
- Increased urine specific gravity
- Dry mucous membranes
- Depressed fontanelles
- Poor skin turgor
- Lethargy
- Refusal to eat
- Distended abdomen
- Weakness
- Absence of tearing and salivation

Remember, each patient's therapy must be adjusted to his individual needs and tolerance levels. When replacing fluid and electrolytes, the type and amounts used may vary from one age-group to another. Nutritional requirements also change with changing growth patterns.

---

pump even if the needle becomes dislodged. Carefully examine the insertion site for signs of infiltration.

Check the patient for fluid overload and dehydration each time you inspect the I.V. site. (See *Fluid and Nutritional Balance: Meeting Infants' and Children's Needs.*) Record intake and output carefully. If flow rate is slower than was ordered, assess the patient's fluid balance and consult the physician before increasing the rate. If an increase is necessary, correct the flow rate *slowly,* especially if the glucose concentration of the solution is greater than 5%; infuse the additional volume as ordered.

Calculation of maintenance fluid requirements is similar to the calculation of pediatric dosages of medication, using body weight (ml/kg/24 hours) and body-surface area (ml/m^2/24 hours). This system is based on the fact that a child needs 100 ml of fluid for every 100 calories expended. (See *Basic Guidelines for Fluid and Nutritional Needs,* p. 300.)

Developmental considerations

In administering I.V. therapy to an infant or child, as in administering medications, the child's age and stage of development must be considered. You must be aware of the child's fears because they will influence your approach to the child and his response. These fears may include fear of bodily injury (pain, mutilation, and death); fear of separation from parents and a familiar environment; fear of the unknown, with its potential for surprise; uncertainty about limits or expected behaviors; and relative loss of control, autonomy, independence, competence, and self-confidence. The degree to which these fears are experienced depends on the child's stage of development and his past experiences with I.V. therapy.

BASIC GUIDELINES FOR FLUID AND NUTRITIONAL NEEDS

Fluid Recommendations

In Newborn Infants

1st day .... 60 to 80 ml/kg
2nd day .... 70 to 90 ml/kg
3rd day .... 80 to 100 ml/kg
4th day .... 100 to 120 ml/kg
5th day and thereafter ....120 to 140 ml/kg

Note: Patent ductus arteriosus or other congenital cardiac conditions may require that fluids be given with greater caution. Also, increased losses may raise fluid requirements.

In Infants and Children

1 to 10 kg .... 100 ml/kg/day
10 to 20 kg .... 1,000 ml plus 50 ml/each kg over 10
20 to 30 kg .... 1,500 ml plus 20 ml/each kg over 20

Note: Increased losses raise fluid requirements. Also, fluid restriction or concurrent disease may limit fluid intake.

Daily Caloric Requirements

0 to 1 year .... 90 to 120 kcal/kg
1 to 7 years .... 70 to 100 kcal/kg
7 to 12 years .... 60 to 75 kcal/kg
12 to 18 years .... 30 to 60 kcal/kg

Caloric requirements may increase:
- 12% for each degree of fever over 37° C. (98.6° F.).
- 20% to 30% with major surgery.
- 40% to 50% with severe sepsis.
- 50% to 100% with long-term failure to thrive.

Nutritional Requirements

Protein
1 to 3 g/kg/day

Carbohydrates
Enough to supply necessary calories and, in combination with fat, to supply 20 to 50 nonprotein calories for every gram of protein

Fats
1 to 4 g/kg/day to provide necessary calories in combination with carbohydrates. If patient's fat intake is restricted, supply 2% to 4% of the calories as linoleic acid to prevent essential fatty acid deficiency.

Electrolytes
Sodium .... 3 to 4 mEq/kg/day
Potassium .... 2 to 3 mEq/kg/day
Chloride .... 2 to 4 mEq/kg/day
Acetate .... 1 to 1.5 mEq/kg/day

Vitamins
Folic acid .... 50 to 75 mcg/kg/day
Vitamin B_{12} .... 5 to 10 mcg/kg/day
Vitamin K .... 150 to 200 mcg/kg/day
MVI .... 0.5 ml/kg/day

Minerals
Phosphate ..... 1 to 3 millimoles/kg/day
Calcium ....300 to 800 mg/kg/day as the gluconate salt
Magnesium .....0.25 to 0.5 mEq/kg/day

Trace elements
Zinc ... 300 mcg/kg/day in infants less than 3 kg; 100 mcg/kg/day over 3 kg
Chromium .... 0.14 mcg/kg/day
Manganese .... .2 mcg/kg/day
Copper .... 20 mcg/kg/day

You can minimize these fears by providing emotional support and honest explanations that are developmentally appropriate. You should also acknowledge the fears and accept them by letting the child know that it is all right to be afraid and to cry. When administering I.V. therapy to an infant, prepare the parents emotionally, and provide comfort for the child. Prepare a toddler or preschooler immediately before the procedure, and a school-age child several hours or a day beforehand, if possible, to allow time for assimilation of information and for asking questions.

Prepare the I.V. therapy equipment out of the child's sight, and perform the venipuncture in a treatment room, so that the child can associate his bed and room with comfort and security. This provides privacy and spares other children unnecessary exposure to the procedure. Involve the parents in comforting (but not restraining) the child during and after the procedure, and make sure they are prepared for the procedure and for their role(s). They should act as liaison between child and nurse, and not the primary information givers or restrainers. Play therapy, using simulated I.V. therapy equipment and dolls, or a coloring book may be used to help a child work out anxieties related to I.V. therapy.

Administering an I.V. infusion

Assemble the equipment outside the patient's room, preferably in a treatment room. Inspect the I.V. solution for clarity and expiration date. Add the prescribed medication to the solution, and label the container with the solution and medication added. Close both clamps on the tubing set. Spike and hang the container on an I.V. pole. Open the clamp between the bag and the volume-control set, and allow 30 to 50 ml of solution to flow into the calibrated chamber. Then tightly close the clamp, and squeeze the drip chamber. Squeezing expels air and creates a vacuum that pulls solution into the drip chamber on release. Release the drip chamber and allow the solution to fill it halfway. Attach the micropore filter to the tubing. Open the clamp on the long tubing below the drip chamber, and allow the solution to flush air from the tubing. When fluid reaches the end of the tubing and all of the air bubbles have been flushed out, close the clamp tightly. Tape all connections to ensure that the tubing does not become disconnected and air does not enter the system (as little as 10 cc of air can cause a fatal embolus). Keep the end of the tubing sterile until you are ready to connect it to the needle or catheter (see also "Administration sets," p. 169).

Cut six 8" to 10" (20- to 25-cm) strips of 1" adhesive tape and three 4" (10-cm) strips of ½" tape. Attach the ends of the tape to the counter surface or the I.V. pole to prevent tangles until ready to use. Place an identification sticker—showing the container number, date, and the patient's name and room number—on the back of the solution bag.

Steps
- Check the order and confirm the identity of the child.
- Explain the procedure to him, in language he can understand (if he is old enough to understand) and to his parent(s).
- Transport the child to the treatment room.
- Obtain assistance from at least one other staff member to help restrain the child during the procedure.
- Reassure the child; tell him another staff member is going to help him hold still.
- To minimize anxiety, you may want to allow the older child to sit up during I.V. insertion.
- Wash your hands.
- Select the insertion site for the needle or catheter. (If it is a scalp vein, shave a small area around the site to provide adequate visualization. Reassure the parents that the hair will grow back quickly. Then place a rubber band around the patient's head to help dilate the temporal vein.)
- Cleanse the insertion site and perform venipuncture in the same manner as for an adult. (See "Inserting a peripheral line," p. 195.)
- When you see venous return in the butterfly needle tubing or catheter stylet hub, attach the I.V. infusion tubing and open the clamp on the long tubing to allow solution to flow into the vein. A 3" (8-cm) connector, such as T or J tubing, may be attached after the stylet is removed; that ensures less manipulation of the I.V. catheter when changing solutions.

PROTECTING AN I.V. SITE

Protecting a child's I.V. site can be a challenge. An active child can easily dislodge an I.V. needle, possibly injuring himself. In minimizing this risk, the first step is securely taping the needle or catheter in place. For details on taping techniques, see Chapter 13, Performing I.V. Therapy Procedures, p. 195.

The next step is patient teaching. If the child is old enough to follow directions, teach him not to touch the equipment, and ask him to protect the site from jostling. If he is ambulatory, show him how to push his I.V. pole to prevent stress on the line. His cooperation reduces the risk of complications.

If possible, use a catheter instead of a needle. A flexible catheter is less likely to perforate the vein wall.

On this page are some other protective measures. But no matter which one you choose, remember these points:
• Never tape the protective cover so tightly to the patient's skin that you occlude blood flow.
• Try to use a clear, protective cover so you can frequently examine the I.V. site for complications, such as infection or infiltration. If the cover is not clear, remove it hourly to inspect the site.
• Restrain the extremity as needed.

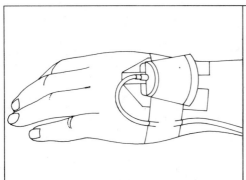

Medicine cup
Take a clean, empty medicine cup made of clear plastic, and cut it in half lengthwise. Using nonallergenic tape, tape the half-cup over the I.V. site. As you can see, the I.V. taping protects his skin from the cup's edges.

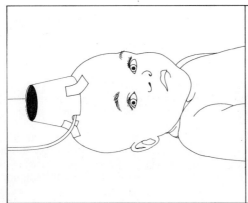

Paper cup
Consider using a small paper cup to protect a scalp site. First, cut off the cup's bottom. Then, cut a small slot through the top rim to accommodate the I.V. tubing. Place the cup upside down over the insertion site, so the I.V. tubing extends through the slot. Then, secure the cup with strips of tape, as shown in this illustration. The opening you cut in the cup allows you to examine the site without disturbing it. *Note:* You may also protect a scalp site by placing a stockinette on the infant's head.

continued

PROTECTING AN I.V. SITE *(continued)*

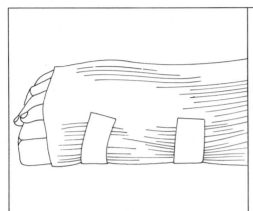

Stockinette and armboard
Obtain some 4" stockinette and cut a piece that is the same length as your patient's arm. Slip the stockinette over your patient's arm, and place that arm on an armboard. Then, grasp the stockinette at both sides of his arm, and stretch it underneath the armboard. Securely tape the stockinette underneath the armboard, as shown.

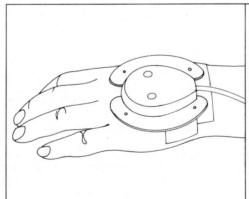

Posey I.V. shield
First, peel back the strips covering the adhesive backing on the bottom of the shield. Position the shield over the site, so that the I.V. tubing runs through one of the shield's two slots. Then, firmly press the shield's adhesive backing against the child's skin. You can easily observe the site's condition through the clear plastic shield.
  Suppose the shield is too large to fit securely over the site? Cut off the shield's narrow end, just below the two air holes. Now, you can easily shape the shield to your patient's arm.

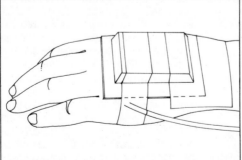

Needle container
If you are using a butterfly needle, make a protective cover out of the needle's plastic container. As you see, this protective device is similar to the medicine cup device.

- Secure the wings of the butterfly needle with ½" adhesive tape, using the crossover technique. To do this, pull a strip of tape into a V. With the sticky side up, slide it under the wings of the butterfly needle so the arms of the V remain exposed approximately 2" (5 cm). Then press the wings down on the tape to secure them. Next, fold the arms back diagonally so they crisscross over the needle. Finish by placing another strip of tape horizontally across the X formed by the bands of tape. A sterile dressing may be applied to the site, according to institutional policy.
- Tape the patient's arm to the padded armboard with 1" adhesive tape to minimize movement, diminish tension on the vein, and decrease the risk of dislodging the needle. Place gauze under the tape wherever it will touch the skin to prevent irritation and skin breakdown. (In young children, the armboard may be applied prior to venipuncture to stabilize the site.)
- Adjust the flow of solution to the correct rate. Keep the clamp between the solution bag and the volume-control set closed until you are ready to add solution to the chamber.
- Protect the I.V. site to prevent accidental dislodging of the needle. (See *Protecting an I.V. Site*, pp. 302-303.)
- Pin the padded armboard to the sheet of the crib or bed, or tape it to a small sandbag pinned to the sheet, to discourage movement.
- Position the solution bag at the appropriate height to maintain a continuous drip. Use a mechanical infusion pump to facilitate a more precise flow rate, particularly for very small children and those sensitive to fluid overload, such as patients with cardiac disorders. *Always* use a volume-control set, even if a pump is used, to minimize the risk of fluid overload in case of accidental detachment of the tubing from the pump.
- Keep the clamp on the long infusion tubing close to the drip chamber and be sure it is out of the child's reach; if extension tubing is used to allow the child greater mobility, securely tape the connection.
- Add solution hourly from the I.V. bag to the volume-control set. To decrease the risk of fluid overload, never place more than 10 to 20 ml extra in the volume-control set each hour. Also assess the infusion site at least hourly for signs of infiltration (swelling, redness, and warmth).
- If a child's food and fluid intake is restricted, provide frequent mouth care. Offer a pacifier to an infant. Assess the state of hydration frequently by observing skin turgor, moistness of the oral mucosa, urinary output and specific gravity, and, in an infant, the state of the anterior fontanelle.
- Keep accurate intake and output and daily weight records.
- Use appropriate restraints to prevent dislodging the needle. Usually, if the needle is inserted into an arm vein, restrain the child's other arm. If it is inserted into a foot vein, restrain the other foot and both arms.
- Check the restraint sites *at least* hourly and provide meticulous skin care, as needed, to prevent breakdown.
- In an older child, secure the device in a way that allows the child to continue play activities.
- To allay anxiety, give a simple explanation to the child who must be restrained while asleep.
- In your notes, record the date and time of insertion, type and amount of parenteral solution, type and gauge of needle, insertion site, and indications of the patient's state of hydration. Document the condition of the infusion site, patency of the I.V. system, and application of restraints. Note the specific gravity of the patient's urine, and record hourly fluid intake and output on the intake and output sheet. Record parenteral infusions on the I.V. record sheet.
- For I.V. therapy that continues several days or longer, change the tubing and solution bag regularly, according to institutional policy, to prevent infection. Label each with the date and time it is replaced.
- If a solution containing a new medication is started, be sure to change the I.V. tubing or flush it with a compatible solution.
- Encourage the child to talk or "play out" feelings.
- Because the child may need to be restrained or positioned in bed, provide appropriate stimulation, activity, and diversions.
- Teach the child (if old enough) and the parents the signs of I.V. complications (such as infiltration, phlebitis, and infection). Tell them to report signs to the nurse immediately.

- In discontinuing an I.V. infusion, follow the principles and techniques used with adult patients.

Parenteral nutrition

Parenteral nutrition, administered through a central or peripheral vein, is given to patients who cannot or will not take adequate food orally and to patients with hypermetabolic conditions who need I.V. supplementation. The latter group includes premature infants and children who have burns or other major trauma, intractable diarrhea, malabsorption syndromes, GI abnormalities, emotional disorders such as anorexia nervosa, and congenital abnormalities.

Solution components
Parenteral nutrition should not only reverse catabolism but also promote normal growth and development. Overall, a child has greater need than an adult for protein, carbohydrate, fat, electrolytes, trace elements, vitamins, and fluid. (See *Basic Guidelines for Fluid and Nutritional Needs*, p. 300.) Accurate calculations of components and correct formulation of parenteral nutrition for children help prevent solution incompatibilities, which impair efficient delivery of nutrients.

Protein is supplied primarily as crystalline amino acids. Adequate nonprotein calories must also be furnished so that amino acids are not metabolized for energy but rather utilized for protein synthesis. Nonprotein calories are supplied as dextrose solutions or fat emulsions, both of which have limitations.

Dextrose, started at a concentration of 5% or 10%, is gradually increased according to the patient's tolerance. Peripheral veins can accept dextrose concentrations as high as 12.5%; phlebitis can develop at higher concentrations. These higher concentrations are administered through central venous lines. Central veins can accept solution concentrations as high as 50%.

Fats, supplied as 10% or 20% emulsions, are administered both peripherally and centrally. Their use is limited by the child's ability to metabolize them. For example, an infant or child with a diseased liver cannot efficiently metabolize fats. Some fats, however, must be supplied to prevent essential fatty acid deficiency and to support normal growth and development. A minimum of calories (2% to 4%) must be supplied as linoleic acid—an essential fatty acid found in lipids.

In the infant, fats are essential for normal neurologic development. Nevertheless, fat solutions may decrease oxygen perfusion and may adversely affect infants with pulmonary disease. That risk can be minimized by supplying only the minimum fat needed for essential fatty acid requirements and not the usual intake of 40% to 50% of the patient's total calories.

Fatty acids can also displace bilirubin bound to serum albumin, causing a rise in free, unconjugated bilirubin and an increased risk of kernicterus. However, fat solutions may interfere with some bilirubin assays and cause falsely elevated levels. To avoid this, a blood sample should be drawn 4 hours after infusion of the lipid emulsion, or, if the emulsion is introduced over 24 hours, the blood sample should be centrifuged before the assay is performed.

Special precautions
- I.V. lines should be used exclusively for nutrient solutions unless all other routes for medication are exhausted. If drugs must be administered through the parenteral line simultaneously with nutrient solutions, first consult the pharmacist for compatibility information. To prevent interactions and precipitation, ask about additives that can be mixed with the solution. Only heparin can be added to a fat emulsion, and no other drug should be introduced at the same time.
- Dextrose-protein solutions should be filtered. Fluids used in parenteral nutrition should be free of microorganisms and particulate matter, but contamination is possible. Therefore, use a 0.22-micron aerophobic filter to prevent inadvertent administration of all microorganisms (except viruses) and particulate matter. Since air cannot pass through the filter after it is primed, it prevents an air embolus from forming if the line has to be changed or the pump breaks down. (Note: Because fats cannot be filtered, the lipid emulsion should be piggybacked into the line below the filter.)

- Administer solutions at the prescribed rate. If the flow rate falls behind, do not adjust to compensate. Consult the physician, and with his permission, increase the rate only as much as 5% per hour, if necessary. Rate changes may quickly cause metabolic problems such as hyperglycemia and hypoglycemia in children.
- Increasing the rate or making up for behind-schedule feedings can result in dextrose overload and subsequent osmotic diuresis, leading to rapid dehydration. Monitor intake and output closely, and be alert for disturbances in fluid balance.
- Considering the patient's size, initially monitor electrolyte, blood urea nitrogen (BUN), and blood glucose levels daily, and cholesterol level weekly. To prevent osmotic diuresis, check for glycosuria every 6 hours. After these levels are stabilized, laboratory monitoring can be done less often.
- Since infection is a serious complication of parenteral nutrition, monitor vital signs closely for early indications of sepsis. Glycosuria > 2% may also be an accurate early indicator of sepsis.
- Scrutinize the catheter site for infection, inflammation, and infiltration.
- Change the tubing down to the catheter hub every 24 hours.
- Initial the dressing, and label it with the time and date it is changed.

Blood transfusion

Transfusing blood and blood products in children is very similar to transfusing in an adult. (See Chapter 16, Blood and Blood Component Transfusion.) The major differences lie in the approach to the patient, the size of the equipment used (24G or 22G thin-walled catheter or 23G or 21G butterfly needle), the rate of infusion, and the volume infused. Transfusing blood in newborns, however, requires highly specialized training because their physiologic requirements differ vastly from those of the normal infant, child, or adult.

One transfusion procedure unique to the newborn is exchange transfusion. Used to treat hemolytic disease of the newborn and performed by a physician with a nurse assisting, exchange transfusion is a sterile procedure that replaces a newborn's blood with an equal amount of compatible donor blood to remove excess bilirubin and prevent kernicterus. A two-volume exchange replaces about 85% of the newborn's blood and lowers the bilirubin level in blood by about 50%. It does not remove bilirubin in tissue and extravascular spaces, and this bilirubin migrates back into the plasma.

Exchange transfusion usually requires umbilical catheterization and is usually performed when the bilirubin level increases more than 1 mg/dl each hour, or reaches 20 mg/dl in a normal full-term newborn or 15 to 16 mg/dl in a premature or weak newborn. It is not performed when the bilirubin level can be lowered by other treatment, such as phototherapy.

Albumin may be given prior to exchange transfusion to bind bilirubin so that it can be extracted during the exchange.

Preservatives in donor blood may lower calcium and dextrose levels. These must be monitored closely during exchange transfusion and during regular transfusion.

Review Questions

1. Name four factors that affect drug dosage in children.

2. What are some factors that affect absorption of orally administered medication? How and why do they affect absorption?

3. In topical application of drugs, how do rate and completeness of absorption in a child compare with the rate and completeness in an adult? Explain why.

4. True or false: Intramuscular administration is a good route in children because absorption of the medication is complete.

5. True or false: Because a child has fewer protein-binding sites than an adult, many drugs are *less bound* to plasma proteins and therefore have a more intense pharmacologic effect.

6. True or false: A water-soluble drug's concentration and effect would be greater in an infant than in an adult.

7. A newborn's ability to metabolize a drug depends on what *three* things?

8. Why should the dosage of a medication such as an antibiotic be reduced in an infant?

9. What is the most common method of calculating pediatric dosages? What is the most accurate method?

10. Other than administering the correct dose, what is the most important consideration in giving an oral medication to an infant?

11. Other than administering the correct dose, what is one of the most important considerations in giving an injection to an infant?

12. List three ways to facilitate medication administration in toddlers and older children.

13. Usually, the _____ is the preferred site for giving an I.M. injection to an infant.

14. When giving eardrops, pull the pinna _____ and _____ in the child under age 3, and _____ and _____ in the child over age 3.

15. How can you prevent a child from quickly closing his eyes before eye medication is instilled?

16. What are three indications for I.V. therapy in children?

17. What is the usual site selected for insertion of an I.V. line in infants and children?

18. What measures should be taken to prevent dislodging the needle?

19. What is the purpose of using a volume-control set and an infusion pump when administering I.V. solutions?

20. What are the indications for parenteral nutrition in children?

21. Because children are smaller than adults, their requirements for protein, carbohydrates, fat, elecrolytes, trace elements, vitamins, and fluid are lower than those of adults. True or false?

22. What is the risk associated with peripheral infusion of highly concentrated dextrose solutions?

23. What serious complication of parenteral nutrition in children would most likely necessitate removal of the catheter?

24. If the flow rate of a feeding solution falls behind the ordered rate, you should increase it by more than 5% per hour to ensure that the child receives the prescribed amount of nutrients. True or false?

25. What is the purpose of neonatal exchange transfusion?

Selected References

American Association of Critical Care Nurses. *Critical Care Nursing of Children and Adolescents.* Edited by Oakes, A.R. Philadelphia: W.B. Saunders Co., 1981.
Chow, M.P., et al. *Handbook of Pediatric Primary Care,* 2nd ed. New York: John Wiley & Sons, 1984.
Drugs, 2nd ed. Nurse's Reference Library. Springhouse, Pa.: Springhouse Corp., 1984.
Hamilton, P.M. *Basic Pediatric Nursing,* 4th ed. St. Louis: C.V. Mosby Co., 1982.
Hilt, N., and Cogburn, S. *Manual of Orthopedics.* St. Louis: C.V. Mosby Co., 1980.
Howry, L.B., et al. *Pediatric Medications.* Philadelphia: J.B. Lippincott Co., 1981.
Latham, H.D., et al. *Pediatric Nursing,* 3rd ed. St. Louis: C.V. Mosby Co., 1977.
Pagliaro, L.A., and Lenin, R.H. *Problems in Pediatric Drug Therapy.* Hamilton, Ill.: Drug Intelligence Pubs., 1979.
Procedures. Nurse's Reference Library. Springhouse, Pa.: Springhouse Corp., 1985.
Scipien, G., et al. *Comprehensive Pediatric Nursing,* 3rd ed. New York: McGraw-Hill Book Co., 1986.
Whaley, L.F., and Wong, D. *Nursing Care of Infants and Children.* St. Louis: C.V. Mosby Co., 1979.
Yaffe, S.J., ed. *Pediatric Pharmacology.* New York: Grune & Stratton, 1980.

Geriatric Drug and I.V. Therapy

When providing drug and I.V. therapy for elderly patients, you should understand patterns of drug use in the elderly, age-related pharmacokinetic and physiologic changes that may affect drug dosage and I.V. therapy techniques, common adverse reactions, and how to improve compliance in the elderly. Although the principles and procedures of drug administration and I.V. therapy are essentially the same for patients of any age, these factors require changes in approach and technique, which are covered in this chapter.

Medication consumption patterns

Medication consumption increases with age. In fact, the elderly consume more prescription and nonprescription drugs than the young because they have a greater variety of diseases requiring one or more medications. An elderly patient with congestive heart failure, for example, may take three prescription drugs: digoxin, to improve cardiac contractility; a diuretic such as furosemide, to help eliminate excess body fluid; and potassium chloride, to replace potassium lost due to the diuretic's action.

Other diseases common to the elderly, such as arthritis and angina pectoris, also may require multiple medications. Besides major diseases, elderly persons may take medication for aches and pains, constipation and other gastrointestinal (GI) complaints, insomnia, and various skin disorders.

An older person's socioeconomic status, personal health, and living environment (extended-care facility or community living, for example) may affect his drug use. In particular, elderly patients in nursing homes take between four and seven medications concurrently; elderly outpatients usually take between two and four different medications. (For the medications taken most frequently by the elderly, see *Geriatric Drug Use: A Closer Look.*)

Physiologic changes affecting drug action

As a person ages, he undergoes gradual anatomic and physiologic changes. Some of these age-related changes may alter the therapeutic and toxic effects of medications.

Body composition
Proportions of fat, lean tissue, and water in the body change with age. Total body mass and lean body mass tend to decrease, and the proportion of body fat tends to increase. Varying from person to person, these changes in body composition affect the relationship between a drug's concentration and its distribution in the body. For example, a water-soluble drug such as gentamicin is not distributed to fat, and since the elderly person has relatively less lean tissue, more drug remains in the blood.

Gastrointestinal function
In the elderly, decreases in gastric acid secretion and GI motility slow gastric emptying and transit of intestinal contents. The precise influence of these changes has yet to be determined; however, it now appears that they do not significantly alter absorption of drugs taken by mouth. Some drugs, however, are not well absorbed in the elderly. Digoxin is one of these. Since the

GERIATRIC DRUG USE: A CLOSER LOOK

According to a recent survey by the National Center for Health Statistics, the drug types shown in this pie chart were most often ordered for geriatric patients. The figures given for each slice of the pie indicate the percentage distribution for each drug.

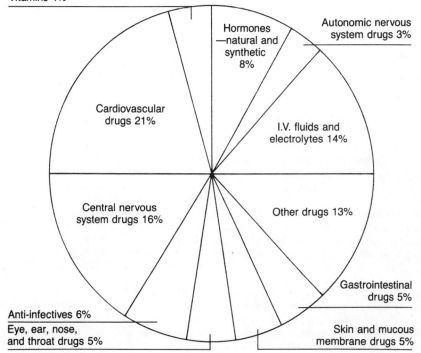

- Vitamins 4%
- Hormones—natural and synthetic 8%
- Autonomic nervous system drugs 3%
- Cardiovascular drugs 21%
- I.V. fluids and electrolytes 14%
- Central nervous system drugs 16%
- Other drugs 13%
- Anti-infectives 6%
- Eye, ear, nose, and throat drugs 5%
- Gastrointestinal drugs 5%
- Skin and mucous membrane drugs 5%

Ten most commonly ordered drugs for females age 65 and older
1. Digoxin (Lanoxin)
2. Furosemide (Lasix)
3. Triamterene and hydrochlorothiazide (Dyazide)
4. Propranolol (Inderal)
5. Methyldopa (Aldomet)
6. Vitamin B_{12}
7. Digoxin (all brands)
8. Ibuprofen (Motrin)
9. Insulin
10. Hydrochlorothiazide (all brands)

Ten most commonly ordered drugs for males age 65 and older
1. Furosemide (Lasix)
2. Digoxin (Lanoxin)
3. Propranolol (Inderal)
4. Digoxin (all brands)
5. Isosorbide (Isordil)
6. Triamterene and hydrochlorothiazide (Dyazide)
7. Aspirin
8. Hydrochlorothiazide (all brands)
9. Hydrochlorothiazide (HydroDIURIL)
10. Prednisone

Source: National Center for Health Statistics

range between sub-therapeutic, therapeutic, and toxic blood levels of digoxin may be very narrow, slight changes in degree of absorption can have a significant effect.

Hepatic function

The liver's ability to metabolize certain drugs decreases with age. That is probably the result of diminished blood flow to the liver, associated with an age-related decrease in cardiac output. When an elderly patient takes certain sleep medications, such as secobarbital, reduced hepatic metabolism of the drug may produce a hangover effect because of central nervous system depression. Elimination of these medications is highly dependent on the liver.

Decreased hepatic function may cause:
- more intense drug effects due to higher blood levels
- longer-lasting drug effects due to prolonged blood concentrations
- greater incidence of drug toxicity.

Renal function

Although an elderly person's renal function is usually sufficient to eliminate excess body fluid and waste products, his ability to eliminate some medications may be reduced by 50% or more. Many medications commonly used by the elderly, such as digoxin, are excreted primarily through the kidneys. If renal excretion of the drug is decreased, high blood concentrations may result. Digoxin toxicity, therefore, is relatively common.

Drug dosages can be modified to compensate for age-related decreases in renal function. Aided by laboratory tests, such as blood urea nitrogen (BUN) and serum creatinine, clinical pharmacists and physicians can adjust medication dosages and dose frequency so that the patient receives the desired therapeutic benefits without risk of toxicity. Observe your patient for signs of toxicity. A patient taking digoxin, for example, may experience anorexia, nausea, and vomiting.

Adverse drug reactions

Compared with younger people, the elderly reportedly experience twice as many adverse drug reactions relating to greater drug consumption, poor compliance, and physiologic changes.

Signs and symptoms of adverse drug reactions—confusion, weakness, and lethargy—are often mistakenly attributed to senility or disease. (See *Senility or Side Effects?*) If an adverse reaction is not identified, the patient may continue to receive the drug. Furthermore, he may receive unnecessary additional medication to treat complications caused by the original medication.

Although any medication can cause adverse reactions, most of the serious reactions in the elderly are caused by relatively few medications. Be particularly alert for toxicity resulting from diuretics, digoxin, corticosteroids, sleep medications, and nonprescription drugs.

Diuretic toxicity

Because total body water decreases with age, normal doses of potassium-wasting diuretics such as hydrochlorothiazide and furosemide may result in fluid loss and even dehydration in an elderly patient. These diuretics may deplete serum potassium, causing weakness. They may also raise blood uric acid and glucose levels, complicating preexisting gout and diabetes mellitus.

Digoxin toxicity

As the body's renal function and rate of excretion decline, digoxin concentrations in the blood may build to toxic levels, causing nausea, vomiting, diarrhea, and—most serious—cardiac dysrhythmias. Try to prevent severe toxicity by observing your patient for early signs, such as appetite loss, confusion, or depression.

Corticosteroid toxicity

Elderly patients on corticosteroids may experience short-term effects, including fluid retention and psychological manifestations ranging from mild euphoria to acute psychotic reactions. Long-term toxic effects, such as osteoporosis, can be especially severe in elderly patients who have been taking prednisone or related steroidal compounds for months or even years. To prevent serious toxicity, carefully monitor patients on long-term regimens. Observe them for subtle changes in appearance, mood, and

SENILITY OR SIDE EFFECTS?

Myth: *All elderly patients who exhibit symptoms associated with old age (such as drowsiness, forgetfulness, and confusion) are senile.*

Fact: *Many symptoms attributed to senility are actually side effects of drugs commonly prescribed for the elderly.*

Elderly patients themselves may assume that adverse drug reactions are due simply to aging. If the physician does not warn them about side effects, they may ignore them or suffer through them needlessly. To help distinguish drug effects from senility in an elderly patient:
• Check the patient's medication to be sure he is getting the lowest effective dose. You can help the physician determine the lowest effective dose by monitoring the patient for therapeutic and adverse effects until steady-state blood concentrations have been attained, and by documenting your observations.
• Teach the patient to watch for possible side effects of his medications. Tell him to contact his physician if they occur.
• Suggest that he have a thorough physical examination to rule out undiagnosed conditions, such as cardiac disease and nutritional deficiencies, that can contribute to senility.
• Review all his medications for possible drug interactions that may cause symptoms that mimic senility. Watch for these:

Symptoms	Possible Causes
Confusion	Methyldopa
Depression	Reserpine
Anorexia	Digoxin
Weakness	Certain diuretics, such as furosemide and hydrochlorothiazide, which can deplete body potassium
Lethargy and drowsiness	Various tranquilizers, analgesics, and sleep medications, including chlorpromazine and pentobarbital
Ataxia	Inappropriately high doses of flurazepam and other sedatives or hypnotics
Forgetfulness	Barbiturates
Constipation	Medications with anticholinergic properties, such as belladonna-containing drugs, narcotics, and tricyclic antidepressants
Diarrhea	Various oral antacid preparations containing magnesium hydroxide
Gastrointestinal distress	Oral iron preparations or antiarthritic medications, such as aspirin, ibuprofen, or indomethacin

mobility, as well as for signs of impaired healing and fluid and electrolyte disturbances.

Sleep medication toxicity
In some cases, sedatives or sleeping aids such as flurazepam cause excessive sedation or residual drowsiness.

Nonprescription drug toxicity
When aspirin and aspirin-containing analgesics are used in moderation, toxicity is minimal, but prolonged ingestion may cause GI irritation and gradual blood loss resulting in severe anemia. Although anemia from chronic aspirin consumption can affect all age-groups, the elderly may be less able to compensate because of their already reduced iron stores.

Laxatives may cause diarrhea in elderly patients who are extremely sensitive to drugs such as bisacodyl. Chronic oral use of mineral oil as a lubricating laxative may result in lipid pneumonia due to aspiration of small residual oil droplets.

Noncompliance

Approximately one-third of the elderly fail to comply with their prescribed drug therapy. They may fail to take prescribed doses or to follow the correct schedule, or they may take medications prescribed for previous disorders, discontinue medications prematurely, or use p.r.n. medications indiscriminately. An age-related decline in sensory acuity is one reason for patient noncompliance. For example, the elderly patient with impaired vision may have difficulty reading prescription instructions. With hearing loss, the patient may not understand oral instructions. Physical disabilities such as those produced by arthritis may hinder him from opening childproof containers.

Since the patient may have received instructions for taking his medications during a time of stress or anxiety, review the amount, time, and frequency of doses with him. Explain how he should take each medication—whether with food or water, or by itself. *And make sure he understands your instructions.*

Proper nursing care can help manage, reduce, or overcome many drug therapy prob-

HELPING THE ELDERLY PATIENT TAKE MEDICATION

For the patient's drug therapy to be effective, he must take his medications exactly as his physician directs, particularly when taking several medications at one time. Here are some helpful hints you may give him:
• Suggest that he label empty jars, extra prescription bottles (he can get these from his pharmacist), or envelopes with the times of day or the days of the week he must take medication. He should use a separate container for each time and fill these containers each morning with the appropriate dose of each medication.
Note: Some drugs may deteriorate when exposed to light. Before he removes drugs from their original containers, have him check with his pharmacist or physician.
• Have him make a medication calendar. Tell him to use a calendar that has enough space to fill in the names of the drugs he needs to take each day. Then, tell him to put a check mark next to the name of the drug after he takes each dose.
• Show him how to make a chart listing:
—name of drug
—what it is for
—what it looks like (shape, color)
—directions for taking the drug
—precautions or side effects
—time of day to take the drug.
  Have him hang this chart near his medicine cabinet.
• Tell him to set the alarm clock or have him ask a relative or friend to remind him when to take his medications.
• Suggest that he use one of the aids pictured on the following page, depending on his specific needs.

Geriatric Drug and I.V. Therapy

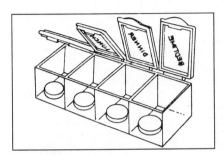

One-day Pill Reminder
Purpose:
• To help the patient determine if he has taken all the medications prescribed for a single day.
Description:
• Plastic device with four medication compartments marked breakfast, lunch, supper, and bedtime. The initial letter of each word is also marked in braille on each compartment.
Special considerations:
• Family member or visiting nurse must remember to fill device with ordered medications at the beginning of each day.
• Not appropriate for large numbers of tablets or capsules.

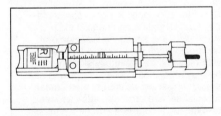

Dos-Aid Syringe Filling Device
Purpose:
• To precisely measure insulin doses (especially appropriate for a patient with vision impairment).
Description:
• Plastic device designed for use with a disposable U-100 syringe and an insulin bottle. The device is set to accommodate the syringe's width; then the plunger is positioned at the point determined by the dose and the stop tightened. When set, the patient can draw up the precise dose ordered for each injection.
Special considerations:
• Not for mixed or variable doses of insulin.
• Settings must be checked and adjusted when syringe size or type is changed.
• Screws may become loose after repeated use of device; instruct the patient to regularly check them.
• Needle can be contaminated easily.

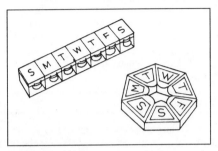

Seven-day Pill Reminder
Purpose:
• To help the patient remember if he has taken all the tablets and capsules prescribed for each day of the week.
Description:
• Both plastic devices shown here have seven medication compartments, marked with the initials for each day of the week (in both braille and letters).
Special considerations:
• Family member or visiting nurse must remember to fill with ordered medications at the beginning of each week.
• Not appropriate for large numbers of tablets and capsules, or tablets and capsules that must be taken at specific times each day.
• Useful if patient takes a medication every other day, rather than daily.

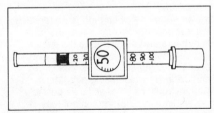

Monoject Scale Magnifier
Purpose:
• To help a vision-impaired diabetic patient read syringe markings and independently fill his own syringe.
Description:
• Plastic magnifier snaps onto syringe barrel.
Special considerations:
• May not be appropriate for an arthritic patient, who may have difficulty attaching the device.

lems in the elderly patient. (See *Helping the Elderly Patient Take Medication,* p. 312, and *Improving Compliance in the Elderly.*) Offer to review his medication regimen with him. Ask the patient or his family about the medications he currently takes. When necessary, call the patient's pharmacy and his physician(s) to get a complete medication history. Give the patient whatever help you can, and refer him to the pharmacist if he needs further information about his medications and their effects.

I.V. therapy

Although the same basic principles apply to patients of all ages, several points must be taken into consideration when administering I.V. therapy to the geriatric patient. The veins in elderly patients may be hardened and sclerosed, or fragile and easily torn. They may also be tortuous, making venipuncture difficult. Therefore, the I.V. insertion site may be difficult to select. It must be selected carefully, and a needle or catheter of appropriate type and size (for example, a 23G butterfly needle) must be chosen. (See *Commonly Used Peripheral I.V. Devices,* p. 183.)

The site must be protected adequately, especially in the confused or forgetful patient, and frequent assessments of the site should be made to prevent or minimize the risk of complications.

Monitoring the I.V. infusion is especially important in the elderly. Because they are often taking medications or have disorders that affect fluid and electrolyte levels, a normal fluid and electrolyte balance is more difficult to maintain. In addition, they may be more susceptible to fluid overload due to varying degrees of cardiac dysfunction. Carefully calculate and monitor flow rates, and observe the patient for signs and symptoms of electrolyte imbalance and fluid overload.

IMPROVING COMPLIANCE IN THE ELDERLY

An elderly patient may want to follow his physician's orders but be hindered by age-related physical problems or financial problems. To help him overcome these and improve his compliance, ask these questions:
* *Can he hear well enough to understand his instructions?* To make sure the patient hears and understands his dosage instructions, eliminate background noise during teaching sessions. Speak slowly and distinctly while facing him. Make your instructions as specific as possible.

Keep in mind that the patient may be embarrassed to admit that he cannot hear well. To make sure he understands you, ask him to repeat the instructions you give him. Writing down the instructions may help, too.
* *Can he open his medication bottles easily?* If he has arthritis or Parkinson's disease, he may need standard caps instead of childproof ones. Remind him to ask the pharmacist for standard caps whenever he needs his prescriptions refilled.
* *Is he on a fixed income?* If so, he may try to make his medications last longer.

Stress the importance of following the physician's orders exactly. If necessary, refer him to a social service representative for information on financial aid.
* *What are his eating habits?* Some of his medications may have to be taken with meals. If he habitually skips meals, he may miss those doses. Work with him to plan a realistic schedule, then contact a social service program, such as Meals on Wheels, if necessary, to help him begin eating properly.
* *Can he see well enough to read the medication labels?* If the medication is packaged in an amber container, tape the label on the outside so it will not be obscured by the tinted glass, or ask the pharmacist to package prescriptions in clear bottles (if not contraindicated). Then, the patient can identify his medication by its appearance. You can also print the dosage instructions and schedule on a separate sheet of paper (using large letters) and tape a sample tablet or capsule to the schedule. Your patient, his family, or a visiting nurse can then easily refer to them.

Review Questions

1. List three factors that affect an elderly person's drug usage.

2. Since the proportion of body fat tends to decrease with age, a water-soluble drug is better distributed to an elderly patient's body tissues. True or false?

3. Gastric acid secretion and gastrointestinal motility are decreased in the elderly and may affect the absorption of certain drugs. True or false?

4. Decreased hepatic metabolism of certain medications may affect the intensity of effect, the duration of effect, and the incidence of drug toxicity. True or false?

5. Since an elderly person's renal function is usually sufficient to eliminate excess fluid and waste products, his ability to eliminate some medications remains intact. True or false?

6. What kinds of medications are apt to cause serious adverse drug reactions in the elderly?

7. Name four possible reasons for the high incidence of noncompliance in the elderly.

8. Describe five nursing interventions that may help the elderly patient comply with his prescribed drug regimen.

9. Why may site selection for I.V. therapy in the elderly be difficult?

10. Why is monitoring the I.V. infusion so important in the elderly?

Selected References

Cros, M.R. *Pharmacology for the Elderly— The Nurse's Guide to Quality Care.* New York: Teachers College Press, 1984.

Drugs, 2nd ed. Nurse's Reference Library. Springhouse, Pa.: Springhouse Corp., 1984.

Ebersole, P., and Hess, P. "Drug Use and Abuse," in *Toward Healthy Aging.* St. Louis: C.V. Mosby Co., 1981.

Appendices

A Guidelines for I.V. Drug Administration 318

B Standard Infusion/Piggyback List 330

C Answers to Review Questions 331

Index 343

Appendix A

Guidelines for I.V. Drug Administration

The following is a sample list of drugs approved by one institution (Quakertown Community Hospital in Pennsylvania) for the administration of I.V. medications by nurses. This example may be useful in determining similar policies in other institutions. Information is included on the type of I.V. administration, with pertinent comments/restrictions and guidelines for their use.

Three categories of nursing staff are used:
A. Staff nurses in any hospital area
B. Certified oncology nurses
C. Staff nurses in the intensive care unit (ICU) or step-down unit (SDU) or in the emergency room (ER), operating room (OR), or recovery room (RR)—where appropriate monitoring is used.

Under each type of I.V. drug administration (continuous infusion, piggyback, etc.) the word *Yes* or *No* appears, signifying whether nurses may administer the drug by this type of administration. Restrictions are noted with the letter A, B, or C, as above. For example, if only a C appears in the column under Push, only those nurses in the ICU, SDU, ER, OR, or RR could administer the drug by I.V. push.

Definitions of Types of I.V. Drug Administration

Continuous infusion—I.V. injections greater than 100 ml that are administered at a constant rate. Drugs in this category may be added to a given infusion (except where potential incompatibility exists) by a pharmacist

DRUGS FOR I.V. ADMINISTRATION

Generic Name	Trade Name	Continuous Infusion	Intermittent Infusion VCS	PB	Push
acetazolamide	Diamox	Yes	No	Yes	Yes
acyclovir	Zovirax	No	Yes	Yes	No
albumin	Albuminar, Buminate	Yes	No	Yes	No
amikacin	Amikin	Yes	No	Yes	No
aminocaproic acid	Amicar	Yes	Yes	Yes	No
aminophylline		Yes	Yes	Yes	No
ammonium chloride		Yes	No	No	No
amphotericin B	Fungizone	Yes	No	No	No
anticancer drugs (see cancer chemotherapy)					
ascorbic acid (vitamin C)		Yes	No	No	No
atropine sulfate		No	No	No	Yes (C)
bretylium tosylate	Bretylol	Yes (C)	Yes (C)	Yes (C)	Yes (C)

and subsequently administered by a nurse. In the absence of a pharmacist or in an emergency, a nurse may admix a drug in this category. Ideally, a pharmacist should prepare *all* continuous infusions, except plain solution and solutions containing potassium chloride and/or multivitamins.

Intermittent infusion—I.V. injections less than 100 ml that are given in 15 minutes to one hour. Depending on the drug (noted on the chart below), intermittent therapy may be administered in one of three ways:

- *I.V. Push (Push)*—a relatively rapid injection of a drug given either through an injection port site (Y-site) in the I.V. tubing or through a heparin lock. Nurses are not permitted to administer an I.V. push injection directly into a vein because of the potential hazards of extravasation or drug reaction.
- *Volume-control set (VCS)*—an I.V. injection of up to 100 ml given in 15 minutes to 1 hour, using a burette chamber device (Buretrol, Soluset). The tubing leading from this device is generally connected to an injection port site on the primary I.V. line. When a VCS is employed, a separate device must be used for each drug. The VCS is labeled with the drug name, dosage, date, and time it was hung. Currently, the practice has become that the pharmacy routinely prepares intermittent infusions of drugs (piggybacks, see below), so that it is less frequently necessary to use a VCS in the inpatient area. However, a VCS may still be used in the emergency room, pediatric unit, or in some inpatient areas.
- *Piggyback (PB)*—an intermittent infusion of up to 100 ml given in 15 minutes to 1 hour, using a minibottle or minibag with an appropriate diluent (see *Standard Infusion/Piggyback List, Appendix B*, p. 330).

Various comments or restrictions may be listed below that correspond to the listed drug. Be sure to consult this list for any drugs you are not familiar with, or consult the pharmacist for further information.

Note—Drugs not appearing in the table below are not approved for administration by nurses. "No" signifies that the drug may not be administered by nurses using the indicated method.

Comments/Restrictions
Infusion concentrations of 7 mg/ml or lower are recommended. Given over 1 hour.
Infusion vehicles include D_5W, $D_{10}W$; NSS for 25% only.
PB only over 30 minutes.
VCS or PB for loading dose. Infusion pump required.
VCS or PB for loading dose. Infusion pump required.
Infuse slowly.
A 1-mg test dose should be given by physician before first dose. If possible, avoid central line administration. Protect bag (not tubing) from light.
C only except during code situation. Patient must be on EKG monitor.
Infusion pump recommended for constant infusion. Patient must be on EKG monitor. C only except during code situation.

DRUGS FOR I.V. ADMINISTRATION *(continued)*

Generic Name	Trade Name	Continuous Infusion	Intermittent Infusion VCS	PB	Push
calcium chloride		Yes	Yes	Yes	Yes (C)
calcium gluconate		Yes	Yes	Yes	Yes (C)
cancer chemotherapy	varied	Yes (B)	Yes (B)	Yes (B)	Yes (B)
cephalosporin antibiotics		Yes	Yes	Yes	No
chloramphenicol	Chloromycetin	Yes	Yes	Yes	No
cimetidine	Tagamet	No	Yes	Yes	No
clindamycin	Cleocin	Yes	Yes	Yes	No
colchicine		No	No	No	Yes
conjugated estrogens	Premarin	Yes	No	No	Yes
corticotropin		Yes	No	No	No
co-trimoxazole	Bactrim Septra	Yes	No	No	No
dexamethasone	Decadron Hexadrol	Yes	Yes	Yes	Yes
dextrans	Rheomacrodex	Yes	No	No	No
dextrose 50%		No	No	No	Yes
diazepam	Valium	Although officially it cannot be recommended, concentrations of <0.1 mg/ml (<10 mg/100 ml) may be used provided they are prepared in glass bottles and diluted in D_5W or NSS only. Use of an inline filter is required. (C only)	No	No	Yes (C)
diazoxide	Hyperstat	Yes (C)	No	No	Yes (C)
digoxin	Lanoxin	No	No	No	Yes
diphenhydramine hydrochloride	Benadryl	Yes	Yes	Yes	Yes
dobutamine	Dobutrex	Yes (C)	No	No	No

Comments/Restrictions

During codes or other emergency may be given I.V. push by A.

During codes or other emergency may be given I.V. push by A.

Cancer chemotherapy may be administered only by a physician or a certified oncology nurse.

Given after dilution with sterile water for injection to a total of 10 ml. Rate of 0.5 mg/min into running I.V. line only.

Slowly through the tubing of running I.V.

Dilute with D_5W to 125 ml/amp. Diluted solution is stable for only 6 hours.

Can be given at 2 mg/min with first dose administered with physician in attendance. Up to 5 mg can be given as follow-up doses by RN with patient being monitored over a 15-minute period.

Push rapid injection (10 seconds preferred). Physician must specify the period of time blood pressure is to be continuously monitored and the desired limits.

Maximum dose of 0.25 mg given over 1 minute.

Preferred to be given P.O. or I.M.

Physician must specify concentration and rate of flow and must indicate in writing the blood pressure and other parameters to be maintained. Precipitates in basic solutions. Protocol recommends continuous blood pressure monitoring.

DRUGS FOR I.V. ADMINISTRATION (continued)

Generic Name	Trade Name	Continuous Infusion	Intermittent Infusion VCS	PB	Push
dopamine	Intropin	Yes (C)	No	No	No
epinephrine		Yes (C)	No	No	Yes (C)
erythromycin		Yes	Yes	Yes	No
ethacrynic acid	Edecrin	No	Yes	Yes	No
furosemide	Lasix	No	Yes	Yes	Yes
gentamicin sulfate	Garamycin	Yes	No	Yes	No
glucagon	Glucagon	Yes			Yes
heparin		Yes	No	No	Yes
histamine		Yes	No	No	No
hydralazine hydrochloride	Apresoline	Yes	Yes	Yes	Yes (C)
hydrocortisone sodium, succinate or phosphate	Solu-Cortef	Yes	Yes	Yes	Yes
hydromorphone	Dilaudid	No	No	No	Yes (C)
insulin, regular		Yes	No	No	Yes
iron dextran	Imferon	Yes	No	No	No
isoproterenol	Isuprel	Yes (C)	No	No	Yes (C)
leucovorin		No	No	No	Yes (C)
levothyroxine	Levothroid Synthroid	No	No	No	Yes
lidocaine hydrochloride	Xylocaine	Yes	No	No	Yes (C)
magnesium sulfate		Yes	No	No	Yes (C)

Comments/Restrictions

Physician must indicate in writing the blood pressure parameters to be maintained. Precipitates in basic solutions. Protocol recommends continuous blood pressure monitoring, except during code.

Patient must be monitored by EKG.

NSS is to be used as diluent. Doses of 500 mg or greater should be further diluted in 150 ml NSS unless patient is fluid-restricted.

D_5W is to be used as diluent. Give over several minutes through running I.V. only.

Push for doses up to 80 mg given over 1 minute. VCS or PB for doses above 80 mg given at 4 mg/min. NSS is preferred diluent. Do not refrigerate.

PB over 30 minutes, never as I.V. push.

Push up to 10,000 units. Continuous infusion by infusion pump—unless low concentration to keep the line patent—provided partial thromboplastin time test is appropriate. Protocol recommended.

Physician must specify concentration and rate of flow and must indicate in writing the blood pressure and other parameters to be maintained. Physician must administer first dose.

Physician must specify concentration and rate of flow and must indicate in writing the blood pressure and other parameters to be maintained. Physician must administer first dose. Not more than 5 mg/min. Continuous blood pressure monitoring if push.

Push slowly (over 2 minutes) when phosphate salt is to be administered—anal itch common if injected rapidly.

Regular insulin is *only* insulin given intravenously.

Not more than 23 ml daily.

Physician must specify concentration and rate of flow and must indicate in writing the blood pressure and other parameters to be maintained. Physician must administer first dose. *Note:* Different size and strength of ampules for push and continuous infusion. Continuous blood pressure monitoring required.

I.V. push over a period of 1 minute. Do not add to other I.V. fluids.

Push for loading dose. Loading dose must precede continous infusion therapy. EKG monitoring required.
C only, except during code.

DRUGS FOR I.V. ADMINISTRATION (continued)

Generic Name	Trade Name	Continuous Infusion	Intermittent Infusion VCS	PB	Push
mannitol		Yes	No	Yes	Yes
meperidine	Demerol	No	No	No	Yes (C)
mephentermine sulfate	Wyamine Sulfate	Yes (C)	No	No	No
metaraminol bitartrate	Aramine	Yes (C)	No	No	No
methyldopa	Aldomet	Yes	No	Yes	No
methylergonovine maleate	Methergine	Yes	No	No	No
methylprednisolone	Solu-Medrol	Yes	Yes	Yes	Yes
metoclopramide	Reglan	No	Yes	Yes	Yes
metronidazole	Flagyl R.T.U.	No	No	Yes	No
morphine		Yes	No	No	Yes (C)
naloxone	Narcan	Yes (C)	No	No	Yes (C)
nitroglycerin	Tridil Nitro-Bid I.V.	Yes (C)	No	No	No
nitroprusside	Nipride	Yes (C)	No	No	No
norepinephrine bitartrate (levarterenol)	Levophed	Yes (C)	No	No	No
oxytocin	Pitocin	Yes	No	No	No
penicillin antibiotics		Yes	Yes	Yes	No
pentazocine	Talwin	No	No	No	Yes
phenobarbital sodium		Yes	Yes	Yes	No
phenylephrine	Neo-Synephrine	Yes	No	No	No

Comments/Restrictions

Blood administration set must be used.

Continuous administration for more than 48 hours not recommended.

Physician must specify concentration and rate of flow and must indicate in writing the blood pressure and other parameters to be maintained. Physician must administer first dose. Continuous blood pressure monitoring required.

Physician must specify concentration and rate of flow and must indicate in writing the blood pressure and other parameters to be maintained. Physician must administer first dose. Continuous blood pressure monitoring required.

Physician must specify concentration and rate of flow and must indicate in writing the blood pressure and other parameters to be maintained.

Postpartum (emergency room patients only).

Push over at least 1 minute.

10 mg over 1 to 2 minutes.

Infuse over 30 to 60 minutes.

Continuous infusion by protocol only. Initial bolus doses by physician.

Continuous infusion for the reversal of high dose (200 mg/kg) fentanyl anesthesia. Usually discontinued within 12 to 16 hours postanesthesia. Sudden reversal of narcotic may lead to hypertensive emergency and vomiting, resulting in possible aspiration.
Physician must be present for suspected overdose in potential opiate addict.
I.V. push except for code situation, C only.

A glass bottle must be used—follow protocol.

Infusion pump required. Physician must specify concentration and flow rate and must indicate in writing the blood pressure and other parameters to be maintained. Protect bottle (not line) from light. Prepare with D_5W only. Continuous blood pressure monitoring required.

Use D_5W only. Continuous blood pressure monitoring required.
C only, except during code.

Postpartum emergency room patients only.

For doses greater than 5 million units, dilute to 250 ml unless patient is fluid-restricted.

Up to a maximum of 30 mg at one time.

Physician must specify concentration and rate of flow and must indicate in writing the blood pressure and other parameters to be maintained. Physician to administer first dose.

DRUGS FOR I.V. ADMINISTRATION (continued)

Generic Name	Trade Name	Continuous Infusion	Intermittent Infusion VCS	PB	Push
phenytoin	Dilantin	No	Yes	Yes	Yes
phytonadione	Aqua-MEPHYTON	Yes	No	No	No
potassium chloride		Yes	No	Yes	No
potassium phosphate		Yes	No	No	No
procainamide	Pronestyl	Yes (C)	Yes (C)	Yes (C)	Yes (C)
prochlorperazine	Compazine	Yes	No	No	Yes (B,C)
propranolol	Inderal	No	No	No	Yes (C)
protamine sulfate		No	No	No	No
quinidine gluconate		Yes (C)	No	No	Yes (C)
sodium acetate		Yes	No	No	No
sodium bicarbonate		Yes	No	No	Yes
sodium iodide		Yes	No	No	No
sodium phosphate		Yes	No	No	No
streptokinase	Kabikinase Streptase	Yes (C)	No	No	No
tetracycline		Yes	Yes	Yes	No
theophylline (see aminophylline for loading dose)		Yes	Yes	Yes	No
thiamine		Yes	No	No	No
tobramycin	Nebcin	No	No	Yes	No

Comments/Restrictions

Push at 50 mg/min maximum. Although officially not recommended, phenytoin has been given successfully after dilution in NSS in a VCS. However, crystallization can occur and should be monitored. The drug must not be diluted in D_5W. If possible, avoid central line administration. Dilution volume is 5 mg/ml or less.

Never push.

Severe hypokalemia (K<2.0)—Up to 40 mEq/100 ml may be given over 1 hour provided the patient is monitored by EKG, an infusion pump is used, and a repeat K is done postinfusion. *Moderate hypokalemia* (K>2.0≤3.0)—Up to 20 mEq/100 ml may be given over 1 hour provided the patient is continuously observed, an infusion pump is used, and a repeat potassium is done postinfusion. Under other circumstances a concentration of >60 mEq/100 ml is not recommended. However, exceptions are allowed in fluid-restricted patients, provided an infusion pump is used and serum K is continuously observed at least once for every 120 mEq administered.

Same as for potassium chloride.

Infusion pump preferred for continuous infusion. EKG must be monitored.

Must be given by physician (ER physician).

Physician must specify concentration and rate of flow and must indicate in writing the blood pressure and other parameters to be maintained. Physician administers first dose. EKG must be monitored.

For infusion, up to 100 mEq/liter. Blood gas level monitoring is essential, except during codes or other emergencies.

Infusion pump only. Protocol must be used.

Protocol recommended.

PB over 30 minutes.

DRUGS FOR I.V. ADMINISTRATION (continued)

Generic Name	Trade Name	Continuous Infusion	Intermittent Infusion		
			VCS	PB	Push
tolazoline	Priscoline	Yes	No	No	Yes
trace elements	MTE-4	Yes	No	No	No
trimethaphan camsylate	Arfonad	Yes (C)	No	No	No
urea		Yes	No	No	No
vancomycin	Vancocin	Yes	No	Yes	No
vasopressin	Pitressin	Yes (C)	No	No	No
verapamil hydrochloride	Calan	Yes (C)	No	No	Yes (C)

investigational drugs

new drugs

Comments/Restrictions

Blood pressure must be monitored hourly.

Rate should not exceed 4 ml/min.

Has been used intraarterially as well as I.V. for GI bleeding. Infusion pump required. Physician must specify in writing the blood pressure and other parameters to be maintained.

Push slowly over 2 minutes. Physician must be present; EKG monitoring required.

Only with prior approval of Pharmacy and Therapeutics Committee and Institutional Review Board (except in emergencies). As a rule, investigational I.V. medications to be administered by a physician.

New drugs and old ones not on list may be administered only with prior approval of Pharmacy and Therapeutics Committee. In the absence of such approval, temporary approval may be given to committee chairman in conjunction with pharmacy director or their designees.

Reprinted with permission from *Pharmacy Practice News (Intravenous Therapy News)*. New York: McMahon Publishing Co., March 1985.

Appendix B

STANDARD INFUSION/PIGGYBACK LIST

The following is a sample list of standard volumes and diluents approved by one institution (Quakertown Community Hospital in Pennsylvania) for I.V. piggybacks and drug infusions. These guidelines may be useful in determining similar policies in other institutions.

Drug	Dose	Solution	Volume of Solution (ml)
aminophylline	1 g	D_5W (dextrose 5% in water)	500
ampicillin	500 mg 1 g 2 g	NSS (normal saline solution) NSS NSS	50 100 100
carbenicillin	all strengths	D_5W	100
cefazolin	500 mg 1 g	D_5W D_5W	50 50
cefoxitin	1 g 2 g	D_5W D_5W	50 50
chloramphenicol	all strengths	D_5W	100
cimetidine	200 mg 300 mg	D_5W D_5W	100 100
clindamycin	all strengths	D_5W	100
erythromycin	all strengths	NSS	150
gentamicin	all strengths	D_5W	100
heparin	25,000 units	½ NSS	500
insulin (regular)	100 units	NSS	500
morphine	100 mg	D_5W	500
nafcillin	1 g 2 g	D_5W D_5W	100 100
penicillin G potassium	all strengths	D_5W	100
theophylline	800 mg	D_5W	500
ticarcillin	all strengths	D_5W	100
tobramycin	all strengths	D_5W	100
vancomycin	500 mg	D_5W	100

Reprinted with permission from *Pharmacy Practice News (Intravenous Therapy News)*. New York: McMahon Publishing Co., March 1985.

Appendix C

ANSWERS TO REVIEW QUESTIONS

Chapter 1—The Nursing Process in Medication Administration and I.V. Therapy

1. D
2. C
3. B
4. A
5. D
6. D

Chapter 2—Legal Risks and Responsibilities in Administering Drug and I.V. Therapy

1. The five rights are:
- the right drug
- the right patient
- the right time
- the right dosage
- the right route.

2. The two rights that should be added include:
- the patient's right to know
- the patient's right to refuse.

3. A *prescription drug* is any drug restricted from regular commercial purchase and sale.

4. The two federal laws that govern the use of drugs in the United States are the Comprehensive Drug Abuse Prevention and Control Act (incorporating the Controlled Substances Act), which regulates those drugs thought to be most subject to abuse; and the Food, Drug, and Cosmetic Act, which restricts interstate shipment of drugs not approved for human use and outlines the process by which drugs are tested and approved.

5. *Dispensing* refers to taking a drug from the pharmacy supply and giving or selling it to another person. *Administering* means actually introducing the drug into the patient's body.

6. The four steps to follow when taking an oral drug order from a physician are:
1) Write down the order exactly as the physician gives it.
2) Repeat the order back to him so that you are sure you heard him correctly.
3) Record in ink the type of drug, the dosage, the time you administered it, and any other information your facility's policy requires.
4) Sign or initial your notes.

7. The three Rs of risk management are rapport, record, and report.

8. The written experimental protocol provided by a research team.

9. The five sources to use when questioning a drug order are:
- standard drug reference
- charge nurse
- pharmacist
- prescribing physician
- prescribing physician's chief of service.

10. The legal basis for nursing practice in I.V. therapy is determined by state nurse practice acts, joint policy statements, and institutional policy. Institutional policy is the final determinant of what a nurse may or may not do. These statutes and policies provide legal protection for the nurse as long as she acts correctly and within the limitations they set up.

Chapter 3—Principles of Pharmacology

1. *Pharmacokinetics* refers to the characteristic actions and movement of a drug, and its pattern of absorption, distribution, metabolism, and excretion.

2. Any three of the following:
- rate of gastric emptying
- GI motility
- pH of GI tract
- presence of food in GI tract
- presence of antacids in GI tract
- fluid intake
- blood flow
- drug form
- amount and type of inert ingredients
- enteric coating.

3. B
4. C
5. D
6. *Half-life* is the amount of time required

for the blood concentration of a drug to decrease by 50%. It is significant in determining optimum dosage regimens, such as loading dose, maintenance dose, and duration of time between doses.

7. *Pharmacodynamics* refers to the process by which a drug combines with cell receptors to exert its effect.

8. Any three of the following:
- underlying pathologic conditions
- route of administration
- dosage form
- drug-drug interactions
- drug-diet interactions
- psychological considerations
- patient compliance.

9. *Potentiation* is an enhanced pharmacologic response occurring from the simultaneous use of two drugs. *Antagonism* is a reduced or absent pharmacologic response to a drug caused by the presence of a second drug.

10. B
11. B
12. First and third trimesters

Chapter 4—Medication Orders and Distribution Systems

1. False
2. True
3. False
4. True
5. True
6. True
7. True
8. True
9. True
10. The incomplete orders are:
    A. Route of administration is missing.
    D. Frequency of administration is missing.
11. All of the following:
- name and dosage of medication
- route of administration
- time and frequency of administration
- physician's signature.
12. "q.i.d." is four times a day, which means the medication is to be given four times while the patient is awake. "q6h" means the medication must be given exactly every 6 hours.

Chapter 5—Calculations and Measurements

1. 60 mg
2. 15 gr
3. 1,000 mcg
4. 60 gtt
5. $\frac{1}{150}$ gr
6. 1 mg
7. 0.5 g
8. 2½ gr
9. 0.015 g
10. 120 mg
11. 2½ tablets
12. 1 tablet
13. 2 tsp
14. 0.6 ml
15. 0.4 ml
16. 5 ml, so that each ml contains 600,000 units
17. 0.5 ml
18. 0.5 ml
19. 0.25 ml
20. 0.8 ml

Chapter 6—Preparation and Administration Guidelines

1. True
2. False
3. False
4. False
5. False
6. True
7. True
8. False
9. False
10. True
11. True
12. True
13. True
14. False
15. True
16. False
17. True
18. True
19. False
20. True
21. True
22. All three of the following:
- when taking the drug container from the shelf or cart bin

- before pouring the medication
- after pouring the medication.

23. All of the following:
- the plunger
- inside of syringe barrel
- syringe tip.

24. All of the following:
- the patient's name and room number
- type of I.V. solution
- type and amount of medication added
- date and time of preparation.

25. *Incompatibility* is an undesired physical or chemical reaction between a drug and a solution or another drug.

26. All of the following:
- Wear gloves and glasses or safety goggles.
- Wear a gown.
- Hold the medication vial so her hand is between the vial's stopper and her face.

27. All of the following:
- Verify the medication order on the cardex with the physician's order in the chart.
- Review the package insert regarding considerations in preparing the drug.
- Have someone check dosage calculations.
- Label the syringe with the patient's name and room number and the drug's name and dosage.

28. C
29. B
30. B
31. D
32. A
33. C
34. D
35. D
36. D

Chapter 7—Administering Oral Medications

1. The syringe is placed in the pocket between the cheek mucosa and the second molar, to minimize the risk of aspiration.
2. Acid or iron preparations should be administered through a straw, to avoid staining the teeth.
3. Unpleasant medications can be made more palatable by any five of the following ways:
- Give through a straw.
- Disguise the taste by diluting with another liquid.
- Give through a syringe.
- Have the patient numb his taste buds by sucking on ice chips beforehand.
- Pour medication over ice, or chill it beforehand.
- Have the patient hold his nose as he swallows.
- Offer hard candy or gum after the medication, or have the patient gargle or rinse his mouth.

4. Proper positioning of a nasogastric tube may be checked by auscultation of an air bubble entering the stomach after instillation of 10 cc of air through the tube. The appearance of gastric contents upon gentle aspiration of the tube with the syringe confirms patency and proper positioning.

5. Approximately 30 ml of the diluted medication is poured into the syringe at one time during instillation through a nasogastric or gastrostomy tube.

6. The flow rate is regulated by raising or lowering the level of the syringe.

7. Instill about 10 ml of water through the tube; a smooth flow of water confirms patency.

8. Nasogastric and gastrostomy tubes should be irrigated after medication instillation to prevent obstruction of the tubes. 50 ml of water should be used to irrigate a nasogastric tube; 30 ml of water should be used to irrigate a gastrostomy tube.

9. The flow of medication can be facilitated by positioning the patient in an upright (Fowler's or semi-Fowler's) position during instillation and for 30 minutes after instillation, *or* by placing the patient on his right side with the head of the bed slightly elevated.

10. Liquids should be at room temperature to prevent abdominal cramping.

11. All of the following are contraindications for administering oral medications:
A. nausea, vomiting, inability to swallow, decreased level of consciousness, unconsciousness
B. absent bowel sounds, obstruction of the tube, improper positioning of the tube, vomiting around the tube

C. absent bowel sounds, obstruction of the tube

Chapter 8—Parenteral Administration of Medication

1. All of the following:
   - risk of nerve damage
   - risk of giving I.V. instead of I.M.
   - risk of bleeding from blood vessel.
2. The five I.M. injection sites are:
   - ventrogluteal
   - deltoid
   - dorsogluteal
   - vastus lateralis
   - rectus femoris.
3. A
4. B
5. Any *two* of the following:
   - Encourage the patient to relax the muscle to be injected.
   - Avoid extrasensitive areas.
   - Wait until the skin antiseptic is dry.
   - Always use a new needle.
   - Draw 0.2 cc of air into the syringe.
   - Dart the needle in rapidly and withdraw it rapidly.
   - Aspirate to be sure the needle is not in a blood vessel.
   - Massage the relaxed muscle.
   - Numb the area before injecting.
6. C
7. A
8. C
9. All of the following:
   - deposits of unabsorbed drugs
   - reduction in desired pharmacologic effect of drug
   - abscess formation or tissue fibrosis.
10. C
11. D
12. The two angles are 45° and 90°. If the fat fold is less than 1", the 45° angle is used; if the fat fold is more than 1", the 90°angle is used. Also, heparin is always injected at a 90° angle.
13. D
14. The needle is inserted at a 15° angle, bevel up, ⅛" into the skin layers.
15. No wheal formation indicates that the needle was placed too low in the skin, and the antigen was injected too deeply. Withdraw the needle, and administer another dose at least 2" from the first site.
16. True
17. B
18. The volume-control set with a membrane filter
19. All three of the following:
   - eliminates the need for multiple venipunctures
   - maintains a continuous I.V. infusion
   - allows intermittent administration of medication.
20. A heparin flush is the instillation of dilute heparin into the heparin lock after administration of a medication; this is done to prevent occlusion of the needle caused by clotting. Normal sterile saline solution is used to flush the heparin lock before and after the administration of the medication, in case the heparin and the medication are incompatible.
21. All three of the following:
   - no blood return on aspiration
   - resistance on injection
   - puffiness or pain at needle insertion site.
22. *Bolus* refers to the concentration or amount of a drug. *I.V. push* is a technique for rapid intravenous injection of a drug.
23. Both of the following:
   - to deliver an antineoplastic drug through a catheter in a major artery directly into a localized, inoperable tumor
   - to deliver vasopressin to the site of gastrointestinal bleeding.
24. Any five of the following:
   - twitching, paresthesia, motor weakness—improper catheter placement
   - vasospasm, arteritis—foreign bodies in the medication or catheter
   - pain or numbness in extremity, or severe visceral pain—clotting in catheter
   - swelling, bleeding around site—internal bleeding from heparin accumulation around site
   - dilated blood vessels (determined by X-ray)—weakened vessel walls from catheter pressure
   - local swelling, drainage at insertion site—infection from fluid or equipment contamination; infrequent dressing changes; lack of aseptic technique

- labored breathing, respiratory collapse—air embolism or air bubbles in line, caused by a disconnection or an empty infusion bottle.

25. The purpose of an intrathecal injection is to allow direct administration of medication into the subarachnoid space of the spinal canal. The purpose of an intraarticular injection is to deliver drugs directly into the synovial cavity of a joint to relieve pain, help preserve function and prevent contractures, and delay muscle atrophy.

26. CNI is indicated when the patient's physical condition makes traditional routes of administration ineffective or when around-the-clock administration of oral, injectable, or rectal narcotics no longer controls the pain.

27. A 1-hour dose of the narcotic is given by I.V. push to provide quick, short-term relief of pain until the CNI takes effect.

28. Narcan should be administered in *small* doses—0.2 to 0.8 mg every 3 to 4 minutes—to restore respiratory function *without* reversing all the analgesic effects.

29. The implantable infusion device needs no dressing changes, and needs only monthly heparinization. It causes less restriction of everyday activity. It also reduces the impact on body image and the risk for infection.

30. The system must be flushed with saline solution *after* each drug and *before* heparinization to prevent incompatibilities, and it should be flushed with heparin after each use to prevent occlusion.

Chapter 9—Application of Medication to the Eye, Ear, Nose, and Throat

1. C
2. In the conjunctival sac, moving from the inner to outer canthus
3. D
4. It may prevent drainage of secretions and create undue pressure in the ear canal.
5. Oily medications are not instilled into the nose because ciliary activity would be inhibited, the risk of respiratory infection would be increased, and accidental inhalation may result in development of lipoid pneumonia.
6. Supine with a pillow under his shoulders so that his head tilts back over the shoulders, or sitting upright with his head tilted back.
7. Two ways to position the patient include:
- Proetz position—patient is supine with his shoulders elevated and his head tilted back over the edge of the bed
- Parkinson position—patient is supine, shoulders elevated, and head turned toward affected side, hanging slightly over the edge of the bed.
8. The dropper should be positioned just above or in front of the nostril, with its tip directed toward the midline of the nose.
9. The correct position is upright. Applying throat medications to a patient who is not sitting up increases the risk of aspiration.
10. The patient should refrain from eating or drinking for 30 minutes. If the medication has an anesthetic effect, the patient should refrain for 1 hour because the anesthetic will inhibit his gag reflex.

Chapter 10—Topical Application of Medication

1. *Topical* refers to giving a medication by placing it on the skin or mucous membranes. The routes of administration include transdermal, vaginal, rectal, sublingual, buccal, instillation, irrigation, and inunction.
2. The first step is to remove any residue of previously applied medication. Removal of residue prevents skin irritation from accumulation of medication on the skin, and it facilitates absorption of freshly applied medication, thereby maximizing its therapeutic effects.
3. Therapeutic baths cleanse the skin; relieve inflammation and pruritus; soften and remove crusts, scales, and old medication; and soothe and relax the patient. They are used primarily for their antipruritic and emollient effects.
4. Because pruritus seems worse at night, give a therapeutic bath before bedtime to promote restful sleep, unless ordered otherwise.
5. A. True
   B. False
   C. True
   D. True

6. Skin medication should not be used on mucous membranes because absorption is much quicker through mucous membranes than through skin.
7. Sublingually and transdermally
8. Transdermal nitroglycerin applied to the skin supplies a constant, controlled dose of medication directly into the bloodstream for prolonged systemic effect.
9. Therapeutic baths produce the following effects:
   A. Colloid baths produce a drying effect.
   B. Oil baths have antipruritic and emollient effects.
   C. Alkaline baths have a cooling effect.
   D. Tar baths leave a film of tar on the skin that works with ultraviolet light to inhibit rapid cell turnover in psoriasis.
10. Dressings may be removed by soaking them with sterile water or saline solution, or by proceeding with the soak and removing the dressing after a few minutes.
11. Buccal and sublingual administration of certain drugs prevents their destruction or transformation in the stomach or small intestine.
12. Alternate sides of the mouth for repeat doses to prevent continuous irritation of the same site.
13. Direct the suppository down initially (toward the spine), and then up and back (toward the cervix).
14. The purpose of warming the solution is to relieve inflammation and pain and to minimize patient discomfort.
15. Insertion of rectal medication is contraindicated in patients with potential cardiac dysrhythmias because of possible vagal stimulation upon insertion. It may also be contraindicated in patients with recent rectal or prostate surgery because of the risk of local trauma or discomfort during insertion.
16. The patient is placed on his left side in Sims' position.
17. This position facilitates the solution's flow by gravity into the descending colon. Alternative positions include placing the patient on his back, on his right side, or in the knee-chest position (for commercially prepared small-volume solutions).
18. Stop the flow of solution. Then, hold the patient's buttocks together or firmly press toilet tissue against the anus. Instruct him to gently massage his abdomen and to breathe slowly and deeply through his mouth to help relax abdominal muscles and promote retention.
19. Warming the solution to room temperature prevents vesical spasms during instillation.
20. The risk of infection is decreased by eliminating the need to disconnect the catheter and drainage tube repeatedly. Continuous bladder irrigation, by providing a continuous flow of medication, allows for maximum contact between the medication and the affected tissue, thereby maximizing the effects of the medication.

Chapter 11—Inhalation Administration of Medication

1. Drugs are absorbed directly through the linings of the respiratory tract or through the alveoli.
2. Use of a hand-held inhaler requires that the patient be able to form an airtight seal around the device, and that the patient have the coordination and clear vision necessary to assemble the device.
3. In order for a drug to be inhaled, certain machines or devices must be used to produce a mist containing tiny droplets of the drug.
4. Any four of the following:
   - nasal inhaler
   - turbo-inhaler
   - metered-dose nebulizer
   - side-stream nebulizer
   - mini-nebulizer
   - IPPB machine.
5. These positions facilitate maximum lung expansion and promote aerosol dispersion.
6. *Intermittent positive pressure breathing* (IPPB) delivers room air or oxygen into the lungs at a pressure higher than atmospheric pressure.
7. It is believed that IPPB treatments deliver aerosolized medications deeper into the air passages.
8. Instruct the patient to hold his breath for a few seconds after full inspiration.
9. The IPPB treatment may induce nausea, and a full stomach reduces lung expansion.
10. IPPB treatment increases intrathoracic pressure and may temporarily decrease cardiac output and venous return, resulting

Appendix **337**

in tachycardia, hypotension, and headache. Monitoring also detects changes from a reaction to the medication used.

Chapter 12—Preparing for I.V. Therapy

1. C
2. D
3. False
4. Isotonic
5. Hypertonic
6. B
7. D
8. C
9. E
10. A
11. 3 hours × 60 minutes = 180 minutes
Drops/minute = volume of solution × drop factor ÷ time in minutes
Answer: 83 drops/minute = 250 ml × 60 drops/ml ÷ 180 minutes
12. Vented
13. 0.22
14. False
15. Controller
16. Volumetric nonperistaltic pump
17. False
18. 21G or 23G butterfly or a 22G to 24G over-the-needle catheter
19. Implantable central port or silastic catheter
20. E

Chapter 13—Performing I.V. Therapy Procedures

1. Any five of the following:
- Obtain blood samples for laboratory tests.
- Administer continuous or intermittent medication.
- Administer blood or blood components.
- Maintain or correct fluid and electrolyte balance.
- Administer a bolus preparation.
- Nourish a patient who cannot eat normally.
- Monitor a CVP.
- Administer an intravenous anesthetic.
- Keep a vein open in case of emergency.
- Perform a phlebotomy.

2. The only *positive* identification of an individual is provided by his identification bracelet. You may use all methods mentioned, but the name bracelet is the most important.

3. The following techniques should be used:
  A. Insertion of a peripheral line—aseptic
  B. Removal of a peripheral line—aseptic
  C. Insertion of a heparin lock—aseptic
  D. Conversion of an I.V. line to a heparin lock—aseptic
  E. Cutdown—sterile
  F. Removal of a cutdown catheter—sterile
  G. Insertion of a central venous line—sterile
  H. Removal of a central venous line—sterile
  I. Insertion of an arterial line—sterile
  J. Removal of an arterial line—sterile
  K. Culturing a removed central venous or arterial catheter—sterile.

4. Insertion of a central venous line. With jugular vein insertion, the catheter may be misdirected toward the brain instead of into the vena cava; a chest X-ray will show this.

5. There are two pros: the tape sticks more effectively to the skin and is more easily removed; the venipuncture site is cleaner. One contraindication: shaving may cause microabrasions, exposing the skin tissue to bacterial invasion.

6. The name is Allen's test. The purpose is to tell you whether or not the patient will receive enough blood through the ulnar artery to supply the hand if the radial artery is occluded.

7. Some of the most common complications associated with the following include:
  A. Subclavian vein insertion—pneumothorax is the most common complication, also air embolism
  B. Jugular vein insertion—catheter may be misdirected toward the brain instead of into the vena cava; air embolism
  C. Arterial line insertion—thrombosis, bleeding and hematoma, air embolism, systemic infection, arterial spasm.

8. The date, needle or catheter size, time, and your initials

9. This removes air from the system, preventing formation of an air embolus.

10. Hemorrhage can occur very quickly as a result of a disconnection in the line.

Chapter 14—Maintaining I.V. Therapy

1. True
2. D
3. False
4. 100 drops/minute
5. 25 drops/15 seconds
6. Four things to check when an I.V. infusion has stopped running can include:
- Is the I.V. container empty?
- Is the I.V. infiltrated?
- Is the needle or catheter patent?
- If a filter is being used, is it the proper type and size?
- Is/are the flow clamp(s) open?
- Is the tubing kinked?
- Is the temperature of the solution too low?
- Is the proper administration set being used?
- Is the taping too tight?

7. G
8. E
9. F
10. B
11. I
12. J
13. D
14. A
15. C
16. H
17. True
18. Methotrexate, dopamine, vincristine, vancomycin, dactinomycin
19. False
20. True
21. True
22. True

Chapter 15—Parenteral Nutrition

1. A
2. B
3. D
4. True
5. D
6. True
7. C
8. B
9. Symptoms of hypokalemia include:
- muscle cramps and weakness
- nausea
- vomiting
- paresthesias
- dysrhythmias with ventricular asystole fibrillation occurring when serum potassium levels fall below 2 mEq/liter.

10. D
11. Site care for TPN should be performed at least three times weekly (once weekly for transparent dressings) and whenever the dressing becomes wet, nonocclusive, or soiled.
12. Any three of the following:
- infusions of blood and blood products
- bolus injections of drugs
- simultaneous administration of I.V. solutions
- measurement of central venous pressure
- aspiration of blood for routine laboratory tests
- addition of medication to an I.V. hyperalimentation solution container
- use of three-way stopcocks.

13. False
14. True
15. Patient monitoring during TPN therapy involves:
- observing for signs and symptoms of complications
- interpreting laboratory results and reporting abnormal findings
- taking vital signs every 4 to 8 hours
- monitoring the flow rate
- testing urine for glucose and acetone
- recording intake and output
- taking daily weight.

16. True
17. True
18. The benefits of home parenteral nutrition include:
- decreased cost for patient and hospital
- shorter hospital stay for patient
- patient may return to daily activities between infusions

19. False
20. True

Chapter 16—Blood and Blood Component Therapy

1. D
2. Maintain blood volume, maintain oxygen-carrying capacity, maintain coagulation
3. Component therapy provides deficiency-specific therapy, expands the potential usefulness of a single blood donation, and helps ease the chronic shortage of blood. The

risks of viral hepatitis and exposure to sensitizing agents or drugs in blood are also reduced.
4. An *antigen* is a substance that can trigger an immune response and induce the formation of a corresponding antibody.
5. An *antibody* is an immunoglobin molecule synthesized in response to a specific antigen.
6. Antigens
7. The types of antigens present or absent on the surfaces of RBCs
8. Blood type O. Type O lacks A and B antigens.
9. Blood type AB. Type AB blood has neither anti-A nor anti-B antibodies.
10. To establish compatibililty and minimize the risk of a hemolytic reaction.
11. *Rh-positive* means that the Rh antigen, $Rh_0(D)$ factor, is present on the surface of the RBCs. A person with Rh-positive blood does not carry anti-Rh antibodies.
12. The five major nursing responsibilities are to:
- know state/institutional policies regarding who is permitted to transfuse blood
- match the right blood to the right patient
- inspect the blood prior to administration to detect abnormalities
- be skilled in the proper technique of blood administration
- observe the patient during and after administration for signs of reaction
13. True
14. True
15. True
16. False
17. To minimize any transfusion reaction
18. The steps, in order, include:
  1) Stop the transfusion.
  2) Change the I.V. tubing.
  3) Start saline at KVO rate to maintain venous access.
  4) Place the patient supine with legs elevated (if appropriate), and monitor vital signs as indicated by the type and severity of the reaction.
  5) Notify the physician.
  6) Compare blood containers to corresponding patient identification forms to ensure transfusion was of the correct blood.
  7) Notify blood bank of possible reaction.
  8) Collect blood and urine samples.
  9) Send samples and all blood containers to blood bank.
  10) Administer medications and prepare for further treatment, as ordered.
19. In *plasmapheresis*, blood withdrawn from a patient is separated into plasma and formed elements. The plasma may be discarded and the formed elements mixed with a plasma replacement fluid and returned to the patient, or it can be filtered to remove the disease mediator and then returned to the patient with the formed elements.
20. *Autotransfusion* is the collection, filtration, and reinfusion of the patient's own blood.
21. It eliminates disease transmission, transfusion reactions, isoimmunization, and the necessity of adding anticoagulants. It can also overcome religious objections to blood transfusion. It delivers blood that has normal levels of 2, 3-DPG, potassium, ammonia, and clotting factors. It delivers blood that has a normal pH and viable platelets.
22. After traumatic injury and before, during, and after surgery
23. Any three of the following:
- malignant neoplasms
- intrathoracic or systemic infections
- coagulopathies
- enteric contamination
- excessive hemolysis
- use of an antibiotic at the site that is not suitable for I.V. administration.

Chapter 17—Pediatric Drug and I.V. Therapy

1. Absorption, distribution, metabolism, and excretion
2. Factors that affect oral administration include:
- the pH of neonatal gastric fluid
- various infant formulas or milk products
- gastric emptying time
- transit time through the small intestine
- the child's activity level.

The pH of neonatal gastric fluid is neutral or slightly acidic; it becomes more acidic as the infant matures. Certain medications are *better* absorbed and others are not absorbed as well in an acidic environment. Various infant formulas *raise* the pH of gastric fluid, impeding absorption of certain medications. Children have a longer gastric emptying time and a longer transit time through the small intestine, thereby increasing absorption of the medication. Because blood is shunted from the GI tract during exercise, drug absorption from the GI tract is decreased.

3. Faster and more completely absorbed in a child. A child's keratin and epithelial layers are much thinner than an adult's.

4. False. The intramuscular route is not a good route because absorption is erratic and unpredictable.

5. True. Only unbound, or free, drug has a pharmacologic effect.

6. True. Volume of extracellular fluid, through which the drug travels to its receptors, is greater in children than adults.

7. The integrity of his hepatic enzyme system, his intrauterine exposure to the drug, and the nature of the drug

8. An infant's renal system is immature and cannot excrete drugs completely. Unless drug dosage is reduced, toxicity may result.

9. The most *common* method of calculating dosages is based on body-surface area (mg/m^2). The most *accurate* method is to use drug information provided by the manufacturer, giving the recommended dose per kilogram (or pound) of body weight.

10. The most important consideration is positioning the infant to prevent aspiration.

11. One of the most important considerations is to restrain the infant adequately to avoid giving the injection in the wrong site or to prevent dislodging, contaminating, or breaking the needle.

12. Any three of the following:
- Establish that there is no choice about taking or receiving the medication.
- When possible, use visual aids and allow the child to play by pretending to give the medication to a doll, a parent, or you.
- When appropriate, provide honest explanations.
- Try to continue any rituals of medication administration that the child is familiar with from home.
- Praise the child afterward, and reward him with a sticker or badge if available.

13. Vastus lateralis muscle

14. Downward, back; upward, back

15. Have the child close his eyes while you retract his lower eyelid; this prevents him from looking at the dropper or applicator as it comes toward his eye.

16. Any three of the following:
- administration of drugs
- replacement of electrolytes
- delivery of parenteral nutrition
- maintenance of fluid balance

17. The usual site is a peripheral vein in the hand, wrist, or foot.

18. Tape the patient's arm to a padded armboard, protect the I.V. site, and use appropriate restraints to prevent dislodging the needle.

19. The purpose of using the volume-control set and the infusion pump is to prevent circulatory overload.

20. The purpose of parenteral nutrition in children is to reverse catabolism and promote normal growth and development.

21. False

22. Phlebitis can develop with high concentrations of dextrose. Central veins are used to deliver high concentrations of dextrose.

23. Sepsis

24. False

25. The purpose of neonatal exchange transfusion is to remove excess bilirubin and prevent kernicterus by replacing a newborn's blood with an equal amount of donor blood.

Chapter 18—Geriatric Drug and I.V. Therapy

1. Any three of the following:
- Elderly persons consume more prescription and nonprescription drugs because they have a greater variety of diseases that require one or more medications.
- An older person's socioeconomic status may affect drug usage.
- An older person's personal health may affect drug usage.
- An older person's health care environment may affect drug usage.
- An older person's physicians and nurses may influence drug usage.

2. False
3. True
4. True
5. False
6. Diuretics, digoxin, corticosteroids, sleep medications, and nonprescription drugs
7. Any four of the following:
- an age-related decline in sensory acuity
- physical disabilities
- stress or anxiety

- financial problems or limitations
- poor eating habits
8. Any five of the following:
- Review the patient's instructions with him, keeping the instructions as specific as possible.
- Eliminate background noises during teaching sessions and have the patient repeat the instructions back to you.
- Write the instructions down.
- Suggest he ask the pharmacist for standard caps instead of child-proof ones.
- Refer him to a social service representative for information and assistance in getting financial aid, if necessary.
- Assist him with planning a realistic schedule for taking his medication.
- Make a medication chart or calendar to help him remember what to take and when.
- Use a commercial aid such as a one-day pill reminder to help him remember his medications and when to take them.

9. The veins in the elderly may be hardened or sclerosed, or fragile and torn easily. They may also be tortuous.

10. Fluid and electrolyte balance may be difficult to maintain because these patients may be taking medication that alters electrolyte levels, and they may have disease conditions that affect fluid *and* electrolyte balance. They may also be more susceptible to fluid overload caused by varying degrees of cardiac dysfunction.

INDEX

A

Abbreviations, used in medication orders, 48
Absorption of drugs
  factors affecting, 33
  process of, 26-28
Acquired immunodeficiency syndrome (AIDS), transfusions as cause of, 261
Admixture(s)
  definition of, 76
  preparation of, 76-79
Age, as factor in drug action, 36
Albumin, components and uses of, 271
Alcohol, advantages and disadvantages of, 196
Allen's test, procedure for performing, 207
Allergy(ies), transfusions as cause of, 261
Ampule(s), withdrawing from, 68-69
Anaphylactic shock, responding to, 39
Anaphylaxis, drugs used to reverse, 40-41
Anthropometric measurement(s), procedure for taking, 233
Antibody, definition of, 257
Antigen, definition of, 256
Apothecaries' system, 52, 53, 54
Application, topical
  of medication, 138-158
  review questions, 157-158
Armboard(s), for restraining I.V. sites, 175-177
Arterial line
  insertion of, 206-207
  removal of, 207-208
Ascorbic acid injection, for subcutaneous treatment of extravasation injuries, 220
Autotransfusion
  complications of, 282
  procedure for performing, 277-282

B

Bath(s), therapeutic, procedure for, 142-143
Bladder, instilling medication to, 154-155
Bladder irrigation, continuous
  administration of medication by, 155-157
  set-up for, 156
Blood
  composition and physiology of, 256-260
  donor, testing of, 260
  transfusion of, 262-266
    under pressure, 265
  whole, components and uses of, 270
Blood component therapy, 256-283
  components of and their uses, 270-271
  nursing responsibilities in, 260-262
  review questions, 283
Blood donation(s), procedures for encouraging, 266
Blood donor(s), selection and screening of, 260
Blood group
  ABO, 257-258
  Rh, 258-260
Blood type compatibility, and transfusion, 259
Blood-warming device(s), procedure for using, 263

C

Calculations, and measurements, for dispensing drugs, 52-59
Cartridge-injection system, preparation of, 73
Catheter position, 186
Catheter(s)
  cutdown
    assisting with, 201-203
    removal of, 204
  for peripheral lines, 185
Cell(s)
  packed, components and uses of, 270
  washed, components and uses of, 270
Central venous line
  insertion of, 205-206
Chemical name, 26, 28
Children
  drug administration and I.V. therapy for, 286-307. See also Drug administration, in children.
  restraining procedures for, 296
Circulatory overload, transfusions as cause of, 261
Citrate toxicity, transfusions as cause of, 261
Continuous narcotic infusion (CNI), management of, 113-116
Controller(s), procedure for setting up, 179-181
Cryoprecipitate, components and uses of, 271
Cutdown catheter
  assisting with, 201-203
  removal of, 204

D

Disk(s), transdermal, application of, 141
Distribution of drugs, process of, 28-29
Dressings, wet, application of, 144
Drug abuse, 12
Drug accumulation, steady state of, 35
Drug action, factors affecting, 36-38
Drug administration
  in children, 287-297
    calculation and monitoring of dosages in, 288-289
    developmental considerations in, 288
    injections, 292-295
    oral, 290
    physiologic considerations in, 286-288
    review questions, 306-307
  in elderly, 308-314
    adverse reactions, 310-312
    guidelines for, 312-313
    improvement of, 314
    noncompliance in, 312-314
    physiologic changes affecting, 308-310
    review questions, 315
    side effects of, 311
  errors in, how to avoid, 11
  refusal to participate in, 12

Drug control laws, 8-10
Drug distribution systems, 49-51
  review questions for, 51
Drug effects, 38-43
Drug experimentation, responsibility in, 10-12
Drug infusion(s), and I.V. piggybacks, list of, 330
Drug names, 26
Drug orders
  questioning of, 13
  taking and carrying out of, 9
Drugs
  and breast-fed infants, 45
  and lactation, 44
  and pregnancy, 43-44
  buccal and sublingual, most commonly used, 146
  chemotherapeutic, preparation of, for administration, 72
  classification of, 26
  compatibility of, combined in a syringe, 70-71, 72-73
  controlled, administration of, 14
  definition of, 8
  dispensing of, liability for, 10
  for reversing anaphylaxis, 40-41
  forms of and routes of administration, 26, 29
  generic vs. trade-name, 27
  I.V. administration of, guidelines for, 318-329
    compatibility chart for, 74-75
  routes of administration, comparison of, 30-32
  transdermal, application of, 141
  types of, 63

E

Eardrop(s), procedure for instilling, 132-133
Elderly
  drug and I.V. therapy for, 308-315. *See also* Drug administration, in elderly.
  medication consumption patterns of, 308
Enema(s)
  retention and irrigating
    procedure for, 150-154
    types of, 151
Equianalgesia, 115-116
Excretion of drugs, process of, 32-34
Extravasation injury(ies)
  administration of infusions with high risk of, 218-221
  patients at high risk for, 218
  treatment of, 219-221
    subcutaneous, suggested antidotes for, 220
Eye medication disk(s), insertion and removal of, 129
Eye medication(s), administration of, 128-132
Eye patch, application of, 131

F

Flow rate, calculation of, 181-183
Fluid balance, guidelines for, in children, 299-300
Fluid system, procedure for setting up, 177-179

G

Gamma globulin, administration of, 268
Gastrostomy tube(s), medication administration via, 88-91
Generic name, 26, 28
Granulocyte(s), components and uses of, 270

H

Half-life, 32, 34
Hand, dorsum of, superficial veins of, 189
Hemoglobin solutions, advantages and disadvantages of, 267
Hemolysis
  acute transvascular, 261
  delayed extravascular, 261
Heparin injection, guidelines for, 94
Heparin lock
  conversion of I.V. line to, 201
  infusion of drug through, 110-111
  insertion of, 200-201
Hepatitis, transfusions as cause of, 261
Household measure, 52, 54
HPN. *See* Parenteral nutrition, home.
Hyaluronidase, for subcutaneous treatment of extravasation injuries, 220
Hydrocortisone sodium succinate, for subcutaneous treatment of extravasation injuries, 220
Hyperalimentation therapy, N.I.T.A. standards for, 23

I

I.V. drug compatibility chart, 74-75
I.V. push injection, medication administration by, 111-113
I.V. therapy. *See* Intravenous therapy.
Immunohematology, 256-260
Implantable fusion port, infusion of drug through, 116-120
Incident report(s), 14-19
  risk-management strategy following, 18-19
  routing of, 16-17
Infant(s)
  breast-fed, drugs and, 45
  I.M. injections for, administration of, 293-294
  liquid medications for, administration of, 291
  oral medication for, administration of, 290-291
Infusion port, implantable, 187
Infusion(s), devices for, selection of, 176
Inhalant(s), administrations of, in children, 297
Inhalation administration
  of medication, 159-166
  review questions, 166
Inhaler(s)
  hand-held, procedure for using, 159-161
  nasal, procedure for using, 160-161
  turbo, procedure for using, 160
  types of, 160
Injection(s). *See also* specific types.
  administration of, in children, 292-295
  into muscle tissues, guidelines for amounts of solutions for, 293
Injury(ies). See specific types.
In-line filters, 174
Insulin, injection of, guidelines for, 94
Insulin infusion pump, use of, 97-99
Intermittent positive-pressure breathing (IPPB), administration of medication by, 164-165
Intraarterial infusion, management of, 120-121
Intraarticular injection(s)
  assisting with, 123-125
  sites of, 124

Intradermal injection(s)
  procedure for, 92-93
  sites of, 93
Intramuscular injection(s)
  procedure for, 99-105
  reducing pain of, 103
  sites of, 100-101
Intrathecal injection(s), assisting with, 122-123
Intravenous administration set, basic, 172
Intravenous connection, taping of, 107
Intravenous controllers and pumps, 175
Intravenous devices
  central, 184-187
  peripheral, commonly used, 183-184
Intravenous infusion, 105-120
  piggyback set for, 106
Intravenous therapy
  administration equipment for, 169-177
  administration of, infusions with high risk of extravasation injury, 218-221
  alarm going off during, what to check, 214
  complications
    arterial line, 229
    central venous line, 226-228
    prevention of, 217-218
  components of, 168
  documentation of, 192
  factors affecting flow rate during, 210-211
  flow rate during, maintenance of, 211-214
  geriatric, 314
    review questions, 315
  home, 221
    N.I.T.A. standards for, 22
  legal implications of, 15
  line patency during, maintenance of, 215
  maintenance of, 210-231
    review questions, 230
  nursing practice in, N.I.T.A. standards for, 19-21
  pediatric, 297-307
    administration of, 301-305
    anatomic considerations of, 297-298
    developmental considerations in, 299-301
    physiologic considerations of, 298-299
    review questions, 306-307
    sites of, protection of, 302-303
  peripheral
    local complications of, 222-223
    systemic complications of, 224-225
  preparation for, 168-194
    review questions, 192-193
  procedures for, 195-209, 212-213
    review questions, 208-209
  sites and systems, maintenance of, 215-217
  standard, uses and special considerations of, 234-235
  team concept in, 210
Iodine, advantages and disadvantages of, 196
Isolation, administering medication to patients in, 62

L

Lactation, drugs and, 44
Lawsuits, drug-related, common bases of, 10
Legal issues, 8-24
  review questions, 24
Liability, protecting oneself from, 13
Lotion, application of, 138-139

M

Measurement systems
  and calculations
    for dispensing drugs, 52-59
    review questions, 58-59
  conversions in, 52-55
Medication administration
  documentation of, 79
  measurement systems for, 52-59
  nurse's role in, 8
Medication cardex, 79
Medication identification check(s), 61
Medication orders, 47-49
  abbreviations used in, 48
  review questions, 51
Medications. *See also* Drugs.
  bladder, instillation of, 154-157
  buccal and sublingual, administration of, 145-146
  ear, instillation of, 132-133
    in children, 295-296
  eye, administration of, 128-132, 296
  inhalation administration of, 159-166
    review questions, 166
  liquid
    administrations of, to infants, 291
    graduated medication cup calibrations for, 56
    measuring procedures for, 63
    types of, and nursing considerations, 64-65
  mucous membrane application of, 145-147
  nasal, instillation of, 133-136
    in children, 295
  oral
    absorption of, factors affecting, 33
    administration of, 84-91
    preparation of, 61-66
  parenteral
    preparation of, 66-75
    administration of, 92-127
  powdered, reconstitution of, 69-72
  preparation and administration guidelines for, 60-82
    review questions, 79-81
  rectal, administration of, 148-150
  responsibility for knowing about, 12-13
  throat, administration of, 136-137
  topical, application of, 138-158
    in children, 297
    pros and cons, 139
    review questions, 157-158
  vaginal, insertion of, 146-147
Metabolism, of drugs, process of, 29-32
Metric system, 52, 54
Mucous membrane(s), application of medication to, 145-157

N

Nasal medication(s), instillation of, procedure for, 133-136
Nasogastric tube(s), medication administration via, 85-89
National Intravenous Therapy Association (N.I.T.A.) standards
  for home I.V. therapy, 22
  for hyperalimentation therapy, 23
  for I.V. nursing care, 19-21

Nebulizer(s)
  administration of medication with, 162-164
  metered-dose, procedure for using, 159-160
  types of, 162-163
Needle(s)
  for peripheral lines, 185
  selection of, for administration of parenteral medications, 67
Nose drop(s), instillation of, patient positioning for, 134
Nursing diagnosis, definition of, 4
Nursing process, 2-7
  diagnosis in, 4
  evaluation in, 6
  implementation phase of, 5-6
  patient assessment in, 2-4
  planning phase in, 4-5
  review questions, 7
Nutrition
  as factor in drug action, 36
  parenteral. *See* Parenteral nutrition therapy.
Nutritional assessment, 232
Nutritional balance, guidelines for, in children, 299

O

Ointment(s)
  application of, 139
  removal of, 140
  transdermal, application of, 141

P

Pain medication flow sheet, 114
Parenteral administration, of medication, 92-127
  less common routes of, 93
  review questions, 125-127
Parenteral medication(s), preparation of, 66-75
Parenteral nutrition
  in children, 305-306
  home (HPN)
    checklist for, 247
    preparing patient for, 247-249
Parenteral nutrition therapy, 232-255. *See also* Total parenteral nutrition.
  review questions, 253-254
  types of, 234-235, 236
Paste, application of, 139-140
Peripheral line(s)
  insertion of, 195-200
  removal of, 200
Peripheral vein nutrition
  administration of, 249-53
  uses and special considerations of, 234-235
Pharmacodynamics, process of, 35-36
Pharmacokinetics, principles of, 26-34
Pharmacology
  principles of, 26-45
  review questions, 44-45
Phentolamine, for subcutaneous treatment of extravasation injures, 220
Piggyback set, 106
Piggyback(s), I.V., and drug infusions, list of, 330
Plasma
  components and uses of, 271
  transfusion of, 267-272
Plasma fractions, transfusion of, 267-272
Plasma protein binding, effect on drug action, 29
Plasma protein fraction, components and uses of, 271
Plasmapheresis, procedure for performing, 275-277
Platelet(s), components and uses of, 271
Potassium toxicity, transfusions as cause of, 261
Povidone-iodine, advantages and disadvantages of, 196
Powder, application of, 138-139
Pregnancy
  categories of, F.D.A.-assigned, 43
  use of drugs during, 43-44
    guidelines for, 44
Pressures, maintenance of, during I.V. therapy, 211
Primary line, infusion of drug through, 105
Protein-sparing therapy, uses and special considerations of, 234-235
Prothrombin, components and uses of, 271
Pump(s)
  infusion, checklist for preventing problems with, 180
  procedure for setting up, 179-181

R

Ready injectable, preparation of, 73
Restraint(s), at I.V. sites, 175-177
Reconstitution, of powdered medications, 69

S

Secondary line, infusion of drug through, 105
Sepsis, as complication of TPN therapy, 239-241
Sex, as factor in drug action, 36
Shampoo, medicated, procedure for giving, 140-142
Skin, applying medication to, 138-140
Skin preparations, common, guide to, 196
Soak(s), medicated, procedure for applying, 143-145
Sodium bicarbonate, for subcutaneous treatment of extravasation injuries, 220
Sodium edetate, for subcutaneous treatment of extravasation injuries, 220
Sodium thiosulfate, for subcutaneous treatment of extravasation injuries, 220
Solutions, I.V.
  abbreviations for, 169
  types of, 168-169, 170-171
Subcutaneous infusion, of medication, 96
Subcutaneous injection(s)
  procedure for, 93-99
  sites of, 95
Suppository(ies)
  rectal
    administration of, in children, 296-297
    insertion of, 149-150
  vaginal, insertion of, 147
Syphilis, transfusions as cause of, 261
Syringe(s)
  compatibility of drugs combined in, 70-71, 72-73
  filling procedures, 68
  selection of, for administration of parenteral medications, 66-68

T

Therapeutic plasma exchange (TPE, plasmapheresis)
  care following, 276
  procedure for performing, 275-277

Therapy. See specific types.
Throat medication(s), application of, 136-137
Total parenteral nutrition (TPN)
  administration of, 238-239
  and central venous line, 234-235
  complications of, 239-243
    catheter insertion, 239
    mechanical, 242-43
    metabolic abnormalities, 241-242
    sepsis, 239-241
  cyclic, 246
  drug compatibility and, 239
  equipment preparation and site care for, 243-245
  home, complications of, 250-251
  indications for, 236
  infusion line and, 238
  monitoring of, 245-247
  solution components of, 236-238
TPE. *See* Therapeutic plasma exchange.
TPN. *See* Total parenteral nutrition.
Trade name, 26, 28
Transfusion reaction(s)
  complications of, 261
  management of, 272-275
  recognizing, 273
Transfusion sets, 269
Transfusion therapy. *See* Blood component therapy.
Transfusion(s)
  blood
    in children, 306
    under pressure, 265
  blood type compatibility and, 259
  massive, complications of, 274
  of plasma and plasma fractions, 267-272
  of whole blood and packed cells, washed cells, and WBCs, 262-266

U

Upper body, peripheral and central veins of, 190

V

Vaginal irrigation, administration of medication by, 147-148
Vaginal medication(s), insertion of, 146-147
Vein(s)
  peripheral and central, of upper body, 190
  superficial, of dorsum of hand, 189
Venesection (cutdown), assisting with, 201-203
Venipuncture, preparation for, 183-191
Venipuncture site(s)
  central, 191
  methods of taping, 198
  peripheral, 188
Volume control set, 174
  use of, 108-110

W

Weight, as factor in drug action, 36
Wet dressings, application of, 144

Y

Y-connector administration set, 252

Z

Z-track injection, procedure for, 104